Acquired Brain Injury

Dong (Dan) Y. Han, PsyD, is the chief of University of Kentucky Neuropsychology Service's Clinical Section, and associate professor of Neurology, Neurosurgery, and Physical Medicine and Rehabilitation at the University of Kentucky College of Medicine. He is also the director of neurobehavioral studies at the Sports Medicine Research Institute of University of Kentucky. He is the past president of the Lexington Board of Brain Injury Alliance, current chair of the Scientific and Medical Advisory Board of the Association of the U.S. Army, and the president of the International Society of Neurogastronomy. He is the recipient of the Honor the Fallen Soldier Patriot Medallion by the Association of the U.S. Army, Flexner Master Educator Award, Jack Runyon Service Award, and the Founder's Award by the International Society of Neurogastronomy. Dr. Han is a funding recipient by federal and state mechanisms, foundational grants, and clinical trials involving studies of brain–behavior relationships and curriculum development. He has presented continuing-education seminars to physicians, psychologists, social workers, and nurses on all aspects of acquired brain injury. His work in translational neuroscience has been featured in *Newsweek, National Geographic, The Wall Street Journal,* and *New Scientist.*

Acquired Brain Injury
Clinical Essentials for Neurotrauma and Rehabilitation Professionals

Dong (Dan) Y. Han, PsyD
Editor

SPRINGER PUBLISHING COMPANY
NEW YORK

Copyright © 2017 Springer Publishing Company, LLC
All rights reserved.

No part of this publication may be reproduced, stored in a retrieval system, or transmitted in any form or by any means, electronic, mechanical, photocopying, recording, or otherwise, without the prior permission of Springer Publishing Company, LLC, or authorization through payment of the appropriate fees to the Copyright Clearance Center, Inc., 222 Rosewood Drive, Danvers, MA 01923, 978-750-8400, fax 978-646-8600, info@copyright.com or on the Web at www.copyright.com.

Springer Publishing Company, LLC
11 West 42nd Street
New York, NY 10036
www.springerpub.com

Acquisitions Editor: Nancy S. Hale
Compositor: S4Carlisle Publishing Services

ISBN: 978-0-8261-3136-2
e-book ISBN: 978-0-8261-3137-9

16 17 18 19 20 / 5 4 3 2 1

The author and the publisher of this Work have made every effort to use sources believed to be reliable to provide information that is accurate and compatible with the standards generally accepted at the time of publication. The author and publisher shall not be liable for any special, consequential, or exemplary damages resulting, in whole or in part, from the readers' use of, or reliance on, the information contained in this book. The publisher has no responsibility for the persistence or accuracy of URLs for external or third-party Internet websites referred to in this publication and does not guarantee that any content on such websites is, or will remain, accurate or appropriate.

Library of Congress Cataloging-in-Publication Data

Names: Han, Dong Y., editor.
Title: Acquired brain injury : clinical essentials for neurotrauma and rehabilitation professionals / [edited by] Dong (Dan) Y. Han.
Other titles: Acquired brain injury (Han)
Description: New York : Springer Publishing Company, [2017] | Includes bibliographical references and index.
Identifiers: LCCN 2016031397 | ISBN 9780826131362 | ISBN 9780826131379 (e-book)
Subjects: | MESH: Brain Injuries | Rehabilitation—methods | Brain Injuries—psychology | Case Reports
Classification: LCC RC387.5 | NLM WL 354 | DDC 617.4/81044--dc23 LC record available at https://lccn.loc.gov/2016031397

Special discounts on bulk quantities of our books are available to corporations, professional associations, pharmaceutical companies, health care organizations, and other qualifying groups. If you are interested in a custom book, including chapters from more than one of our titles, we can provide that service as well.

For details, please contact:
Special Sales Department, Springer Publishing Company, LLC
11 West 42nd Street, 15th Floor, New York, NY 10036-8002
Phone: 877-687-7476 or 212-431-4370; Fax: 212-941-7842
E-mail: sales@springerpub.com

Printed in the United States of America by Gasch Printing.

*This book is dedicated to Robin, Aeryn, and Jaesun.
I thank God every day for you.*

Contents

Contributors   ix
Preface   xiii
Acknowledgments   xv

1. **Mild Traumatic Brain Injury: An Overview**   *1*
   James B. Hoelzle and Kathryn A. Ritchie

2. **Moderate to Severe Brain Injury**   *21*
   P. Tyler Roskos and Lauren R. Schwarz

3. **Cerebrovascular Injuries**   *41*
   Luke Bradbury, Matthew Jensen, and Justin Sattin

4. **Brain Tumors**   *61*
   Sharoon Qaiser and Donita Lightner

5. **Neuroinfection**   *73*
   Julia Novitski, Kathleen Elverman, Donna Kwan, Evan Schulze, and Christopher Grote

6. **Neurotoxic and Metabolic Injuries**   *95*
   Bruce J. Diamond, Joseph E. Mosley, Katherine Makarec, and Krista Dettle

7. **Hypoxia/Anoxia**   *127*
   Jill Z. Stuart, Thomas J. Farrer, and Alex L. Heintzelman

8. **Electrical and Lightning Brain Injuries**   *143*
   Shravan Parikh, Joseph Fink, Maia Feigon, and Neil Pliskin

9. **Acquired Brain Injury Secondary to Substance Use Disorder**   *167*
   Benjamin A. Pyykkonen

10. **Post–Acquired Brain Injury Headaches** *185*
    Mauricio F. Villamar and Jonathan H. Smith

11. **Post–Acquired Brain Injury Epilepsy** *203*
    Erin Plumley, Robert J. Kotloski, and Bruce Hermann

12. **Post–Acquired Brain Injury Movement Disorders** *229*
    Hannah L. Combs, Kathryn J. Dunham, Brittany D. Walls, and Amelia J. Anderson-Mooney

13. **Acquired Brain Injury in Children** *245*
    Ana C. Albuja and Robert Baumann

14. **Acquired Brain Injury in the Elderly** *261*
    Thomas J. Farrer and Jill Z. Stuart

15. **Psychosocial Characteristics of Acquired Brain Injury** *279*
    Leslie Guidotti Breting, Courtney Nelson, and Thomas Cothran

16. **Acquired Brain Injury Rehabilitation: Clinical Essentials** *299*
    Silke Bernert and Dong (Dan) Y. Han

17. **Feigning Issues in Brain Injury** *321*
    David T. R. Berry, Brittany D. Walls, Chelsea M. Bouquet, and Elizabeth R. Wallace

Index *331*

Contributors

Ana C. Albuja, MD Department of Neurology, University of Kentucky, Lexington, Kentucky

Amelia J. Anderson-Mooney, PhD Departments of Neurology and Neurosurgery, University of Kentucky, Lexington, Kentucky

Robert Baumann, MD Departments of Neurology and Pediatrics, University of Kentucky, Lexington, Kentucky

Silke Bernert, MD Department of Physical Medicine and Rehabilitation, University of Kentucky, Lexington, Kentucky

David T. R. Berry, PhD Department of Psychology, University of Kentucky, Lexington, Kentucky

Chelsea M. Bouquet, MS Department of Psychology, University of Kentucky, Lexington, Kentucky

Luke Bradbury, MD Department of Neurology, University of Wisconsin, Madison, Wisconsin

Leslie Guidotti Breting, PhD Department of Psychiatry, Northshore University Health System, University of Chicago, Evanston, Illinois

Hannah L. Combs, MS Department of Psychology, University of Kentucky, Lexington, Kentucky

Thomas Cothran, MS Department of Psychiatry, Northshore University Health System, University of Chicago, Evanston, Illinois

Krista Dettle, PhD Department of Psychology, William Paterson University, Wayne, New Jersey

Bruce J. Diamond, PhD Department of Psychology, William Paterson University, Wayne, New Jersey

Kathryn J. Dunham, PsyD Department of Neurology, University of Kentucky, Lexington, Kentucky

Kathleen Elverman, MS Department of Behavioral Sciences, Rush University, Chicago, Illinois

Thomas J. Farrer, PhD Department of Psychiatry & Behavioral Sciences, Duke University, Durham, North Carolina

Maia Feigon, PhD Department of Psychiatry, University of Chicago, Chicago, Illinois

Joseph Fink, PhD Department of Psychiatry, University of Chicago, Chicago, Illinois

Christopher Grote, PhD Department of Behavioral Sciences, Rush University, Chicago, Illinois

Dong (Dan) Y. Han, PsyD Departments of Neurology, Neurosurgery, and Physical Medicine and Rehabilitation, University of Kentucky, Lexington, Kentucky

Alex L. Heintzelman, BS Department of Psychiatry & Behavioral Sciences, Duke University, Durham, North Carolina

Bruce Hermann, PhD Department of Neurology, University of Wisconsin, Madison, Wisconsin

James B. Hoelzle, PhD Department of Psychology, Marquette University, Milwaukee, Wisconsin

Matthew Jensen, MD Department of Neurology, University of Wisconsin, Madison, Wisconsin

Robert J. Kotloski, MD, PhD Department of Neurology, William S. Middleton Veterans Memorial Hospital, Madison, Wisconsin; Department of Neurology, University of Wisconsin, Madison, Wisconsin

Donna Kwan, MA Department of Behavioral Sciences, Rush University, Chicago, Illinois

Donita Lightner, MD Department of Neurology, University of Kentucky, Lexington, Kentucky

Katherine Makarec, PhD Department of Psychology, William Paterson University, Wayne, New Jersey

Joseph E. Mosley, MA Department of Psychology, William Paterson University, Wayne, New Jersey

Courtney Nelson, BS Department of Psychiatry, Northshore University Health System, University of Chicago, Evanston, Illinois

Julia Novitski, PhD Department of Behavioral Sciences, Rush University, Chicago, Illinois

Shravan Parikh, BS Department of Clinical Psychology, Adler University, Chicago, Illinois

Neil Pliskin, PhD Department of Psychiatry, University of Illinois, Chicago, Illinois

Erin Plumley, PsyD Department of Neurology, University of Wisconsin, Madison, Wisconsin

Benjamin A. Pyykkonen, PhD Department of Psychology, Wheaton College, Wheaton, Illinois

Sharoon Qaiser, MD Department of Neurology, University of Kentucky, Lexington, Kentucky

Kathryn A. Ritchie, BA Department of Psychology, Marquette University, Milwaukee, Wisconsin

P. Tyler Roskos, PhD Department of Physical Medicine and Rehabilitation, Wayne State University, Detroit, Michigan

Justin Sattin, MD Department of Neurology, University of Wisconsin, Madison, Wisconsin

Evan Schulze, MS Department of Behavioral Sciences, Rush University, Chicago, Illinois

Lauren R. Schwarz, PhD Department of Psychiatry, Saint Louis University, St. Louis, Missouri

Jonathan H. Smith, MD Department of Neurology, University of Kentucky, Lexington, Kentucky

Jill Z. Stuart, PhD Department of Psychiatry & Behavioral Sciences, Duke University, Durham, North Carolina

Mauricio F. Villamar, MD Department of Neurology, University of Kentucky, Lexington, Kentucky

Elizabeth R. Wallace, BS Department of Psychology, University of Kentucky, Lexington, Kentucky

Brittany D. Walls, BA Department of Psychology, University of Kentucky, Lexington, Kentucky

Preface

Acquired Brain Injury: Clinical Essentials for Neurotrauma and Rehabilitation Professionals is a clinically relevant reference guide for health care trainees, medical providers, and active allied health professionals who work with patients and clients suffering from all aspects of insults to the brain. Not limited to traumatic brain injuries, this text provides easy-to-follow formatting in providing information involving all aspects of acquired injuries to the brain and related clinical outcomes. The main objective of this book is to lay out the foundational information and practice-oriented essentials for the audience, in order that they may utilize this as a handy reference tool for clinical encounters with those with brain injuries.

This handbook lays out in each chapter an overview of a subtype of brain injury, accompanied by history, pathophysiology, etiology, epidemiology, clinical presentation, other diagnostic considerations, treatment, prognosis, and clinical synopsis. Useful case studies are also provided for most conditions described in this book. This book differs from other texts of brain injury by utilizing a format of inclusiveness of all subtypes of brain injury and their clinical sequelae. This format is intended to be useful for practice-oriented audiences including clinical trainees, early-career professionals, and all levels of clinicians who encounter patients with acquired insults to the brain.

Acknowledgments

The editor would like to acknowledge all of the contributing authors, and the dedication and support of Sarah Phillips, Sarah Holtzclaw, Iyabo Erinkitola, and Gina Mullins.

CHAPTER 1

Mild Traumatic Brain Injury: An Overview

JAMES B. HOELZLE
KATHRYN A. RITCHIE

OVERVIEW

Although historically considered a common and relatively benign injury, mild traumatic brain injury (mTBI), or concussion,[1] has recently received extensive media attention. Once described by the Centers for Disease Control and Prevention (National Center for Injury Prevention and Control, 2003) as a "silent epidemic," mTBI is now regularly discussed across disciplines and demographics. News stories routinely describe empirical research and atypical case studies suggesting there are possible short- and long-term risks associated with youth participation in contact sports. A great deal of attention has also been directed toward the Department of Veterans Affairs, focusing on how care is provided to service men and women who have sustained traumatic brain injuries while deployed overseas. Interestingly, committed fans of the National Football League are even drawn to controversies surrounding concussions, and some have a sophisticated understanding of medical protocols that are in place to protect players and determine when it is safe to return to play. It is clear that there is nothing "mild" about mTBI and our interest in it.

---

[1] Although the terms "mTBI" and "concussion" are often used interchangeably, we acknowledge that some researchers disagree with this position. For example, McCrory et al. (2009) describe that structural imaging results are uniformly normal following a concussion, but this is not necessarily true after an mTBI.

Although the literature suggests that a great majority of individuals recover from mTBI over the course of weeks to several months (e.g., Carroll et al., 2004), many clinicians recognize that recovery processes vary significantly from patient to patient, and a meaningful percentage of individuals who seek medical care in the postacute phase of recovery attribute a wide range of difficulties to mTBI. The body of literature describing risk factors, associated symptoms, and outcome from mTBI is quickly growing and sometimes appears to be contradictory. The present chapter is structured to provide sufficient background information to recognize some unique challenges associated with diagnosis and treatment of mTBI. A brief historical overview provides background and in part explains why well-respected and knowledgeable researchers and clinicians have reached different conclusions regarding the significance and outcomes associated with mTBI. The neurobiological mechanisms underlying mTBI, risk factors associated with extended recovery, and debates regarding recovery course and long-term cumulative impact of mTBI will also be discussed. Collectively, this information should help clinicians identify issues that might confound diagnosis and recovery from mTBI. Additionally, this information may be useful to share with patients when formulating treatment plans and discussing prognosis.

HISTORY

Although the term "concussion" has come to define the transient sequelae of symptoms associated with mTBI, particularly in the sports literature, it has been used colloquially for centuries, and its meaning has evolved over time. As early as 900 CE, the Latin term *commotio cerebri* was used in medical literature to convey a disruption in brain function without lesions or fracture (McCrory & Berkovic, 2001). In the generations that followed, the term "concussion," likely derived from the Latin *concutere*, or "to shake," was used to refer to an acute set of symptoms caused by "shaking" of the brain (McCrory & Berkovic, 2001).

Throughout the 20th century, the dominant perspective in the medical literature was that in most cases concussions were harmless and did not bear any long-standing effects on behavior (Bigler, 2008). In fact, any persisting symptoms associated with concussion were considered psychological relics of involvement in an accident or litigation, termed "accident neurosis" (Miller, 1961). The focus of concussion research in the 21st century, and perhaps the most elusive aspect of concussion research, has been to determine whether concussion results in transient functional disturbance with no enduring damage or whether there is lasting pathological damage via axonal shearing (McCrory & Berkovic, 2001). More recent research has also aimed to identify a minimum necessary biomedical threshold of impact to produce mTBI and evaluate potential long-term implications associated with the cumulative effects of multiple concussions.

A significant number of challenges are associated with studying mTBI. For one, there have been only a few controlled, prospective studies of the acute injury characteristics of mTBI (McCrea, 2008). Those that do exist often have small sample sizes, or low generalizability for various reasons. For example, studies that include individuals involved in accidental falls or motor vehicle accidents (MVAs), in the absence of eyewitnesses, may inaccurately report event parameters or acute injury characteristics (e.g., loss of consciousness; posttraumatic amnesia) that help quantify injury severity. Additionally, symptom reporting may be influenced by secondary gain issues and ongoing litigation. The significance of this issue cannot be understated. For example, after controlling for injury severity and premorbid factors, individuals involved in litigation report more significant symptoms, social dysfunction, and poorer outcome relative to those who are not pursuing compensation (see, for example, Feinstein, Ouchterlony, Somerville, & Jardine, 2001; Paniak et al., 2002).

A positive development in understanding mTBI and the natural course of recovery was the recognition that observing athletic participation is in many ways an ideal and rigorous natural laboratory. It is well documented that a significant number of athletes will sustain a concussion while participating in their respective sports. Postinjury neurocognitive performance relative to preseason baseline performances allow one to fully appreciate and quantify neurocognitive issues associated with mTBI. Additionally, injuries occur in individuals who are most likely young and healthy, and motivated to recover quickly. In other words, many of the confounding factors that are associated with MVAs (e.g., litigation) and unreported falls (e.g., no collateral information defining injury parameters) are not present in athletes who sustain concussion (McCrea, 2008).

For decades, research has been conducted to quantify the effects of sports-related concussion. Belanger and Vanderploeg (2005) conducted a meta-analysis of this literature and reported that it is common to observe decreased neurocognitive functioning in athletes during the first 24 hours postinjury. Encouragingly, full neuropsychological recovery is typically observed within 7 to 10 days in athletes. Although beyond the scope of the current work, collectively, this study, those contributing to it, and many others have made it possible to develop evidence-based guidelines for injury diagnosis, evaluation, and return-to-play decisions (e.g., Echemendia, Giza, & Kutcher, 2015; McCrea, Broshek, & Barth, 2015). Nevertheless, despite these positive developments, some researchers have questioned whether information obtained during sports concussion research can be generalized to nonathletes. For example, some have correctly pointed out that athletes likely have a variety of protective factors, which may include both physiological (i.e., better developed neck musculature) and psychological attributes (i.e., motivation to return to play, symptom underreporting), that increase the likelihood of rapid and positive recovery (Rabinowitz, Li, & Levin, 2014).

PATHOPHYSIOLOGY

Numerous attempts have been made to identify the minimum threshold of force (g-force) necessary for mTBI. Innovative technology has been developed to record linear head acceleration at impact and makes clear that a positive relationship exists between magnitude of impact and the probability of mTBI. Although it has been proposed that a range of 80 to 100 g is a minimal biomedical threshold sufficient to cause mTBI (McCrea, 2008), Zhang, Yang, and King (2004) established that there is a 25% chance of mTBI with 66 g, 50% chance with 82 g, and 80% chance with 106 g. Additionally, it is recognized that the addition of rotational forces greatly increases the odds of mTBI (Ommaya & Gennarelli, 1974).

Despite a seemingly plausible threshold of mechanical force for injury, there is not clear evidence that affect magnitude (linear or rotational acceleration), or affect location, is meaningfully related to acute clinical outcome (Guskiewicz et al., 2007). Once an injury threshold is exceeded, a neurometabolic cascade of complex physiological events may adversely affect cerebral functioning for days to weeks by affecting intracellular and extracellular concentrations of potassium, sodium, calcium, and magnesium ions (Giza & Hovda, 2004). A complex chain of ionic, metabolic, and physiological events is thought to render neurons dysfunctional as opposed to destroyed (McCrea, 2008). There is a strong desire to pursue "objective" hallmark neurophysiological sequelae of mTBI using traditional and novel neuroimaging methods. Although this has proven to be somewhat challenging, attempts to do so have resulted in a better understanding of the relationship between injury severity and outcome. It is important to recognize that although CT scans are commonly obtained in emergency departments (EDs) to rule out hemorrhagic lesions or structural injury, the method has poor sensitivity to detect abnormalities typically associated with mTBI. Advanced MRI and DTI approaches appear to be more effective in detecting neuropathology associated with mTBI, including miniscule hemorrhages and diffuse axonal injury (e.g., Belanger, Vanderploeg, Curtiss, & Warden, 2007; Chastain et al., 2009). fMRI research also provides evidence that structures mediating working memory are affected by mTBI (e.g., McAllister, Flashman, McDonald, & Saykin, 2006). In terms of patient outcome, there is an important distinction between normal and abnormal imaging. The latter results in a classification of "complicated mTBI" and increases the risk for delayed or incomplete recovery (e.g., Iverson, Brooks, Collins, & Lovell, 2006).

ETIOLOGY

A major challenge in studying mTBI is the heterogeneous nature of injuries sustained (Cassidy et al., 2004). As the majority of mTBIs are associated with various types of accidents, many factors can complicate recovery, including other orthopedic and neurological injuries, involvement in litigation, and premorbid psychiatric factors. These issues are typically less relevant in the context of sports-related concussion (SRC). As such, the scientific literature typically distinguishes mTBIs into sport and nonsport etiologies, but the degree to which the etiologies are interrelated is uncertain (Rabinowitz et al., 2014).

Traumatic brain injury (TBI) is most frequently attributed to blunt-force trauma or closed-head injury. Blunt-force trauma occurs when the head hits a fixed object or when a moving object strikes the head. Blunt-force trauma occurs most commonly because of

MVAs, accidental falls, assaults, sports injury, or other accidents (Roberts & Roberts, 2011). In most instances of blunt-force trauma, the force of the impact is transferred from the skull to the brain, without breaking the skull, though an impact can still be considered a closed-head injury if the skull is fractured and the meningeal covering of the brain is not punctured (Lezak, Howieson, Bigler, & Tranel, 2012). Throughout the life span, most TBIs are due to accidental falls (35.2%). According to the CDC, the second most common etiology is due to MVAs (16.5%), followed by being hit by or against an object (16.5%), and assaults (10%) (Faul, Xu, Wald, & Coronado, 2010).

Military combat also presents a common etiology for mTBI. Although blunt-force trauma has long been understood as a source of combat-related mTBI, in light of Operation Iraqi Freedom (OIF) and Operation Enduring Freedom (OEF), recent research attention has focused on the symptom sequelae associated with blast-related mTBI. As OIF and OEF have presented new warfare tactics, including exposure to improvised explosive devices (IEDs), an understanding of blast-related TBI is somewhat less developed relative to other areas of TBI research. Noteworthily, there is some neuroimaging evidence that suggests the neuropathology of blast-related TBI may differ from that of blunt-force trauma (Warden et al., 2009).

SRC also constitutes a sizable proportion of all mTBIs reported annually. In American collegiate athletes, 6.2% of all sports injuries were mTBIs (Covassin, Swanik, & Sachs, 2003). Team contact sports such as hockey and football may have the highest rates of SRC per year, though there is great in-sport variability in the estimated incidence of concussion in individual sports (Schulz et al., 2004).

EPIDEMIOLOGY

TBI is one of the most common health conditions in the United States, with prevalence estimates between 1.4 and 3 million cases per year (Summers, Ivins, & Schwab, 2009). It is estimated that mTBIs make up 70% to 90% of all TBI cases reported to EDs annually (Cassidy et al., 2004). Because of its high prevalence rate and associated societal cost, TBI is a very significant public health concern.

Because of the unique factors associated with mTBI, it is somewhat challenging to determine epidemiological rates and risk factors associated with the condition. A systematic review of incidence and risk factors associated with mTBI reveals great heterogeneity among published mTBI studies based on inclusion criteria and the manner in which mTBI is operationalized (Cassidy et al., 2004). Because there is not a universally agreed-upon definition of mTBI (described in greater detail in the following sections), it is difficult to estimate true incidence and prevalence rates, especially in less severe cases of mTBI. Another factor complicating accurate epidemiological rates is the fact that mTBI is severely underreported (McCrea, 2008). Most incidence rate studies rely only on ED reports, but one study has estimated that approximately 25% of the population did not seek medical attention after sustaining mTBI (Sosin, Sniezek, & Thurman, 1996). Although review of the literature suggests incidence rates of 100 to 300/100,000 adults, studies that included self-reported mTBI observed incidence rates as high as 600/100,000 (Cassidy et al., 2004). It will be interesting to see whether these incidence rates increase in the future with greater societal awareness of mTBI.

Though it has been difficult to determine distinct risk factors across the heterogeneous literature, some crude epidemiological trends have emerged. For instance, male patients account for approximately two-thirds (59%) of all reported cases (American Psychiatric Association [APA], 2013; Summers et al., 2009). Additionally, mTBIs exhibit a unique, bimodal age distribution, occurring most frequently in late childhood and adolescence, and then again in later adulthood (APA, 2013; McCrea, 2008) (see Chapters 13 and 14). This pattern indicates that mTBI affects people across the life span and that there are many developmental considerations to take into account when assessing for and treating concussions. Finally, a higher incidence of mTBI is reported by minorities; however, it has been difficult to distinguish whether these observed differences can be attributed to race or other risk factors for mTBI, such as socioeconomic status (McCrea, 2008).

As previously noted, another common cause of mTBI is SRC. The Centers for Disease Control and Prevention reported an annual incidence of approximately 300,000 SRCs, though this number is likely a conservative estimate because as many as half of all SRCs remain unreported (McCrea, Hammeke, Olsen, Leo, & Guskiewicz, 2004). Cumulatively, SRC is responsible for about 20% of all reported TBIs annually (Bailey, McCrea, & Barth, 2013). It is certainly plausible that this number will increase in the future as athletes, coaches, parents, and athletic trainers become more aware of symptoms associated with concussion. The incidence of mTBI is also high within the military population as it is the most common injury associated with recent military involvement (Hoffer, Donaldson, Gottshall, Balaban, & Balough, 2009). In fact, between 2000 and 2012, more than 244,000 military personnel were diagnosed with TBI, and 80% of the injuries were considered mild in nature (Defense and Veterans Brain Injury Center, 2012).

CLINICAL PRESENTATION

Typically, after sustaining an mTBI, individuals experience a pattern of neuropsychological and physiological impairments for a brief period of time (e.g., Carroll et al., 2004; Gasonique, 1992). These neuropsychological deficits may manifest as difficulty paying attention at school or work, feeling overwhelmed by new information, and being unable to quickly and efficiently problem solve. Problems such as forgetfulness, impulsivity, and disorganization are often reported in the days following an injury. Physiologically, those who have sustained an mTBI often report experiencing headaches, dizziness, smell and taste changes, sensitivity to light and/or noise, and fatigue as well. These acute sequelae of symptoms often occur directly after the injury, but dissipate within days (McCrea, 2008). In most cases, individuals fully recover from their symptoms within a few weeks to a few months (APA, 2013).

Many symptoms reported following a concussion overlap with various mood disorders (which also potentially affect neurocognitive functioning). This makes it challenging to diagnose and understand symptoms associated with mTBI. Nonspecific general emotional distress, depression, and anxiety are commonly reported following a concussion (e.g., McAllister, 2011). Furthermore, posttraumatic stress disorder is frequently a comorbid diagnosis (e.g., Mayou, Black, & Bryant, 2000). The presence of a premorbid psychiatric condition, or the development of one subsequent to mTBI, increases the likelihood of a delayed recovery.

DIAGNOSTIC CONSIDERATIONS

Broadly, TBI is the result of brain injury occurring because of impact or acceleration or deceleration (Lezak et al., 2012). TBI injury severity is conventionally graded with the labels "mild," "moderate," or "severe" on the basis of diagnostic factors, particularly a score on the Glasgow Coma Scale (GCS). The GCS is a rapid assessment rating scale that quantifies TBI severity on the basis of neurological factors such as degree of consciousness or presence of posttraumatic amnesia (PTA). Although GCS is useful predictor of outcome in cases of severe TBI, the crude measurement is less useful in diagnosing mTBI and associated symptoms because of a ceiling effect (Nelson, Janecek, & McCrea, 2013). In other words, the GCS measures acute physical symptoms (e.g., unconsciousness) that may or may not occur as a result of a concussion, but it does not capture the unique injury characteristics that might complicate recovery from mTBI. This is problematic because about 80% of TBI cases diagnosed annually are considered mild in nature (Krause, McArthur, Silverman, & Jayaraman, 1996).

The fifth edition of the *Diagnostic and Statistical Manual of Mental Disorders* (*DSM-5*; APA, 2013) defines TBI by the following symptom sequelae: loss of consciousness (LOC), posttraumatic amnesia, or neurological indicators such as positive neuroimaging, new or markedly worse seizures, visual field deficits, olfaction impairment, or hemiparesis. However, most experts agree that TBI can occur without experiencing some of the hallmark symptoms, such as LOC (e.g., Ruff et al., 2009).

To address the heterogeneity in mTBI diagnosis, the American Congress of Rehabilitation Medicine Mild Traumatic Brain Injury Committee (1993) offered more specific criteria for diagnosing mTBI. The committee defined mTBI as occurring based on one or more of the following symptoms: LOC, any immediate retrograde or anterograde amnesia, or any disruption in mental state (i.e., confusion or disorientation) in conjunction with other neurological deficits (e.g., hemiparesis). Moderate or severe TBI is defined by experiencing LOC for more than 30 minutes or amnesia for more than 24 hours (American Congress of Rehabilitation Medicine Mild Traumatic Brain Injury Committee, 1993). These diagnostic criteria were echoed by the World Health Organization's Collaborate Task on Mild Traumatic Brain Injury (Holm, Cassidy, Carroll, & Borg, 2005) and eventually supported by the National Academy of Neuropsychology (Ruff et al., 2009).

TREATMENT

Before developing a treatment plan, it is important to explore whether a patient actually had a concussion. If it is erroneously assumed that an individual experienced a concussion, it may significantly affect how neurocognitive and emotional symptoms are perceived and experienced. Once it is established that the parameters of impact were sufficient to cause mTBI and a patient's initial symptoms support a diagnosis, a thorough understanding of premorbid history is essential in developing an effective treatment plan. Substance abuse issues, mood disorders, and other medical or psychiatric conditions have the potential to confound recovery and should be appropriately managed with empirically supported treatments. Additionally, a neuropsychological evaluation may be useful in quantifying cognitive ability. Postinjury performances should be interpreted in light of educational and vocational histories, and clinicians should recognize that it is common for patients to perceive past functioning in an unrealistically positive light. It is equally important to recognize the presence of a single impaired score may reflect normal variability in performance as opposed to a deficit associated with mTBI per se (e.g., Binder, Iverson, & Brooks, 2009). Furthermore, it is invariably useful to obtain collateral information to better understand a patient's current and past functioning.

Providing psychoeducation early during the recovery process can improve outcomes. Specifically, there is compelling evidence that supportive discussions regarding the anticipated course of recovery, common symptoms, and issues that may confound recovery and warrant treatment are beneficial (e.g., Mittenberg, Tremont, Zielinski, Fichera, & Rayls, 1996; Ponsford, 2005). Clinicians should strive to provide this information as early as possible during the recovery process as a patient is less likely to be receptive to this information if he or she has already experienced a course of recovery that is inconsistent with a significant body of literature.

PROGNOSIS

After sustaining mTBI, individuals experience a transient pattern of both neuropsychological and physiological symptoms that typically subside in the weeks following the event. Systematic reviews and meta-analyses on the recovery of cognitive symptoms associated with mTBI have revealed that for most individuals, cognitive symptoms resolve within 90 days, though athletes tend to have a shorter recovery period, typically reporting complete symptom resolution within 1 week (e.g., Iverson, 2005; Karr, Areshenkoff,

& Garcia-Barerra, 2014). When the recovery period is extended to 6 months, it is estimated that approximately 90% or more of patients who experience mTBI make a full recovery of function following acute head trauma (Roberts & Roberts, 2011). Although it is well documented that the majority of individuals recover completely from symptoms within 3 months, there is a "miserable minority" of individuals—which ranges from about 10% to 20% across studies—who continue to experience residual mTBI symptoms (Ruff, 2005; Ruff, Camenzuli, & Mueller, 1996). These individuals are thought to experience postconcussion syndrome (PCS), or the occurrence of cognitive, physiological, and psychological symptoms that persist long after the typical recovery period. Notably, patients sustaining mTBI as a result of SRC are less likely to develop PCS (Bazarian et al., 1999).

Though "PCS" is a term used regularly in the literature, the diagnosis was a research condition in the fourth edition, text revision of the *Diagnostic and Statistical Manual of Mental Disorders (DSM-IV-TR*, APA, 2000) and was excluded from the current edition of the publication, *DSM-5* (APA, 2013). Nevertheless, PCS is currently a diagnostic code available in the *International Classification of Diseases, Tenth Revision (ICD-10*; World Health Organization, 1992).

Although specific definitions vary from source to source, PCS can be broadly defined as a pervasive constellation of symptoms and functional impairments that occur after sustaining a concussion that fall outside of the typical recovery trajectory (McCrea, 2008). The problem with PCS is that its diagnosis relies heavily on self-report of symptoms, which encompass a wide variety of both physiological and emotional factors that are not specific to concussion. In fact, individuals who have never sustained mTBI, nor have ever been diagnosed with psychiatric conditions, endorse PCS symptoms at rates of 37% to 81% (Iverson & Lange, 2003). The same study found that 92% of the healthy sample endorsed enough PCS symptoms to meet *ICD-10* diagnostic criteria. Although more recent studies have indicated that individuals who have sustained mTBI tend to endorse PCS symptoms at a higher rate, no significant differences on symptom endorsement were observed between the mTBI and healthy control group (Garden & Sullivan, 2010). Because the vague symptomatology associated with PCS is relatively common in healthy individuals and not limited to those who experience mTBI, the legitimacy of the condition is passionately debated.

Much research has attempted to explain why some individuals experience lingering postconcussive symptoms, and there are several leading theories. One explanation is that personality dimensions, specifically anxiety sensitivity and alexithymia, influence the likelihood of developing PCS (Wood, O'Hagan, Williams, McCabe, & Chadwick, 2014). Research has also pointed to premorbid psychological functioning as a factor in the development of PCS. For example, McCauley and colleagues (2013) identified that low mood and low levels of resiliency predicted greater PCS symptom endorsement.

Another prospective explanation of PCS is expectation. There is a body of research supporting the idea that an expectancy-guided retrospective recall bias may contribute to the experience of PCS symptoms following mTBI (Ferguson, Mittenberg, Barone, & Schneider, 1999; McCrea, 2008). This phenomenon occurs when those who have experienced mTBI misattribute general symptoms that were experienced before their injury as explicitly due to the injury. Recent studies have suggested that the role of expectation in the onset of PCS symptoms may be better understood through the "good old days" hypothesis, or the idea that after a negative event like mTBI, people may be more likely to misattribute any negative symptoms as a direct result of their injury (Gunstad & Suhr, 2001; Yang et al., 2014).

Despite the fact that the research literature has not isolated a singular cause of PCS, research trends reveal that the onset of PCS symptoms may be moderated by other factors including psychological traits and states, response bias, and expectation. As the vast majority of individuals recover quickly and fully, it may be important to assess for factors beyond acute injury characteristics when recovery is compromised.

It is also important to recognize that issues previously described are not the only factors associated with poor outcome. A host of other issues may contribute to delayed recovery including, but not limited to, age, injury severity (complicated vs. uncomplicated mTBI), litigation, and a history of recurrent mTBI (see McAllister, 2011 for a more comprehensive review). Regarding the latter issue, an investigation of college football players revealed that individuals who reported three or more concussions were three times more likely to sustain another concussion relative to players with no concussion history (Guskiewicz et al., 2003). More promising, there is evidence that individuals with higher educational attainment experience fewer cognitive symptoms as a result of mTBI (Karr et al., 2014; McAllister, 2011; McCrea, 2008).

CLINICAL SYNOPSIS

- mTBI is a significant public health concern. It is estimated that more than 1 million people experience mTBI on an annual basis.
- mTBI is typically defined by one or more of the following symptoms: LOC, any immediate retrograde or anterograde amnesia, or any disruption in mental state (i.e., confusion or disorientation).
- Despite a significant number of cases going unreported, mTBI most frequently occurs in late childhood and adolescence, and then again in later adulthood.
- Neurocognitive symptoms associated with mTBI in the acute stage of injury may include impairments in processing speed, attention, and memory. A great majority of patients experience symptom reduction in the days, weeks, and possibly months following injury.
- A small percentage of patients experiences postconcussive symptoms months and years after injury. It is important to recognize that these symptoms are not specific per se to mTBI and may reflect a host of other factors.
- Early evaluation of mTBI is ideal because it presents the opportunity to provide critical psychoeducational material regarding common symptoms, expected recovery course, and confounding factors.

CASE STUDY

The following case was selected to illustrate: (1) legitimate concerns a patient could have status-post injury, (2) premorbid risk factors, and (3) the advantages of thorough assessment. Patient was a 33-year-old woman who was involved in an MVA and sustained a concussion. She was referred by a primary care physician and evaluated approximately 6 weeks after the MVA. The vehicle she was driving was sideswiped by a semitruck. Details surrounding the event suggested that a minimum biomedical threshold was met for mTBI. Reported acute symptoms included LOC for several minutes and retrograde amnesia for approximately

10 to 15 minutes. She recalled being dazed and confused immediately after the event. She reported having a headache for several days and increased fatigue for approximately 2 weeks. Although she acknowledged difficulties focusing and multitasking immediately after the event, she perceived that cognitive symptoms were becoming more significant. When police and paramedics arrived at the scene of the accident, she denied the offer to be transported to a local medical center for further evaluation.

A thorough psychosocial interview identified both risk and protective factors that would affect her recovery. The patient had an advanced degree in engineering and was competitively employed. In fact, she was recently promoted to a management position. She was in relatively good health, denied past traumatic events, and felt supported by her family and friends. She acknowledged experiencing episodes of depression and anxiety in the past, most commonly associated with major life events and transitions (e.g., attending college, the divorce of her biological parents). She participated in therapy in the past and was uncertain whether it was beneficial. She denied use of illicit substances, rarely consumed alcohol, and was not prescribed medications.

The patient's performances on neuropsychological tests were invariably average to superior across cognitive domains. Most relevant to her concerns, working memory, verbal memory, and visual memory varied from high average to superior. Executive functioning was high average. Nonverbal abilities were more developed than were verbal abilities, though both were technically within normal limits. The neuropsychological profile as a whole was considered consistent with what might have been expected given her background. She also completed an extended self-report measure of emotional functioning and personality. She completed the inventory in a conscientious and open manner. Her overall profile reported excessive health concerns, anxiety, and indifference toward the future. The profile was considered consistent with information obtained during the clinical interview.

The feedback session with the patient lasted more than 1 hour. She was fully engaged with the session and asked numerous questions. She appreciated learning how mTBI is diagnosed and had many questions related to whether or not her immediate symptoms were common. She was relieved to receive feedback regarding her neuropsychological functioning. She acknowledged that the discrepancy between objective data and her subjective appraisal likely reflected anxiety. She questioned whether the clinician believed that she should participate in psychotherapy to develop effective strategies to manage symptoms of anxiety. Treatment goals were established during the feedback session. The most productive aspect of the feedback session was discussion of risk factors that would increase the likelihood of an atypical recovery from mTBI. The patient immediately recognized that she was at risk on the basis of her history of emotional difficulties. This recognition was a relief; for the first time since the MVA she perceived that she had some control over the trajectory of recovery as opposed to worry that she might be chronically disabled. The patient left the feedback session optimistic that better days were in her future and she was hopeful that engaging in psychotherapy would help her function at a higher level.

Clinicians who regularly work with individuals who sustain mTBI in the acute or postacute stage of recovery will recognize that it is somewhat rare for evaluations to end with such a productive, positive, and empowering conversation. Although this is true, it does not mean that clinicians should approach each assessment with hesitation that they will ultimately share information with patients that will not be accepted or result in positive outcomes. Clinicians should take pride in the fact that mTBI has been so thoroughly investigated. Expected outcomes and complicating factors have been consistently identified in the literature and should be openly discussed with patients and guide treatment.

REFERENCES

American Congress of Rehabilitation Medicine Mild Traumatic Brain Injury Committee. (1993). Definition of mild traumatic brain injury. *Journal of Head Trauma and Rehabilitation, 8*(3), 86–87.

American Psychiatric Association. (2000). *Diagnostic criteria from DSM-IV-TR.* Washington, DC: Author.

American Psychiatric Association. (2013). *Diagnostic and statistical manual of mental disorders* (5th ed.). Arlington, VA: American Psychiatric Publishing.

Bailey, C., McCrea, M., & Barth, J. (2013). Athletes and sport-related concussion: Complex issues in medical management. In D. B. Arciniegas, N. D. Zasler, R. D. Vanderploeg, & M. S. Jaffee (Eds.), *Management of adults with traumatic brain injury.* Washington, DC: American Psychiatric Association.

Bazarian, J. J., Wong, T., Harris, M., Leahey, N., Mookerjee, S., & Dombovy, M. (1999). Epidemiology and predictors of post-concussive syndrome after minor head injury in an emergency population. *Brain Injury, 13*(3), 173–189.

Belanger, H. G., & Vanderploeg, R. D. (2005). The neuropsychological impact of sports-related concussion: A meta-analysis. *Journal of the International Neuropsychological Society, 11*(4), 345–357.

Belanger, H. G., Vanderploeg, R. D., Curtiss, G., & Warden, D. L. (2007). Recent neuroimaging techniques in mild traumatic brain injury. *Journal of Neuropsychiatry and Clinical Neurosciences, 19*(1), 5–20. doi:10.1176/jnp.2007.19.1.5

Bigler, E. D. (2008). Neuropsychology and clinical neuroscience of persistent post-concussive syndrome. *Journal of the International Neuropsychological Society, 14*(1), 1–22. doi:10.1017/S135561770808017X

Binder, L. M., Iverson, G. L., & Brooks, B. L. (2009). To err is human: "Abnormal" neuropsychological scores and variability are common in healthy adults. *Archives of Clinical Neuropsychology, 24*(1), 31–46. doi:10.1093/arclin/acn001

Carroll, L. J., Cassidy, J. D., Peloso, P. M., Borg, J., von Holst, H., Holm, L., . . . WHO Collaborating Center Task Force on Mild Traumatic Brain Injury. (2004). Prognosis for mild traumatic brain injury: Results of the WHO Collaborating Center Task Force on Mild Traumatic Brain Injury. *Journal of Rehabilitation Medicine,* (43, Suppl.), 84–105.

Cassidy, J. D., Carroll, L. J., Peloso, P. M., Borg, J., von Holst, H., Holm, L., . . . WHO Collaborating Center Task Force on Mild Traumatic Brain Injury. (2004). Incidence, risk factors and prevention of mild traumatic brain injury: Results of the WHO Collaborating Centre Task Force on Mild Traumatic Brain Injury. *Journal of Rehabilitation Medicine,* (43, Suppl.), 28–60.

Chastain, C. A., Oyoyo, U. E., Zipperman, M., Joo, E., Ashwal, S., Shutter, L. A., & Tong, K. A. (2009). Predicting outcomes of traumatic brain injury by imaging modality and injury distribution. *Journal of Neurotrauma, 26*(8), 1183–1196. doi:10.1089/neu.2008.0650

Covassin, T., Swanik, C. B., & Sachs, M. L. (2003). Sex differences and the incidence of concussions among collegiate athletes. *Journal of Athletic Training, 38*(3), 238–244.

Defense and Veterans Brain Injury Center. (2012). *DoD worldwide numbers for TBI.* Retrieved from http://dvbic.dcoe.mil/dod-worldwide-numbers-tbi

Echemendia, R. J., Giza, C. C., & Kutcher, J. S. (2015). Developing guidelines for return to play: Consensus and evidence-based approaches. *Brain Injury, 29*(2), 185–194. doi:10.3109/02699052.2014.965212

Faul, M., Xu, L., Wald, M. M., & Coronado, V. (2010). *Traumatic brain injury in the United States*. Atlanta, GA: National Center for Injury Prevention and Control, Centers for Disease Control and Prevention.

Feinstein, A., Ouchterlony, D., Somerville, J., & Jardine, A. (2001). The effects of litigation on symptom expression: A prospective study following mild traumatic brain injury. *Medicine, Science and the Law, 41*(2), 116–121.

Ferguson, R. J., Mittenberg, W., Barone, D. F., & Schneider, B. (1999). Postconcussion syndrome following sports-related head injury: Expectation as etiology. *Neuropsychology, 13*(4), 582–589.

Garden, N., & Sullivan, K. A. (2010). An examination of the base rates of post-concussion symptoms: The influence of demographics and depression. *Applied Neuropsychology, 17*(1), 1–7. doi:10.1080/09084280903297495

Gasonique, P. G. (1992). Affective state and awareness of sensory and cognitive effects after closed head injury. *Neuropsychology, 6*(3), 187–196.

Giza, C. C., & Hovda, D. A. (2004). The pathophysiological of traumatic brain injury. In M. R. Lovell, R. J. Echemendia, J. T. Barth, & M. W. Collins (Eds.), *Traumatic brain injury in sports: An international neuropsychological perspective*. Exton, PA: Swets & Zeitlinger.

Gunstad, J., & Suhr, J. A. (2001). "Expectation as etiology" versus "the good old days": Postconcussion syndrome symptom reporting in athletes, headache sufferers, and depressed individuals. *Journal of the International Neuropsychological Society, 7*(3), 323–333.

Guskiewicz, K. M., McCrea, M., Marshall, S. W., Cantu, R. C., Randolph, C., Barr, W., . . . Kelly, J. P. (2003). Cumulative effects associated with recurrent concussion in collegiate football players: The NCAA concussion study. *JAMA, 290*(19), 2549–2555. doi:10.1001/jama.290.19.2549

Guskiewicz, K. M., Mihalik, J. P., Shankar, V., Marshall, S. W., Crowell, D. H., Oliaro, S. M., . . . Hooker, D. N. (2007). Measurement of head impacts in collegiate football players: Relationship between head impact biomechanics and acute clinical outcome after concussion. *Neurosurgery, 61*(6), 1244–1252; discussion 1252–1243. doi:10.1227/01.neu.0000306103.68635.1a

Hoffer, M. E., Donaldson, C., Gottshall, K. R., Balaban, C., & Balough, B. J. (2009). Blunt and blast head trauma: Different entities. *The International Tinnitus Journal, 15*(2), 115–118.

Holm, L., Cassidy, J. D., Carroll, L. J., & Borg, J. (2005). Summary of the WHO collaborating center for neurotrauma task force on mild traumatic brain injury. *Journal of Rehabilitation Medicine, 37*(3), 137–141.

Iverson, G. L. (2005). Outcome from mild traumatic brain injury. *Current Opinion in Psychiatry, 18*(3), 301–317. doi:10.1097/01.yco.0000165601.29047.ae

Iverson, G. L., Brooks, B. L., Collins, M. W., & Lovell, M. R. (2006). Tracking neuropsychological recovery following concussion in sport. *Brain Injury, 20*(3), 245–252. doi:10.1080/02699050500487910

Iverson, G. L., & Lange, R. T. (2003). Examination of "postconcussion-like" symptoms in a healthy sample. *Applied Neuropsychology, 10*(3), 137–144. doi:10.1207/S15324826AN1003_02

Karr, J. E., Areshenkoff, C. N., & Garcia-Barrera, M. A. (2014). The neuropsychological outcomes of concussion: A systematic review of meta-analyses on the cognitive sequelae of mild traumatic brain injury. *Neuropsychology, 28*(3), 321–336. doi:10.1037/neu0000037

Krause, J. F., McArthur, D. L., Silverman, T., & Jayaraman, M. (1996). Epidemiology of brain injury. In R. W. Evans (Ed.), *Neurology and Trauma* (pp. 3–17). Houston, TX: Saunders.

Lezak, M. D., Howieson, D. B., Bigler, E. D., & Tranel, D. (2012). *Neuropsychological assessment* (5th ed.). New York, NY: Oxford University Press.

Mayou, R. A., Black, J., & Bryant, B. (2000). Unconsciousness, amnesia and psychiatric symptoms following road traffic accident injury. *British Journal of Psychiatry, 177*, 540–545.

McAllister, T. W. (2011). Mild brain injury. In J. M. Silver, T. W. McAllister, & S. C. Yudofsky (Eds.), *Textbook of traumatic brain injury* (2nd ed.). Arlington, VA: American Psychiatric Publishing.

McAllister, T. W., Flashman, L. A., McDonald, B. C., & Saykin, A. J. (2006). Mechanisms of working memory dysfunction after mild and moderate TBI: Evidence from functional MRI and neurogenetics. *Journal of Neurotrauma, 23*(10), 1450–1467. doi:10.1089/neu.2006.23.1450

McCauley, S. R., Wilde, E. A., Miller, E. R., Frisby, M. L., Garza, H. M., Varghese, R., . . . McCarthy, J. J. (2013). Preinjury resilience and mood as predictors of early outcome following mild traumatic brain injury. *Journal of Neurotrauma, 30*(8), 642–652. doi:10.1089/neu.2012.2393

McCrea, M. (2008). *Mild traumatic brain injury and postconcussion syndrome: The new evidence base for diagnosis and treatment*. New York, NY: Oxford University Press.

McCrea, M., Broshek, D. K., & Barth, J. T. (2015). Sports concussion assessment and management: Future research directions. *Brain Injury, 29*(2), 276–282. doi:10.3109/02699052.2014.965216

McCrea, M., Hammeke, T., Olsen, G., Leo, P., & Guskiewicz, K. (2004). Unreported concussion in high school football players: Implications for prevention. *Clinical Journal of Sport Medicine, 14*(1), 13–17.

McCrory, P., Meeuwisse, W., Johnston, K., Dvorak, J., Aubry, M., Molloy, M., & Cantu, R. (2009). Consensus statement on concussion in sport—The Third International Conference on Concussion in Sport held in Zurich, November 2008. *The Physician and Sports Medicine, 37*(2), 141–159. doi:10.3810/psm.2009.06.1721

McCrory, P. R., & Berkovic, S. F. (2001). Concussion: The history of clinical and pathophysiological concepts and misconceptions. *Neurology, 57*(12), 2283–2289.

Miller, H. (1961). Accident neurosis. *British Medical Journal, 1*(5230), 919–925.

Mittenberg, W., Tremont, G., Zielinski, R. E., Fichera, S., & Rayls, K. R. (1996). Cognitive-behavioral prevention of postconcussion syndrome. *Archives of Clinical Neuropsychology, 11*(2), 139–145.

National Center for Injury Prevention and Control. (2003). *Report to Congress on mild traumatic brain injury in the United States: Steps to prevent a serious public health problem.* Atlanta, GA: Centers for Disease Control and Prevention.

Nelson, L. D., Janecek, J. K., & McCrea, M. A. (2013). Acute clinical recovery from sport-related concussion. *Neuropsychology Review, 23*(4), 285–299. doi:10.1007/s11065-013-9240-7

Ommaya, A. K., & Gennarelli, T. A. (1974). Cerebral concussion and traumatic unconsciousness: Correlation of experimental and clinical observations of blunt head injuries. *Brain, 97*(4), 633–654.

Paniak, C., Reynolds, S., Toller-Lobe, G., Melnyk, A., Nagy, J., & Schmidt, D. (2002). A longitudinal study of the relationship between financial compensation and symptoms after treated mild traumatic brain injury. *Journal of Clinical and Experimental Neuropsychology, 24*(2), 187–193. doi:10.1076/jcen.24.2.187.999

Ponsford, J. (2005). Rehabilitation interventions after mild head injury. *Current Opinion in Neurology, 18*(6), 692–697.

Rabinowitz, A. R., Li, X., & Levin, H. S. (2014). Sport and nonsport etiology of mild traumatic brain injury: Similarities and differences. *Annual Review of Psychology, 65*, 301–331.

Roberts, R. J., & Roberts, M. A. (2011). *Mild traumatic brain injury: Episodic symptoms and treatment.* San Diego, CA: Plural Publishing.

Ruff, R. (2005). Two decades of advances in understanding of mild traumatic brain injury. *Journal of Head Trauma Rehabilitation, 20*(1), 5–18.

Ruff, R. M., Camenzuli, L., & Mueller, J. (1996). Miserable minority: Emotional risk factors that influence the outcome of a mild traumatic brain injury. *Brain Injury, 10*(8), 551–565.

Ruff, R. M., Iverson, G. L., Barth, J. T., Bush, S. S., Broshek, D. K., & National Academy of Neuropsychology Policy and Planning Committee. (2009). Recommendations for diagnosing a mild traumatic brain injury: A National Academy of Neuropsychology education paper. *Archives of Clinical Neuropsychology, 24*(1), 3–10. doi:10.1093/arclin/acp006

Schulz, M. R., Marshall, S. W., Mueller, F. O., Yang, J., Weaver, N. L., Kalsbeek, W. D., & Bowling, J. M. (2004). Incidence and risk factors for concussion in high school athletes, North Carolina, 1996–1999. *American Journal of Epidemiology, 160*(10), 937–944. doi:10.1093/aje/kwh304

Sosin, D. M., Sniezek, J. E., & Thurman, D. J. (1996). Incidence of mild and moderate brain injury in the United States, 1991. *Brain Injury, 10*(1), 47–54.

Summers, C. R., Ivins, B., & Schwab, K. A. (2009). Traumatic brain injury in the United States: An epidemiologic overview. *The Mount Sinai Journal of Medicine, 76*(2), 105–110. doi:10.1002/msj.20100

Warden, D. L., French, L. M., Shupenko, L., Fargus, J., Riedy, G., Erickson, M. E., . . . Moore, D. F. (2009). Case report of a soldier with primary blast brain injury. *Neuroimage, 47*(Suppl. 2), T152–T153. doi:10.1016/j.neuroimage.2009.01.060

Wood, R. L., O'Hagan, G., Williams, C., McCabe, M., & Chadwick, N. (2014). Anxiety sensitivity and alexithymia as mediators of post-concussion syndrome following mild traumatic brain injury. *Journal of Head Trauma Rehabilitation, 29*(1), E9–E17. doi:10.1097/HTR.0b013e31827eabba

World Health Organization. (1992). *The ICD-10 classification of mental and behavioral disorders: Clinical descriptions and diagnostic guidelines.* Geneva, Switzerland: Author.

Yang, C. C., Yuen, K. M., Huang, S. J., Hsiao, S. H., Tsai, Y. H., & Lin, W. C. (2014). "Good-old-days" bias: A prospective follow-up study to examine the preinjury supernormal status in patients with mild traumatic brain injury. *Journal of Clinical and Experimental Neuropsychology, 36*(4), 399–409. doi:10.1080/13803395.2014.903899

Zhang, L., Yang, K. H., & King, A. I. (2004). A proposed injury threshold for mild traumatic brain injury. *Journal of Biomechanical Engineering, 126*(2), 226–236.

CHAPTER 2

Moderate to Severe Brain Injury

P. TYLER ROSKOS
LAUREN R. SCHWARZ

OVERVIEW

The Centers for Disease Control and Prevention (CDC) defines traumatic brain injury (TBI) as an injury to the head arising from blunt or penetrating trauma or from acceleration/deceleration forces resulting in one or more of the following: decreased level of consciousness, amnesia, objective neurological or neuropsychological abnormalities, skull fractures, diagnosed intracranial lesions, or head injury listed as a cause of death in the death certificate (Coronado, McGuire, Faul, Sugerman, & Pearson, 2013; National Center for Injury Prevention and Control, 2003; Thurman, Sniezek, Johnson, Greenspan, & Smith, 1995). TBI can result in multiple physical, cognitive, emotional/psychological, and social and functional symptoms and deficits. Injuries of greater severity (classified as moderate or severe TBI) tend to require more complex acute and postacute care, as well as result in greater long-term health care costs and morbidity (Draper & Ponsford, 2008; Finkelstein, Corso, & Miller, 2006).

As a resource for clinical professionals and trainees, the goal of this chapter is to provide a brief history of intervention for moderate and severe TBI, as well as a review of our current knowledge regarding the clinical features, intervention strategies, and prognosis for people with these injuries. We will also provide a case example of the theoretical and research-based concepts presented.

HISTORY

Early medical interventions for TBI were focused largely on acute injuries sustained on the battlefield in the context of warfare (Teasdale & Zitnay, 2013). It was not until the latter half of the 20th century and the development of the automobile, increased road traffic, and urban growth, that civilian TBI became more recognized. Most clinical care for TBI patients was within the domain of neurosurgery. The 1970s brought advances in medical technology, such as the computed tomography (CT) scanner (Ambrose, Gooding, & Uttley, 1976), that had a direct impact on the ability to evaluate and treat head injuries. Additionally, the Glasgow Coma Scale (GCS), which is still widely used today to assess injury severity, was developed by Graham Teasdale and Bryan Jennett in 1974. The 1980s and 1990s saw additional notable advancements in evaluation and intervention for acute head injury, including issues such as monitoring of intracranial pressure, use of neuroprotective pharmacological agents, and establishment of standard guidelines for clinical care. These advancements resulted in reduced mortality and improved outcomes from head injury (Teasdale & Zitnay, 2013).

Interdisciplinary brain injury rehabilitation programs began to develop during the 1940s during and after World War II, with the formal recognition of Physical Medicine and Rehabilitation as a medical specialty (Teasdale & Zitnay, 2013). Leaders in the field established early rehabilitation programs over several decades. Furthermore, the Vietnam War era resulted in improved legislation for individuals with disability, including support for community-based rehabilitation. During the 1980s, organizations focused on brain injury awareness, and specialized rehabilitation and advocacy also were established and grew (e.g., Brain Injury Association and the International Brain Injury Association). The TBI Model Systems programs were also established and funded by the National Institute of Disability and Rehabilitation Research (NIDRR), resulting in an increase in collaborative research involving clinical care and outcomes from TBI.

During the 1990s and early 2000s, there was an emphasis on demonstrating the effectiveness and efficacy of rehabilitation programs for TBI. This resulted in more rigorous scientific scrutiny of clinical strategies used by clinicians and the establishment of guidelines for acute care and rehabilitation for TBI (Neurotrauma Foundation, American Association of Neurological Surgeons). There was also increased emphasis on costs of care, lengths of rehabilitation stay, and insurance reimbursement issues during the early 2000s.

Currently, intervention for moderate and severe TBI can involve a complex continuum including the neurosurgical intensive care unit, shock trauma unit, a neurology or trauma floor, acute rehabilitation, nursing home, skilled nursing facility, long-term acute care, outpatient therapy, home health, day programs, residential rehabilitation and residential placement programs (Ivanhoe, Durand-Sanchez, & Spier, 2013). Rehabilitation programs often emphasize a multidisciplinary team approach to address the wide range of symptoms and problems that may develop over the course of acute and postacute rehabilitation care. The Functional Independence Measure (FIM) has also been established as the most widely used outcome measure in rehabilitation settings, and has been used as the gold standard to demonstrate the efficacy of rehabilitation programs for TBI patients across settings and providers (Granger, Cotter, Hamilton, & Fiedler, 1993; Granger, Divan, & Fiedler, 1995).

PATHOPHYSIOLOGY

The acute pathophysiology of moderate and severe TBI is typically viewed as a process involving both primary and secondary focal and diffuse brain injury that results from the initial blunt trauma event (Yokobori & Bullock, 2013). Acceleration and deceleration during blunt trauma can lead to both translational and rotational forces that impact the head, leading to brain injury (Viano, 2013). Additionally, there can be more chronic complications of TBI, resulting in potentially greater morbidity in these patients. These pathophysiological components of TBI are discussed in greater detail in the following subsections.

Primary Injury

Contusions are hemorrhages caused by acceleration–deceleration forces, leading to differential movement between brain and skull or brain matter at gray–white interfaces (Ponsford, Sloan, & Snow, 2013). Often referred to as "coup–contrecoup" injuries, contusions can be seen at the site of impact and at the opposite side of the impact (Gaetz, 2004). The bony skull protuberances located on the frontal bone, sphenoidal ridge, temporal bone, and the edges of the falces often result in contusive injury on the poles of the frontal and temporal lobes (Le & Gean, 2009). Contusions can lead to necrosis and apoptosis (i.e., cell death) owing to reduced supply of blood, oxygen, and glucose.

Tearing of blood vessels as a result of external impact to the head can cause bleeding inside of the skull (i.e., hematomas) and the formation of clots that can compress brain tissue (Gennarelli & Graham, 2005; Ponsford et al., 2013). Subdural hematoma (SDH) results from bleeding between the dura and arachnoid layers of the meninges, and subarachnoid hemorrhage (SAH) refers to bleeding between the arachnoid and pia layers. An intracerebral hematoma (ICH) forms within the brain parenchyma as a result of a tear in deep brain vasculature. Hematomas within the meninges or brain tissue can result in increased intracranial pressure, ischemic brain damage, and obstruction of the flow of cerebrospinal fluid, often requiring neurosurgical intervention.

Diffuse axonal injury (DAI), also known as "traumatic axonal injury" (TAI), is the primary mechanism of injury in a large number of moderate and severe TBIs, and can result in micropathological injury to axons in multiple brain regions (Gaetz, 2004; Meythaler, Peduzzi, Eleftheriou, & Novack, 2001). In DAI, deformation of brain tissue caused by acceleration–deceleration forces during blunt head trauma results in shearing, tearing, and twisting of neuronal axons, as well as local cell death and downstream denervation and wallerian degeneration (a process that occurs when nerve fiber is damaged, in which the part of the axon separated from the neuron's cell body degenerates) over time following injury (Ponsford et al., 2013). Petechial hemorrhage, as well as SAH and intraparenchymal hemorrhage (IPH), can also be associated with DAI because of rotational forces, causing further white matter damage (Povlishock & Katz, 2005). The most common sites of DAI include the subcortical white matter, corpus callosum, gray–white matter junctions, and brain stem.

Secondary Injury

Increased intracranial pressure (ICP) is a common consequence of intracranial injury that can result in reduced cerebral perfusion pressure and blood flow (Gennarelli & Graham, 2005). Disruption in blood flow due to increased ICP can cause diffuse ischemic injury, increases in inflammation, and metabolic dysfunction, leading to neuronal death. Additionally, increased ICP can lead to shifting of brain tissues and/or downward herniation. If not addressed, herniation can result in compression of the brain stem, leading to respiratory arrest and eventual death (Gennarelli & Graham, 2005). Decompressive craniotomy is the most common neurosurgical intervention involving removal of a portion of the skull to allow for reduction in pressure to reverse the process of herniation. Other secondary factors that can lead to greater brain injury include hypoxia, cerebral edema, and infection (i.e., meningitis or cerebral abscess; Long, 2013; Ponsford et al., 2013).

Chronic Complications of TBI

Individuals with moderate or severe TBI are also at risk for a number of neurological complications that can affect functioning and recovery. Hydrocephalus can be caused by disruptions in the flow of cerebrospinal fluid (CSF) in the ventricles (noncommunicating), or can result from blood within the subarachnoid space, preventing proper absorption of CSF (communicating). This can be difficult to diagnose using radiological studies alone because of the presence of ex vacuo dilation of the ventricles in many moderate and severe TBI patients (Long, 2013). Aspects of clinical presentation (e.g., behavioral or cognitive worsening) can be diagnostically useful in determining patients who need treatment, which usually involves neurosurgical placement of a ventriculoperitoneal shunt.

Posttraumatic epilepsy is also a common chronic complication of moderate and severe TBI. When looking over a 5-year period, Annegers, Hauser, Coan, and Rocca (1998) found the following prevalence rates of seizures following TBI: 0.5% for mild injuries, 1.2% for moderate injuries, and 10% for severe injuries. Many patients are treated prophylactically with antiepileptic medications within the first week postinjury to reduce early-onset seizures, but this has not been shown to reduce the risk of late-onset seizure disorder (Ponsford et al., 2013).

ETIOLOGY

The etiology of TBI typically involves an external force (i.e., injury mechanism) that causes injury to the brain. Falls are the most common injury mechanism of TBI overall, especially in children and older adults (Coronado et al., 2013). The CDC reported that from 2006 to 2010, falls accounted for 40% of all TBIs that led to emergency department (ED) visits, hospitalizations, or deaths. Unintentional blunt trauma and motor vehicle accidents (MVAs) account for 15% and 14%, respectively, of all TBI-associated ED encounters (Centers for Disease Control and Prevention [CDC], 2016). MVAs are the most common mechanism of injury in teenagers and younger adults (ages 15–34; Coronado et al., 2013).

Sports-related TBI has also emerged as a public health issue in the United States, with an estimated 1.6 to 3.8 million sports-related TBIs per year. However, moderate or severe TBI cases are a minority of sports-related injuries, with most patients being treated in the emergency department and released (Coronado et al., 2013). TBI has also been a critical health issue in military combat veterans, moderate and severe TBI representing about 10% of cases from 2000 to 2015 (Center for Defense and Veterans Brain Injury, 2015).

EPIDEMIOLOGY

Despite the growing awareness of TBI as a public health concern, the determination of incidence rates has been complicated by factors such as accuracy of diagnosis, cost related to these medical workups, and timeliness of diagnosis (Korley, Kelen, Jones, & Diaz-Arrastia, 2015). To further complicate the matter, many individuals with mild injuries never come to the attention of medical providers. Much of what is known about prevalence rates comes from investigations of EDs. The CDC (2016) reported that in 2010, TBI accounted for 2.5 million ED visits, hospitalizations, or deaths. Specifically, TBI resulted in more than 280,000 hospitalizations and was related to the cause of death in more than 50,000 individuals. In the last decade, the number of individuals seen in the ED for TBI increased by 70%, hospitalization rate increased by 11%, but the rate of death fell by 7%.

Of those individuals hospitalized with TBI, discharge rates vary by severity of injury. More specifically, most patients with mild and moderate injuries are discharged from the hospital and return home; however, those with more severe injuries may be sent from the acute setting into a skilled care facility. The discharge diagnoses include, for example, intracranial injury with and without fracture, concussion, intracranial hemorrhage, contusion, and so forth. Despite discharge, TBI can be a lifelong injury for patients. It is estimated that 80,000 to 90,000 individuals have new onset of disability due to TBI each year, with more than 1 million individuals disabled secondary to TBI (Thurman, 1999; Thurman, Alverson, Dunn, Guerrero, & Sniezek, 1999). It is estimated that the annual economic cost of TBI in the United States is at least $76 billion (Coronado et al., 2013).

Certain members of the population have been found to be at greater risk for experiencing TBI. More specifically, age has been identified as a risk factor, with those between 15 and 24 years old and those over the age of 65 having the highest rates of brain injury (Kraus & Chu, 2005; Sosin, Sniezek, & Thurman, 1996). Children under the age of 5 also have a higher reported incidence rate of TBI (Jager, Weiss, Coben, & Pepe, 2000). An additional risk factor appears to be gender, with males having a 1.6 to 2.8 times greater rate compared with females (Kraus & Chu, 2005). Individuals with a prior history of TBI are also at a 2.8 to 3.0 times increased risk of additional injury (Salcido & Costich, 1992). Several investigations have found higher rates of TBI in individuals of lower socioeconomic status (SES) (Roebuck-Spencer & Sherer, 2008). Finally, alcohol consumption has also been implicated as a risk factor for TBI (Smith & Kraus, 1988).

CLINICAL PRESENTATION AND DIAGNOSTIC CONSIDERATIONS

Severity of Injury

In the evaluation of patients with TBI, severity of injury is one of the most important factors to consider, as this has implications for predictions concerning symptoms, course of recovery, and, ultimately, outcome. Several sources of information are often used to determine severity, including duration of loss of consciousness (LOC)/coma, time to follow commands, length of posttraumatic amnesia (PTA), GCS (Teasdale & Jennett, 1974), and the presence of neuroimaging findings. Concerning LOC, Lezak and colleagues developed a classification index for severity as follows: ≤20 minutes = mild, ≤6 hours = moderate, and greater than 6 hours = severe (Lezak, 1995; Lezak, Howieson, Loring, Hannay, & Fischer, 2004). PTA refers to the time period during which individuals are responsive, but disoriented, confused, and unable to form new memories. Russell and Smith (1961) developed the most frequently used classification ranges, which are as follows: less than 1 hour = mild, 1 to 24 hours = moderate, 1 to 7 days = severe, and greater than 7 days = very severe. This time period can be assessed by asking patients their first and last memory surrounding the injury or more formal measures of orientation such as the Orientation Log (Jackson, Novack, & Dowler, 1998) and the Galveston Orientation and Amnesia Scale (GOAT) (Levin, O'Donnell, & Grossman, 1979). The GCS is tabulated by assessing patients' eye opening, motor movements, and verbal communication. Scores range from 3 to 15; higher numbers are associated with greater levels of functioning. GCS classification ranges are as follows: 13 to 15 = mild, 9 to 12 = moderate, 6 to 8 = severe, and 3 to 5 = very severe. Numerous studies have investigated the distributions of severity of injury. This data has varied significantly according to the severity parameters utilized (Roebuck-Spencer & Sherer, 2008). In general, about 80% of injuries are mild in nature, whereas 10% are moderate, and 10% are severe.

Typical Cognitive Deficits

The deficits patients experience acutely following injury depend largely on severity of injury. In the case of mild TBI (mTBI), typical acute deficits include slowed speed of thought processes, reduced attention span, and memory inefficiency. In a meta-analysis, Schretlen and Shapiro (2003) found that 96% of mTBI patients were asymptomatic at 3 months. Although there is some variability in recovery rate after mTBI, the overall consensus is that barring any complicating factors, individuals who suffer mTBI typically make a good recovery. In contrast, the severity and pattern of deficits in patients with moderate to severe TBI are quite variable and depend not only upon the injury itself, but also on factors such as premorbid level of functioning. In general, patients with moderate to severe TBI often experience deficits in attention, expressive language, speed of processing, memory, and reasoning skills (Roebuck-Spencer & Sherer, 2008).

Physical and Emotional Symptoms

Physical symptoms are commonly associated with TBI. Typical symptoms include headache, dizziness, double vision, light sensitivity (i.e., photophobia), smell and taste changes, and motoric slowing and incoordination. Other motor-related symptoms can arise and are typically associated with brain bleeds/contusions and include dysarthria, dysphagia, imbalance, spasticity, and hemiparesis. Sleep quality is also an area of concern; about 67% of TBI patients have some form of sleep disturbance (including hypersomnia or insomnia) (Kempf, Werth, Kaiser, Bassetti, & Baumann, 2010).

Neurobehavioral symptoms are also quite common in patients with moderate to severe TBI. Oftentimes, patients and family members report these symptoms to be the most distressing. Symptoms can include depression, fatigue, anxiety, irritability, and personality change (Roebuck-Spencer & Sherer, 2008). Impaired awareness of deficits is common in patients with moderate to severe TBI.

Course of Recovery

Patients who have suffered moderate to severe TBIs typically experience recovery in stages. However, there is a significant amount of interindividual variability in progression of recovery. TBI is often associated with impairment in the level of alertness/consciousness. On the severe end of the spectrum, coma represents a time in which patients are completely nonresponsive. Level of alertness/coma is often the first state to improve. It is rare for patients who recover from coma to remain in a persistent vegetative status (<1%, Jiang, Gao, Li, Yu, & Zhu, 2002). Once alertness has improved, individuals may be in a period of confusion. During this time, individuals may have marked impairments in cognition, as mentioned previously. This period is typically referred to as "PTA." The skills of orientation, attention, expressive language, memory, and executive functioning typically recover in the order in which they were listed. The research has been mixed with regard to duration of time for cognitive recovery. Some studies have cited up to 18 months (Levin, 1995); however, more recent investigations have indicated recovery can occur significantly beyond that time frame. With respect to motoric recovery, Walker and Pickett (2007) found that in general, motoric improvements in severely brain-injured patients plateaued at 12 months and that over one third of them continued to manifest impairment at 2 years.

Complication Factors in Recovery

There are certain patient characteristics that have been associated with less than optimal injury recovery. One uncontrollable factor is age. Being over the age of 65 at the time of injury is associated with higher TBI-related mortality and morbidity (Gomez et al., 2000). History of experiencing more than one TBI, even if they are mild in nature, has a tendency to be related to poorer outcome. Other factors related to psychiatric status have been linked with complicating TBI recovery. Alcohol abuse, in particular, has been linked with less than optimal recovery. The development of conditions such as depression, anxiety, and posttraumatic stress disorder (PTSD) has also been linked to suboptimal or prolonged recovery in brain-injured patients. Thus, treatment for TBI must ensure that all aspects of patients are being treated, which include appropriate referrals for mental health interventions.

TREATMENT

Rehabilitation Therapy

The treatment of patients with moderate and severe TBI takes place across a range of settings in order to address the patients' needs at various time points during recovery. The Commission on Accreditation of Rehabilitation Facilities accredits brain injury rehabilitation facilities in the following categories: inpatient, outpatient, home- and community-based, residential, long-term residential, and vocational (Cope & Reynolds, 2005). Although neurosurgeons or trauma surgeons typically manage the acute care of moderate and severe TBI patients, rehabilitation is typically managed by a multidisciplinary team led by a physiatrist and including physical therapists, occupational therapists, speech and language pathologists, social workers, psychologists/neuropsychologists, and nurses (Cope & Reynolds, 2005). Each of these professionals is trained to address specific deficits associated with injury and to provide education and support to patients, as well as their families. Overall, brain injury rehabilitation can promote recovery, reduce comorbidities, and serve to educate patients and families to promote continued progress and recovery after discharge (Ivanhoe et al., 2013).

Cognitive rehabilitation involves development of compensatory and remediation strategies to address cognitive impairments resulting from brain injury, such as memory, attention, and problem-solving deficits (Gordon, 2005). This can involve modifications to the environment, development of individualized compensatory strategies, and other direct interventions designed to improve cognitive skills.

Several reviews and meta-analytic studies have demonstrated the effectiveness of cognitive rehabilitation techniques (e.g., Cicerone et al., 2000; Park & Ingles, 2001). Overall, there is support for intervention for attention, memory, functional communication, and executive deficits following TBI.

Pharmacotherapy

Multiple brain neurotransmitter systems are affected by TBI, with evidence that acute and chronic effects of injury are different. Therefore, the timing of pharmacotherapy is important to consider, with evidence that different treatments may be important in the early versus late phases of recovery (Meythaler & Zafonte, 2013). Overall, there is support for multiple pharmacological agents that can have a beneficial impact on neuro-recovery following injury, depending on the timing of the intervention.

Increases in serotonergic or norepinephrine pathway activation immediately following injury have been associated with greater neuronal cell death and worsening of secondary injury effects (Meythaler & Zafonte, 2013). However, in the postacute and chronic recovery phases from TBI, there is support for the use of selective serotonin reuptake inhibitors (SSRIs) such as sertraline for treating postinjury depression, as well as medications that enhance norepinephrine, such as methylphenidate, in treating attentional disorders (Novack, Banos, Brunner, Renfroe, & Meythaler, 2009; Whyte et al., 1997). Gamma-aminobutyric acid (GABA) has been proposed to be neuroprotective immediately following injury; therefore, GABA agonists such as benzodiazepines may have deleterious effects on neuro-recovery and rehabilitation (Meythaler & Zafonte, 2013). The cholinergic system, which is associated with memory and aspects of motor functioning, has also been a target of pharmacological agents used to promote long-term recovery (i.e., donepezil). Medications that enhance dopamine activity have also been supported to improve recovery outcomes from TBI (i.e., amantadine; Meythaler, Brunner, Johnson, & Novack, 2002).

Psychotherapy and Neurobehavioral Interventions

It has been well established that there is a significant psychosocial impact of TBI, including changes in family and other interpersonal relationships, social activities, and educational and occupational pursuits (Ponsford et al., 2013). Depression, anxiety, and PTSD have also been shown to be common comorbidities in patients with moderate and severe TBI. In addition, behavioral issues, such as emotional dysregulation, impulsivity, poor social pragmatics, irritability/aggression, personality changes, and agitation are common long-term consequences of TBI (Roebuck-Spencer & Sherer, 2008). The use of psychotherapeutic techniques has been demonstrated to be of benefit, beyond that of pharmacological interventions, to address emotional and behavioral issues in this patient population (Pollack, 2005). A primary goal of psychotherapy with TBI patients usually involves restoration of identity and sense of self postinjury, which can include reflection on the preinjury self and participation in new activities to establish meaning and new self-identity (Ponsford et al., 2013; Prigatano, 1999).

PROGNOSIS

Patients and their families often have questions about prognosis for recovery from moderate or severe TBI, and view prognostic information as psychologically important (Junqué, Bruna, & Mataró, 1997). However, measurement and prediction of outcome from moderate and severe TBI has generated a large volume of research and is complex; therefore, clinicians often need to consider many contextual factors when providing such feedback to patients and their families. With knowledge of prognostic factors and typical outcome variables, clinicians can make reasonable estimates of outcome and prognosis to educate patients and their families.

Outcome assessments can include survival rate, physical impairments, functioning in activities of daily living, cognitive functioning, behavioral functioning, return to work, need for supervision/functional independence, and quality of life (Kothari & DiTommaso, 2013). Additionally, a number of variables have been shown to reliably predict outcome, including age, initial GCS score, LOC, duration of PTA, early CT or MRI findings, and neuropsychological testing data (Kothari & DiTommaso, 2013; Sherer et al., 2002). Overall, lower GCS scores, longer duration of PTA, and longer duration of coma are all associated with poorer outcomes. Presence of deep brain lesions on MRI, as well as bilateral brain stem lesions on imaging, has been shown to predict poor outcome. Older age has also been reliably shown to be associated with worse outcome.

Regarding cognitive recovery, Christensen et al. (2008) showed that moderate and severe TBI patients tend to show the steepest recovery over the first 6 months postinjury, whereas their cognitive recovery curve tends to plateau over months 7 to 12 postinjury. Memory and speeded executive functioning skills were the most persistent cognitive deficits at 1 year postinjury.

CLINICAL SYNOPSIS

- Moderate and severe TBI is typically caused by blunt-force or acceleration/deceleration trauma resulting in physical, cognitive, emotional/psychological, and social and functional deficits.
- Evaluation methods and treatment techniques for TBI have evolved over time, with comprehensive, interdisciplinary rehabilitation programs emerging as the current standard of care.
- The pathophysiology of moderate and severe TBI consists of primary and secondary focal and diffuse injury to the brain. There also exist multiple chronic complications that can contribute to morbidity in these patients.
- Most moderate and severe TBIs are caused by falls, with MVAs and other blunt-force trauma representing the majority of the remainder of cases. Sport-related and combat-related injuries also can cause moderate and severe TBI.
- The CDC (2016) reported that in 2010, TBI accounted for 2.5 million ED visits, hospitalizations, or deaths. Specifically, TBI resulted in more than 280,000 hospitalizations and was related to the cause of death in more than 50,000 individuals.
- Several sources of information are used to determine severity of injury including duration of LOC/coma, time to follow commands, length of PTA, GCS, and the presence of neuroimaging findings.
- TBI is associated with significant symptoms including cognitive deficits as well as physical and emotional symptoms. The deficits seen acutely depend largely on the severity of injury, with mTBI being associated with the best prognosis. Factors such as advancing age, alcohol misuse, and development of psychiatric disorders have been linked with less than optimal recovery.

- Comprehensive rehabilitation therapies across many settings and involving a range of specially trained clinical professionals have been shown to be the most effective treatment for moderate and severe TBI. Pharmacological and psychotherapeutic treatments have also been demonstrated to have benefit for addressing the physical, cognitive, behavioral, and emotional consequences of TBI.
- Knowledge of prognosis is important for patients and families. Clinicians must consider many predictive factors and outcome variables when providing feedback to patients and their families regarding their prognosis.

CASE STUDY

When reading the following case example, please consider the following questions: How severe would you grade the patient's TBI? Are his deficits consistent with what you would expect for the severity of his injury? What factors may complicate the patient's recovery? What recommendations would you make for the patient?

The patient is a 45-year-old, right-handed, White man who fell 40 feet from construction equipment while at work. The exact duration of LOC was not known, but likely was at least 15 minutes. He sustained a traumatic subarachnoid hemorrhage. GCS upon presentation to the emergency room (ER) was 10. He had 1 day of PTA. The patient presented for an evaluation 1 year postinjury and complained of memory loss, slowed thinking, and inability to return to work. Past medical history is remarkable for back pain, alcohol and marijuana use, and depression. The patient completed 12 years of education, but did not perform well in the academic setting. He has a history of legal difficulties—he had a number of DWIs. The patient is married and has two children.

On neurocognitive testing, his performances were suggestive of average preinjury intelligence with intact (i.e., high average to low average) skills in the areas of attention, working memory, and visual naming. His performances were variable on measures of speed of processing, verbal fluency, and executive functioning. Performances were consistently impaired on measures of learning, memory, and fine motor coordination. Psychological testing was remarkable for depression and anxiety.

After reading the information just given, take a moment to answer the questions posed at the beginning. Here are some potential answers to the questions: *How severe would you grade the patient's TBI?*—likely a moderate injury based upon GCS of 10, 1 day of PTA, and positive neuroimaging findings. *Are his deficits consistent with what you would expect for the severity of his injury?*—yes, deficits in reaction time, memory, reasoning skills, and fine motor coordination would not be atypical of a patient with a moderate TBI. *What factors may complicate the patient's recovery?*—this patient has a history of drug and alcohol misuse, depression, and chronic pain, all of which have been linked with poorer outcomes. *What recommendations would you make for the patient?*—possible recommendations for the patient include psychiatric treatment, cognitive rehabilitation, and vocational rehabilitation services.

REFERENCES

Ambrose, J., Gooding, M. R., & Uttley, D. (1976). E.M.I. scan in the management of head injuries. *Lancet, 1*(7964), 847–848.

Annegers, J. F., Hauser, W. A., Coan, S. P., & Rocca, W. A. (1998). A population-based study of seizures after traumatic brain injuries. *The New England Journal of Medicine, 338*(1), 20–24. doi:10.1056/NEJM199801013380104

Center for Defense and Veterans Brain Injury. (2015). *DOD numbers for traumatic brain injury worldwide-totals*. Retrieved from http://dvbic.dcoe.mil/dod-worldwide-numbers-tbi

Centers for Disease Control and Prevention (2016). *TBI: Get the facts*. Retrieved from www.cdc.gov/traumaticbraininjury/get_the_facts.html

Christensen, B. K., Colella, B., Inness, E., Hebert, D., Monette, G., Bayley, M., & Green, R. E. (2008). Recovery of cognitive function after traumatic brain injury: A multilevel modeling analysis of Canadian outcomes. *Archives of Physical Medicine and Rehabilitation, 89*(12, Suppl.), S3–S15. doi:10.1016/j.apmr.2008.10.002

Cicerone, K. D., Dahlberg, C., Kalmar, K., Langenbahn, D. M., Malec, J. F., Bergquist, T. F., . . . Morse, P. A. (2000). Evidence-based cognitive rehabilitation: Recommendations for clinical practice. *Archives of Physical Medicine and Rehabilitation, 81*(12), 1596–1615. doi:10.1053/apmr.2000.19240

Cope, N. D., & Reynolds, W. E. (2005). Systems of care. In J. M. Silver, T. W. McAllister, & S. C. Yudofsky (Eds.), *Textbook of traumatic brain injury*. Arlington, VA: American Psychiatric Publishing.

Coronado, V., McGuire, L., Faul, M., Sugerman, D., & Pearson, W. (2013). Traumatic brain injury epidemiology and public health issues. In N. D. Zasler, D. I. Katz, & R. D. Zafonte (Eds.), *Brain injury medicine: Principles and practice*. New York, NY: Demos Medical Publishing.

Draper, K., & Ponsford, J. (2008). Cognitive functioning ten years following traumatic brain injury and rehabilitation. *Neuropsychology, 22*(5), 618–625. doi:10.1037/0894-4105.22.5.618

Finkelstein, E., Corso, P., & Miller, T. R. (2006). *The incidence and economic burden of injuries in the United States*. New York, NY: Oxford University Press.

Gaetz, M. (2004). The neurophysiology of brain injury. *Clinical Neurophysiology, 115*(1), 4–18.

Gennarelli, T., & Graham, D. (2005). Neuropathology. In J. M. Silver, T. W. McAllister, & S. C. Yudofsky (Eds.), *Textbook of traumatic brain injury*. Arlington, VA: American Psychiatric Publishing.

Gomez, P. A., Lobato, R. D., Boto, G. R., De la Lama, A., Gonzalez, P. J., & de la Cruz, J. (2000). Age and outcome after severe head injury. *Acta Neurochirurgica, 142*(4), 373–380; discussion 380–371.

Gordon, W. A. (2005). Cognitive rehabilitation. In J. M. Silver, T. W. McAllister, & S. C. Yudofsky (Eds.), *Textbook of traumatic brain injury*. Arlington, VA: American Psychiatric Publishing.

Granger, C. V., Cotter, A. C., Hamilton, B. B., & Fiedler, R. C. (1993). Functional assessment scales: A study of persons after stroke. *Archives of Physical Medicine and Rehabilitation, 74*(2), 133–138.

Granger, C. V., Divan, N., & Fiedler, R. C. (1995). Functional assessment scales: A study of persons after traumatic brain injury. *American Journal of Physical Medicine and Rehabilitation, 74*(2), 107–113.

Ivanhoe, C. B., Durand-Sanchez, A., & Spier, E. T. (2013). Acute rehabilitation. In D. K. N. Zasler & R. Zafonte (Eds.), *Brain injury medicine: Principles and practice*. New York, NY: Demos Medical Publishing.

Jackson, W. T., Novack, T. A., & Dowler, R. N. (1998). Effective serial measurement of cognitive orientation in rehabilitation: The Orientation Log. *Archives of Physical Medicine and Rehabilitation, 79*(6), 718–720.

Jager, T. E., Weiss, H. B., Coben, J. H., & Pepe, P. E. (2000). Traumatic brain injuries evaluated in U.S. emergency departments, 1992–1994. *Academic Emergency Medicine, 7*(2), 134–140.

Jiang, J. Y., Gao, G. Y., Li, W. P., Yu, M. K., & Zhu, C. (2002). Early indicators of prognosis in 846 cases of severe traumatic brain injury. *Journal of Neurotrauma, 19*(7), 869–874. doi:10.1089/08977150260190456

Junqué, C., Bruna, O., & Mataró, M. (1997). Information needs of the traumatic brain injury patient's family members regarding the consequences of the injury and associated perception of physical, cognitive, emotional and quality of life changes. *Brain Injury, 11*(4), 251–258.

Kempf, J., Werth, E., Kaiser, P. R., Bassetti, C. L., & Baumann, C. R. (2010). Sleep-wake disturbances 3 years after traumatic brain injury. *Journal of Neurology, Neurosurgery and Psychiatry, 81*(12), 1402–1405. doi:10.1136/jnnp.2009.201913

Korley, F. K., Kelen, G. D., Jones, C. M., & Diaz-Arrastia, R. (2015). Emergency department evaluation of traumatic brain injury in the United States, 2009–2010. *Journal of Head Trauma Rehabilitation*. Advance online publication. doi:10.1097/HTR.0000000000000187

Kothari, S., & DiTommaso, C. (2013). Prognosis after severe traumatic brain injury: A practical, evidence-based approach. In N. Zasler, D. Katz, & R. D. Zafonte (Eds.), *Brain injury medicine: Principles and practice*. New York, NY: Demos Medical Publishing.

Kraus, J. F., & Chu, L. D. (2005). Epidemiology. In J. M. Silver, T. W. McAllister, & S. C. Yudofsky (Eds.), *Textbook of traumatic brain injury*. Arlington, VA: American Psychiatric Publishing.

Le, T. H., & Gean, A. D. (2009). Neuroimaging of traumatic brain injury. *Mount Sinai Journal of Medicine, 76*(2), 145–162. doi:10.1002/msj.20102

Levin, H. S. (1995). Prediction of recovery from traumatic brain injury. *Journal of Neurotrauma, 12*(5), 913–922.

Levin, H. S., O'Donnell, V. M., & Grossman, R. G. (1979). The Galveston Orientation and Amnesia Test: A practical scale to assess cognition after head injury. *Journal of Nervous and Mental Disease, 167*(11), 675–684.

Lezak, M. D. (1995). *Neuropsychological assessment* (3rd ed.). New York, NY: Oxford University Press.

Lezak, M. D., Howieson, D. B., Loring, D.W., Hannay, H. J., & Fischer, J. S. (2004). *Neuropsychological assessment* (4th ed.). New York, NY: Oxford University Press.

Long, D. F. (2013). Diagnosis and management of late intracranial complications of traumatic brain injury. In N. D. Zasler, D. I. Katz, & R. D. Zafonte (Eds.), *Brain injury medicine: Principles and practice*. New York, NY: Demos Medical Publishing.

Meythaler, J. M., Brunner, R. C., Johnson, A., & Novack, T. A. (2002). Amantadine to improve neurorecovery in traumatic brain injury-associated diffuse axonal injury: A pilot double-blind randomized trial. *Journal of Head Trauma Rehabilitation, 17*(4), 300–313.

Meythaler, J. M., Peduzzi, J. D., Eleftheriou, E., & Novack, T. A. (2001). Current concepts: Diffuse axonal injury-associated traumatic brain injury. *Archives of Physical Medicine and Rehabilitation, 82*(10), 1461–1471.

Meythaler, J. M., & Zafonte, R. D. (2013). Neuropharmacology: A rehabilitation perspective. In N. D. Zasler, D. I. Katz, & R. D. Zafonte (Eds.), *Brain injury medicine: Principles and practice*. New York, NY: Demos Medical Publishing.

National Center for Injury Prevention and Control. (2003). *Report to Congress on mild traumatic brain injury in the United States: Steps to prevent a serious public health problem*. Atlanta, GA: Centers for Disease Control and Prevention.

Novack, T. A., Banos, J. H., Brunner, R., Renfroe, S., & Meythaler, J. M. (2009). Impact of early administration of sertraline on depressive symptoms in the first year after traumatic brain injury. *Journal of Neurotrauma*, 26(11), 1921–1928. doi:10.1089/neu.2009.0895

Park, N. W., & Ingles, J. L. (2001). Effectiveness of attention rehabilitation after an acquired brain injury: A meta-analysis. *Neuropsychology*, 15(2), 199–210.

Pollack, I. W. (2005). Psychotherapy. In J. M. Silver, T. W. McAllister, & S. C. Yudofsky (Eds.), *Textbook of traumatic brain injury*. Arlington, VA: American Psychiatric Publishing.

Ponsford, J., Sloan, S., & Snow, P. (2013). *Traumatic brain injury: Rehabilitation for everyday adaptive living* (2nd ed.). New York, NY: Psychology Press.

Povlishock, J. T., & Katz, D. I. (2005). Update of neuropathology and neurological recovery after traumatic brain injury. *Journal of Head Trauma Rehabilitation*, 20(1), 76–94.

Prigatano, G. P. (1999). *Principles of neuropsychological rehabilitation*. New York, NY: Oxford University Press.

Roebuck-Spencer, T., & Sherer, M. (2008). Moderate and severe traumatic brain injury. In J. E. Morgam & J. H. Ricker (Eds.), *Textbook of clinical neuropsychology* (pp. 411–429). New York, NY: Taylor & Francis Group.

Russell, W. R., & Smith, A. (1961). Posttraumatic amnesia in closed head injury. *Archives of Neurology*, 5, 4–17.

Salcido, R., & Costich, J. F. (1992). Recurrent traumatic brain injury. *Brain Injury*, 6(3), 293–298.

Schretlen, D. J., & Shapiro, A. M. (2003). A quantitative review of the effects of traumatic brain injury on cognitive functioning. *International Review of Psychiatry*, 15(4), 341–349. doi:10.1080/09540260310001606728

Sherer, M., Novack, T. A., Sander, A. M., Struchen, M. A., Alderson, A., & Thompson, R. N. (2002). Neuropsychological assessment and employment outcome after traumatic brain injury: A review. *Clinical Neuropsychologist*, 16(2), 157–178. doi:10.1076/clin.16.2.157.13238

Smith, G. S., & Kraus, J. F. (1988). Alcohol and residential, recreational, and occupational injuries: A review of the epidemiologic evidence. *Annual Review of Public Health, 9*, 99–121. doi:10.1146/annurev.pu.09.050188.000531

Sosin, D. M., Sniezek, J. E., & Thurman, D. J. (1996). Incidence of mild and moderate brain injury in the United States, 1991. *Brain Injury, 10*(1), 47–54.

Teasdale, G., & Jennett, B. (1974). Assessment of coma and impaired consciousness: A practical scale. *Lancet, 2*(7872), 81–84.

Teasdale, G., & Zitnay, G. (2013). History of acute care and rehabilitation of head injury. In N. D. Zasler, D. I. Katz, & R. D. Zafonte (Eds.), *Brain injury medicine: Principles and practice*. New York, NY: Demos Medical Publishing.

Thurman, D. J. (1999). *Traumatic brain injury in the United States: A report to Congress*. Atlanta, GA: Centers for Disease Control and Prevention.

Thurman, D. J., Alverson, C., Dunn, K. A., Guerrero, J., & Sniezek, J. E. (1999). Traumatic brain injury in the United States: A public health perspective. *Journal of Head Trauma Rehabilitation, 14*(6), 602–615.

Thurman, D. J., Sniezek, J. E., Johnson, D., Greenspan, A., & Smith, S. M. (1995). *Guidelines for surveillance of central nervous system injury*. Atlanta, GA: U.S. Department of Health and Human Services, Public Health Service, Centers for Disease Control and Prevention.

Viano, D. C. (2013). Biomechanics of brain injury. In N. D. Zasler, D. I. Katz, & R. D. Zafonte (Eds.), *Brain injury medicine: Principles and practice*. New York, NY: Demos Medical Publishing.

Walker, W. C., & Pickett, T. C. (2007). Motor impairment after severe traumatic brain injury: A longitudinal multicenter study. *Journal of Rehabilitation Research and Development, 44*(7), 975–982.

Whyte, J., Hart, T., Schuster, K., Fleming, M., Polansky, M., & Coslett, H. B. (1997). Effects of methylphenidate on attentional function after traumatic brain injury: A randomized, placebo-controlled trial. *American Journal of Physical Medicine and Rehabilitation, 76*(6), 440–450.

Yokobori, S., & Bullock, M. R. (2013). Pathobiology of primary traumatic brain injury. In N. D. Zasler, D. I. Katz, & R. D. Zafonte (Eds.), *Brain injury medicine: Principles and practice*. New York, NY: Demos Medical Publishing.

CHAPTER 3

Cerebrovascular Injuries

LUKE BRADBURY
MATTHEW JENSEN
JUSTIN SATTIN

OVERVIEW

Stroke is an enormous public health problem as it is one of the leading causes of both death and disability worldwide. The word "stroke" is used by different groups of people in different ways, often leading to confusion. To avoid this, it can be helpful to distinguish the syndromes from the disorders related to the term.

A stroke syndrome involves the sudden onset of symptoms or signs that match a focal area of the central nervous system, without features suggesting a nonvascular cause. Technically, this includes the spinal cord and retinae, but the word "stroke" is used mainly for events involving the brain. The word "focal" in this context is important, and clinicians often divide syndromes of the central nervous system into those that are focal and those that are nonfocal. A focal syndrome may involve one lobe of the cerebrum or a small area of the brain stem or cerebellum, whereas a nonfocal, or diffuse, brain syndrome usually involves most of the cerebral cortex on both sides. Stroke commonly involves focal brain syndromes and rarely involves diffuse brain syndromes, which are more commonly caused by the large number of conditions that can cause syndromes such as syncope or delirium. Some sudden-onset, focal central nervous system syndromes may appear similar to stroke syndromes, except for features suggesting a nonvascular cause, such as the tonic or clonic motor activity that may occur with seizures.

The disorders that usually cause stroke syndromes are divided into two categories: ischemic stroke and hemorrhagic stroke. Ischemia involves insufficient blood flow, and hemorrhage involves bleeding. Ischemic stroke is more common, and is usually caused by the sudden occlusion of a cerebral artery, most often from a thrombus (blood clot), although there are other mechanisms by which cerebral ischemia may occur. Hemorrhagic stroke is divided into spontaneous intracerebral (also called "intraparenchymal") hemorrhage, which is bleeding into the brain tissue, and spontaneous subarachnoid hemorrhage, which is bleeding into the cerebrospinal fluid that surrounds the brain and spinal cord. Bleeding into these spaces and other intracranial spaces may also occur with trauma, but most clinicians do not use the word "stroke" for traumatic intracranial hemorrhage.

Focal cerebral ischemia may cause a temporary stroke syndrome because of dysfunction of brain tissue from lack of blood flow, but then perfusion may be restored before infarction occurs. Infarction is irreversible tissue injury from ischemia. The term "transient ischemic attack" is used for this situation, but an older and a newer definition are both in common use. The older definition was a stroke syndrome that completely resolves within 24 hours. This definition was developed before modern brain imaging techniques, which then led to the realization that many of the patients had visible cerebral infarction on scans. The new definition is a stroke syndrome that resolves rapidly without evidence of cerebral infarction on testing. Transient ischemic attack is often described to patients as a "mini-stroke."

Many patients have misunderstandings about stroke, often confusing it with cardiac events, or other neurological events such as seizures or "pinched nerves." This is understandable but unfortunate, because it causes many patients to have a delay in presentation to medical attention that may lead to missed treatment opportunities. On the clinical side, it is also not uncommon for stroke patients to be initially misdiagnosed, because there are a large number of stroke syndromes that may occur, often with clinical features that heavily overlap with other disorders. The optimal strategies for tests and treatments of different stroke patient populations are evolving rapidly, and the following information will describe the fundamentals for approaching this increasingly complex area of medicine.

HISTORY

There is historical evidence that stroke was recognized as a cause of death and disability since antiquity. However, because advanced age is one of the strongest risk factors for stroke, its incidence likely has increased gradually over time as life expectancy has increased.

Stroke, like all diseases, was probably attributed to supernatural causes integral with the dominant religion of the people involved. For example, authors have speculated about possible cases of stroke in the Bible, such as when Saul was struck blind on the road to Damascus (Bullock, 1978), or the child of the Shunammite woman: "And he said unto his father, my head, my head. And he said to a lad, carry him to his mother. And when he had taken him, and brought him to his mother, he sat on her knees till noon, and then died" (Mathew & Pandian, 2010).

What could be described as the first medical descriptions of stroke are attributed to the person or people called Hippocrates in the fourth and fifth centuries BCE (Nilsen, 2010). In addition to describing contralateral weakness from traumatic brain injury, there are also descriptions of cases with spontaneous abnormal speech with right-sided paralysis (Nilsen, 2010). The term apoplexy was used for these cases, which translated as "struck with violence," presumably referring to the suddenness of the syndrome onset (Nilsen, 2010). An alternative, and more colorful, translation is "struck with violence as if by a thunderbolt" (Quest, 1990). The word "apoplexy" gradually dwindled into use for hemorrhage into some organs, and the word "stroke" replaced it, initially appearing in English in 1599; the term "cerebrovascular accident" also developed as a synonym at some point (Nilsen, 2010). The Hippocratic writings described cases of attacks of numbness preceding apoplexy, which were likely transient ischemic attacks, and cases of sudden headaches followed by deterioration of consciousness and death, which were likely hemorrhagic stroke (Quest, 1990). Apoplexy was attributed to "heating of cranial vessels with subsequent flow of phlegm or black bile to the head" (Quest, 1990). In the second century BCE, Aretaeus of Cappadocia hypothesized that apoplexy could be caused by abnormal blood flow (Quest, 1990). In the second century CE, Galen proposed that phlegm blocked the flow of animal spirits through brain arteries (Quest, 1990). These ideas largely held for the next millennium, and common treatments included bloodletting, purging, and vomiting based on these humoral concepts of disease (Caplan, 2004; Nilsen, 2010; Quest, 1990).

Multiple developments occurred in the 17th century. Nymman suggested cardioembolism as a cause of apoplexy, Wepfer described brain hemorrhage and cerebral arterial occlusion, and Willis refined cerebrovascular anatomy and described transient ischemic attack. In the 18th and 19th centuries, increasingly accurate distinctions developed about the kinds and causes of stroke through clinical, pathological, and laboratory descriptions by many, including Morgagni, Baillie, Cheyne, Bright, Cooper, Virchow, Serres, Abercrombie, Charcot, Duret, Bouchard, and Osler (Caplan, 2004; Nilsen, 2010; Quest, 1990).

Advances accumulated rapidly during the 20th century, involving too many people to name here (Caplan, 2004; Nilsen, 2010; Quest, 1990). Vascular imaging developed, first with direct injection angiography, then later with catheter angiography, as well as brain imaging with computed tomography and magnetic resonance imaging. Preventive treatments for stroke became widespread, including an understanding of lifestyle risk factors, treatments for vascular risk factors, antithrombotic agents, and surgical treatments such as carotid endarterectomy. All of this history has led up to now, which is the era of expanding acute stroke treatments involving reperfusion for ischemic stroke, as well as critical care and surgical interventions seeking to improve outcomes for both ischemic and hemorrhagic stroke patients.

PATHOPHYSIOLOGY

Stroke occurs because of a disruption of the brain's blood supply. Broadly, there are three general mechanisms by which this disruption occurs; these involve the heart, the blood vessels, or the blood. The specific diseases affecting each of these three components of the cerebrovascular system are discussed in the etiology section.

- *Heart*: Strokes arising because of heart disease are almost always ischemic; they are due to embolism of clot (and rarely, other material) from the heart into a cerebral artery.
- *Blood vessels*: Occlusion of a cervical or cerebral artery causes brain ischemia, whereas blood vessel rupture causes hemorrhage.

- *Blood*: Coagulopathies result in an excessive tendency toward either thrombosis of a cervical or cerebral blood vessel or hemorrhage into or around the brain.

ETIOLOGY

Heart

- *Atrial fibrillation*: The most common cardiac condition leading to stroke is atrial fibrillation. In this condition, the heart's atria do not contract regularly, but rather quiver continuously. Blood flow within the fibrillating atria is turbulent, which can lead to clot formation. Pieces of clot can then break loose, travel into the brain, and lodge in the cerebral circulation; this causes ischemic stroke.
- *Ventricular thrombosis*: Occasionally, thrombus forms in the left ventricle rather than the left atrium and then embolizes into the brain. A common cause of this is myocardial infarction, where the ventricle's contractions are not well coordinated, leading to turbulent blood flow and thrombus formation.
- *Patent foramen ovale (PFO)*: The foramen ovale is an opening between the right and the left atria of the heart. In utero, it is normally patent, allowing deoxygenated blood to bypass the not-yet-functioning lungs and to instead be oxygenated via the placenta. The foramen normally closes at birth, but remains somewhat patent in approximately 25% of people. In a person with a venous thrombus, most commonly a deep venous thrombosis of the leg, the clot may migrate through the venous system and into the right atrium. Instead of being carried into the pulmonary arteries (causing a pulmonary embolism), the clot can instead traverse the PFO, enter the left atrium, and then be carried into the cerebral circulation, causing an ischemic stroke.
- *Endocarditis*: Endocarditis refers to inflammation of the heart's valves. It can be infective or noninfective. Infective endocarditis is caused by a variety of bacteria. It arises when bacteria enter the bloodstream, often because of poor dentition, intravenous drug abuse, or an immunocompromised state. Pieces of infective debris can dislodge from the heart, causing

ischemic stroke. The noninfective endocarditides, often called "marantic" or "Libman–Sacks" endocarditis, are associated with cancer and rheumatological conditions, respectively.

- *Intracardiac tumor*: Much less common than the just-listed conditions are the formation of tumors within the heart. These include papillary fibroelastomas and atrial myxomas. Fragments of the tumor can break loose and travel into the brain, causing vascular occlusion and ischemic stroke.

Blood Vessels

- *Atherosclerosis:* Atherosclerosis is an extremely common disease and a leading cause of stroke. It can occur in any vascular bed (coronary, visceral, peripheral, etc.), and the cerebral circulation is a common site of involvement. Embolization of atheromatous debris or, more commonly, associated thrombus, from the aortic arch, carotid or vertebral arteries, or the intracerebral vessels deeper into the brain leads to ischemic stroke. Atherosclerosis can also cause occlusion of the larger arteries in the neck and brain via thrombosis (i.e., the clot occludes the vessel at that location and does not embolize further).
- *Lipohyalinosis:* Lipohyalinosis is a pathology of the microvasculature—the smallest arteries deep within the brain. The arteries essentially degenerate and either become occluded, leading to small (lacunar) infarcts, or they rupture, leading to intracerebral hemorrhage.
- *Amyloid angiopathy*: Amyloid angiopathy is another pathology of the microvasculature. It is characterized by the deposition of a protein called "amyloid" in the walls of the brain's arteries. It is very similar to the amyloid deposited in the brain parenchyma in patients with Alzheimer's disease, and the two conditions often coexist. The classic manifestation of cerebral amyloid angiopathy is intracerebral hemorrhage, often in lobar locations, as opposed to the hemorrhages of lipohyalinosis, which occur in the basal ganglia, brain stem, thalamus, and cerebellum. Amyloid angiopathy has other, less common, clinical manifestations as well.
- *Saccular aneurysm*: Saccular aneurysms are outpouchings of the larger cerebral vessels that run in the subarachnoid space

at the base of the brain. Rupture of these aneurysms causes subarachnoid hemorrhage.

- *Dissection*: Dissection is a relatively common cause of stroke in younger patients. It involves disruption of the arterial wall, with blood tracking in between the wall's layers and compromising flow through the lumen of the vessel. Clots can form at the site of disruption or elsewhere in the artery because of turbulent blood flow. Dissections can arise as a complication of trauma (e.g., motor vehicle accidents or sports injuries) or spontaneously.
- *Vascular malformation*: These include arteriovenous malformations (AVMs), cavernous angiomas, and developmental venous anomalies. Rupture of these lesions (most commonly, AVMs) leads to intracerebral hemorrhage.
- *Vasospasm*: Vasospasm is a narrowing of the artery owing to contraction of its muscular wall. The impairment of blood flow past the narrowing results in cerebral ischemia. There are two main causes of vasospasm:
  - *Subarachnoid hemorrhage*: One of the most feared complications of aneurysmal subarachnoid hemorrhage is delayed cerebral ischemia. The presence of blood in the subarachnoid space, through which the major cerebral arteries course, results, via an unknown mechanism, in vasospasm and thus cerebral ischemia. This is typically delayed by a few days to a few weeks after the subarachnoid hemorrhage.
  - *Reversible cerebral vasoconstriction syndrome (RCVS):* RCVS is characterized by sudden, severe headache, the absence of subarachnoid hemorrhage, and the finding of arterial narrowing on vascular imaging that normalizes upon repeat imaging. It is associated with many conditions, including various drug exposures, the postpartum state, neurosurgical procedures, and sexual activity, among others.
- *Vasculitis*: Inflammation of the arteries is termed "vasculitis." Vasculitis of the brain can be primary, meaning that it arises alone, or it can be part of a rheumatological disorder such as polyarteritis nodosa, Wegener's granulomatosis, or Churg–Strauss syndrome. When larger arteries are involved, the

inflammation can cause narrowing of the vessels that looks like vasospasm and leads to thrombosis and thromboembolism. Involvement of the microvasculature can cause either vascular occlusion and ischemic stroke or vascular rupture and intracerebral hemorrhage.

Blood

- *Anticoagulation:* The most common coagulopathy is that caused by therapeutic anticoagulation, usually to prevent thromboembolism in patients with atrial fibrillation. When the intensity of anticoagulation is too high, hemorrhage can occur in any brain compartment—usually intracerebral or subdural hemorrhage.

- *Prothrombotic drugs*: Drugs with prothrombotic effects include estrogens (found in oral contraceptives and hormone replacement therapies), testosterone, tamoxifen, bevacizumab, and glucocorticoids. These are associated mostly with venous thromboembolism, including cerebral venous sinus thrombosis.

- *Antiphospholipid antibodies:* Patients with a lupus anticoagulant, particularly anticardiolipin or anti–beta 2-glycoprotein I antibodies, are hypercoagulable. Such antibodies arise in the setting of lupus and other rheumatological conditions, but can also occur alone. Unlike most other hypercoagulable states, antiphospholipid antibodies are most strongly associated with arterial rather than venous thrombosis.

- *Other acquired prothrombotic states:*
  - *Pregnancy:* Pregnancy is a relatively hypercoagulable state, causing mostly venous thromboembolism.
  - *Malignancy:* Malignancy is also a relatively prothrombotic state. It is associated with both venous and arterial thrombosis.
  - *Trauma:* Trauma, especially major trauma, is associated with venous thromboembolism.

- *Hereditary thrombophilias:* These include deficiencies of antithrombin or proteins C or S and mutations in the factor V and prothrombin genes. Such thrombophilias are most closely associated with venous thromboembolism.

CEREBROVASCULAR INJURIES 49

EPIDEMIOLOGY

Nearly 800,000 Americans suffer from a stroke every year, and about 2.7% of adults have a history of stroke. However, these rates vary widely by race and location (Mozaffarian et al., 2015). A total of 4.6% of American Indian/Alaskan Natives, 4.0% of African Americans, 2.5% of non-Hispanic Whites, 2.3% of Hispanics, and 1.3% of Asian/Pacific Islanders have suffered from a stroke. There is a higher incidence of stroke in the southeastern United States as well, which increases the stroke death rate in that region.

Ischemic strokes constitute the large majority of strokes, at 87%, and hemorrhages account for the rest. Approximately 3% of all strokes are subarachnoid hemorrhages. Stroke deaths overall have been declining. From 2001 through 2011, the total number of stroke deaths declined by 21.2%. Stroke had previously been the fourth leading cause of death behind cardiac disease, cancer, and chronic lung conditions, but in 2015, accidental injuries overtook stroke, and stroke is now the fifth leading cause of death.

CLINICAL PRESENTATION

Stroke symptoms, with very few exceptions, begin with the sudden onset of focal neurological deficits, which are confined to a vascular territory. These can include weakness, numbness, dysarthria, language disturbances such as aphasia, double vision, blind spots, balance difficulties, and, less commonly, confusion. Ischemic strokes are mostly painless in their presentation, although patients may report a headache, particularly when the stroke is located in the posterior circulation. Hemorrhagic strokes often involve a great deal of pain as the blood expands and affects the surrounding blood vessels and meninges that contain pain receptors. Increased intracranial pressure is also associated with severe headache pain. Also, unlike most ischemic strokes, hemorrhagic strokes often affect the patient's level of consciousness. A typical large intraparenchymal hemorrhage, for example, will he heralded by a severe, thunderclap headache followed by focal deficits like contralateral weakness and numbness and then decreased consciousness and even coma. If the same area of brain is affected by an ischemic stroke, the same weakness and numbness may occur, but often the patient does not complain of headache and remains conscious.

Cerebral venous thrombosis also is associated with headache, but the neurological deficits are often much more gradual in their onset. A patient will complain of worsening headache over the course of days and then develop other symptoms similar to those noted earlier. These symptoms may start in a very mild manner and wax and wane in their severity, but will generally, if the thrombosis is not treated with anticoagulation, become fixed.

DIAGNOSTIC CONSIDERATIONS

Focal neurological deficits can have a wide range of differential diagnoses, some of which are listed here:

- Seizure (specifically, unilateral weakness in the postictal state, Todd's paralysis)
- Metabolic disorders, mostly glucose abnormalities (hypoglycemia being much more common than hyperglycemia)
- Certain headache syndromes (complicated migraines, hemiplegic migraines)
- Psychogenic weakness (conversion disorder, malingering, Munchausen's syndrome)
- Benign paroxysmal positional vertigo
- Brain tumors
- Demyelinating diseases (multiple sclerosis)
- Peripheral nerve injuries

These can often, with a careful history and examination, be excluded, but often, imaging is needed to definitively rule them out. One of the primary stroke differentials is the rapid onset of deficits with maximal symptoms being within seconds, whereas most of the stroke mimics will cause more gradual evolution of deficits. Findings on the neurological examination that may differentiate between stroke and stroke mimics include nonorganic weakness or language difficulties, sensory symptoms that cannot be explained neuroanatomically, or constellations of symptoms that are not referable to a vascular territory.

TREATMENT

Treatment of stroke can generally be divided into three categories: acute stroke management, rehabilitation, and secondary stroke prevention. In recent years, acute stroke management has undergone many changes, and guidelines are being revised to accommodate new research and therapies. Rehabilitation also has evolved rapidly with a better understanding of neuroplasticity and the therapies that can support healing. As for secondary stroke prevention, data from older studies suggests that the stroke recurrence rate in the 1960s was as high as 7% to 8%, but now is much closer to 3% (Hong, Yegiaian, Lee, Lee, & Saver, 2011).

Acute Stroke Management

Ischemic Stroke
The modern era of acute ischemic stroke treatment began with the approval of intravenous tissue plasminogen activator (IV-tPA) by the U.S. Food and Drug Administration (FDA) in 1996 (The National Institute of Neurological Disorders and Stroke rt-PA Stroke Study Group, 1995). It remains the only FDA-approved medication for treatment of acute stroke and has several absolute and relative contraindications. In 2015, the FDA revised the package insert for IV-tPA to better reflect the evidence supporting possible risks of administering IV-tPA. As a thrombolytic, IV-tPA disrupts blood clots by binding to fibrin and converting plasminogen to plasmin. Because of this action, the risk of hemorrhagic complications is significant, and it must be used with great care.

The primary absolute contraindication is evidence of an intracranial hemorrhage. In order to screen patients with the acute onset of neurological deficits for intracranial hemorrhages, most hospitals have a policy of immediately obtaining a noncontrasted head CT. This was the test used in the original IV-tPA study and remains the standard for hemorrhage screening. A hemorrhage will appear as a bright white area (hyperdensity) on the CT scan, whereas an ischemic stroke will often not be evident at all.

Another commonly encountered contraindication is severe uncontrolled hypertension. If the systolic blood pressure is greater than 175 mmHg or the diastolic blood pressure is greater than 110 mmHg, IV-tPA should be withheld. Unlike other contraindications, however, hypertension can be treated, and if the blood pressure is safely maintained below 175/110 mmHg, it can be administered. Close monitoring of the blood pressure during and after IV-tPA is always warranted, but special care must be given to patients who present with extremely elevated pressure before the drug is given. Other contraindications for IV-tPA can be found in Table 3.1.

TABLE 3.1 CONTRAINDICATIONS FOR INTRAVENOUS TISSUE PLASMINOGEN ACTIVATOR

Contraindication	Examples
Active internal bleeding	Recent GI hemorrhage
Recent intracranial, spinal, or other major surgery	Coronary artery bypass graft; obstetrical delivery; intracranial aneurysm clipping
Some intracranial tumors (those with high risk of bleeding)	Primary tumors (e.g., glioblastomas); metastatic tumors (renal cell cancer, melanomas)
Bleeding diathesis	Thrombocytopenia (platelet count < 100,000/μL)
Recent trauma	Motor vehicle accident; a fall with significant injury to the head
Anticoagulant use	Warfarin (with an INR > 1.7); dabigatran; apixaban; rivaroxaban
Intracranial hemorrhage	Subarachnoid, subdural, or epidural hemorrhage
Current severe uncontrolled hypertension	Repeated systolic BP measurements of >175 mmHg or diastolic measurements of >110 mmHg

GI, gastrointestinal; INR, international normalized ratio.

Some relative contraindications for IV-tPA include advanced age (greater than 77 years), significant liver or kidney disease, pregnancy, and subacute bacterial endocarditis. As with any medication, though, the risk and benefits must be evaluated for each individual patient before a decision is made.

In late 2014, a study called MR CLEAN (Multicenter Randomized Clinical Trial of Endovascular Treatment for Acute Ischemic Stroke in the Netherlands) was published that showed the efficacy of endovascular treatment for acute stroke (Berkhemer, 2015). This trial and subsequent trials with similar design enrolled patients with large vessel occlusions in the anterior circulation (distal internal carotid artery and proximal middle cerebral artery) and randomized them to receive standard care alone or standard care with endovascular clot retrieval. A retrievable stent was used in nearly all of the patients who were randomized to clot retrieval.

These novel devices are designed specifically for the cerebral circulation and have greatly reduced the amount of time to reperfusion when compared with previous endovascular devices. A stent is deployed through the blood clot, and then both the stent and the clot are removed through a large-bore catheter. The results of these studies were dramatic. MR CLEAN, for example, showed an odds ratio of 1.67 for reduction in the modified Rankin scale at 90 days. The number needed to treat for a patient to have less disability was only 3 to 5, and that for a patient to be nondisabled was 7.

Just as in the case of IV-tPA, however, patients who are considered for endovascular therapy must be screened carefully. In addition to a noncontrasted head CT, vascular imaging is often obtained in patients with signs or symptoms of a large vessel stroke. This is most often done with a CT angiogram. (IV contrast is injected in a vein, and when it reaches the arterial phase in the head and neck, a CT scan is obtained.) CT perfusion imaging is also commonly performed to ensure that the area of brain affected by the stroke remains viable to rescue; if the infarct has already been completed, there is no utility in removing the clot.

Hemorrhagic Stroke
Hemorrhagic strokes are managed very differently than ischemic strokes, and the location and etiology of the hemorrhage will determine much of what is done acutely. Hemorrhages are often identified on the initial head CT, and the location (subarachnoid, intraparenchymal, subdural, epidural) will determine the need for any further imaging studies or medications.

Regarding medications, IV-tPA is ruled out immediately. The focus then shifts to blood pressure management and, when necessary, reversal of anticoagulation. Patients with uncontrolled hypertension are at particularly high risk for intracranial hemorrhages, specifically intraparenchymal, subdural, and subarachnoid hemorrhages. They commonly present with systolic blood pressure readings above 180 mmHg, and in order to reduce the risk of further hemorrhaging, this must be lowered. Many hospitals use labetalol as a first-line agent to lower blood pressure, although hydralazine and nicardipine are also used. The current American Heart Association (AHA) guidelines for blood pressure management recommend bringing the systolic level to 140. Care should be taken not to lower the blood pressure too aggressively, though, as that may cause reduced cerebral perfusion to normal brain in the setting of chronically uncontrolled hypertension.

Many patients are on anticoagulation agents for a variety of reasons, and this predisposes them to intracranial hemorrhages. In patients taking warfarin, supratherapeutic international normalized ratios (INRs) of greater than 3 are at particular risk. When an INR is found to be elevated or even if it is in the normal 2 to 3 range in the setting of a hemorrhage, it must be corrected. Currently, many hospitals are able to achieve this with prothrombin complex concentrates, which contain clotting factors that can bring the blood quickly back to normal clotting ability within 1 hour. Where these are not available, fresh frozen plasma from blood donations is used. This also has clotting factors that can reverse the effects of warfarin, but takes much longer and involves administering a large volume of fluid to the patient as well. The new class of novel anticoagulants including dabigatran, apixaban, and rivaroxaban similarly increase the risk of hemorrhage. As of this writing, only dabigatran has a reversal agent that is approved for use by the FDA.

Unlike ischemic strokes, certain hemorrhages may warrant emergency surgical treatment. In the case of hemorrhages causing severe or rapidly worsening signs or symptoms (coma, midline shift, or elevated intracranial pressure), surgery with a decompressive craniotomy may reduce mortality. For cerebellar hemorrhages, where the patient is deteriorating or there are signs of brain stem compression, the AHA recommends decompressive craniotomy as soon as possible.

Subarachnoid hemorrhages may also require urgent surgery to control bleeding. If vascular imaging reveals an aneurysm that appears to have a high risk of further bleeding, the patient may require urgent open surgery for aneurysm clipping or endovascular treatment for aneurysm coiling. In the latter case, small platinum coils are inserted into the aneurysm to relieve pressure and form a stabilizing blood clot.

Venous Sinus Thrombosis

Treatment of blood clots in the venous sinus system is anticoagulation. Even in the setting of hemorrhage due to venous congestion, anticoagulation with heparin or enoxaparin is necessary to begin the process of opening the venous drainage so that the risk of infarction from low flow is reduced. After stabilization, warfarin is often used for longer term anticoagulation. Follow-up imaging with CT angiography or MR angiography is used to ensure that the clot burden has resolved before cessation of anticoagulation.

Rehabilitation

Recovery after a stroke begins as soon as the patient is medically stable enough to tolerate therapy. Physical, occupational, speech, and language therapists are enlisted early in the hospital course to evaluate both the types and intensity of therapy needed for each individual patient. Depending on the size and location of the area of ischemia or hemorrhage, a patient may need a great deal of physical and occupational therapy but very little speech therapy or vice versa. Once the types of therapy necessary are established, the intensity level that will be most helpful but also tolerable by the patient is determined. Some of the more significantly affected patients will be discharged to acute inpatient rehabilitation hospitals, where physiatrists and therapists will spend several hours daily in therapy sessions working with the patient. If the deficits are milder or the patient cannot tolerate several hours of therapy (because of advanced age, medical comorbidities, or very severe strokes), the patient may require subacute rehabilitation in a skilled facility. In this setting, the patient will receive therapy a few days a week and still have necessary nursing care. When the symptoms are very mild, therapies can be done on an outpatient basis or at home from visiting therapists. The duration of any level of therapy is dependent on how much that individual patient will need.

Secondary Stroke Prevention
The stroke recurrence rate after an initial stroke or transient ischemic attack has dropped dramatically over the past several decades, and this has been largely effective in reducing stroke morbidity and mortality. This drop is due largely to the development of medications that, depending on the etiology of the stroke, can greatly reduce the risk of another ischemic or hemorrhagic stroke.

An ischemic stroke can be prevented by determining whether it is a lacunar stroke or a large vessel embolic stroke, and, accordingly, directing medical therapy for that individual. In the case of lacunar strokes, the primary risk factor is hypertension, and several classes of medications can be used to bring the patient's blood pressure within an acceptable range, defined as the systolic being less than 140 mmHg in the current guidelines. Diuretics and ACE inhibitors are commonly used, although in difficult-to-control cases, or when side effects prevent their use, calcium channel blockers, angiotensin receptor blockers, and direct vasodilators can also be used.

Hypercholesterolemia is also a commonly found risk factor in patients with lacunar strokes, and the mainstay of therapy is a daily statin, medications that inhibit HMG-CoA reductase in the liver and prevent the synthesis of low-density lipoproteins (LDL). In the Stroke Prevention by Aggressive Reduction in Cholestrol Levels (SPARCLE) trial, which compared high-intensity atorvastatin

(80 mg per day) with placebo, the group receiving atorvastatin had a reduced risk of fatal and nonfatal strokes with a hazard ratio of 0.84 (Amarenco et al., 2006).

Antiplatelet therapy is also a mainstay of stroke prevention in lacunar strokes. Although many studies have attempted to determine the optimal type and dose of which antiplatelet agent to use, current guidelines recommend a low dose of aspirin (50–100 mg) daily. Alternatively, patients who are allergic or have a sensitivity to aspirin may use clopidogrel or another antiplatelet agent. Dual therapy with aspirin and another agent has generally been shown to increase the risk of bleeding complications but not significantly reduce the risk of ischemic stroke.

Diabetes mellitus, an increasingly common affliction throughout the world, is a risk factor for lacunar strokes, and the American Diabetes Association has several guidelines for glucose management, depending on the severity of the disease. A hemoglobin A_{1c} goal of less than 7% is generally encouraged. Although diet and exercise are helpful, medications such as metformin and insulin are often necessary to achieve that level of glucose control.

Lifestyle modifications are often recommended as well. Smoking cessation, increased physical activity (at least three to four times per week of moderate to vigorous physical activity), and dietary changes are all important. For specific diet recommendations, the Dietary Approach to Stop Hypertension (DASH) and Mediterranean diets have been shown to reduce the risk of recurrent stroke. At a minimum, patients should be counselled to try and reduce the amount of saturated fat, cholesterol, and salt as much as possible.

For large vessel embolic strokes, the most common etiology is atrial fibrillation. Atrial fibrillation can be paroxysmal (generally lasting less than 7 days), persistent (longer than 7 days), and sometimes permanent (refractory to medical or electrical cardioversion). In any of these cases, the longer a patient has atrial fibrillation, the higher the risk of forming a blood clot in the left atrium that can be ejected from the heart and travel to the brain. Warfarin, a vitamin K antagonist that reduces the efficacy of several clotting factors in the blood, had been the primary treatment for several decades. However, the risk of a hemorrhagic complication is significant, particularly when the level of the medication is above the recommended therapeutic threshold. More recently, three novel anticoagulants (apixaban, dabigatran, and rivaroxaban) have all been FDA approved for stroke prevention in the setting of atrial fibrillation.

As previously mentioned in this chapter, only dabigatran currently has a reversal agent. Compared with warfarin, these medications offer the advantage of stable dosing (no need for frequent changes), no need for blood draws to check medication efficacy levels, fewer dietary restrictions, and less medication interactions.

PROGNOSIS

Prognosis after a stroke of any type depends greatly on the location and size of the stroke as well as patient comorbidities. Large vessel strokes can affect significant territories in the brain and can be very difficult to recover from. For example, a patient with a large middle cerebral artery stroke in the left hemisphere can have persistent aphasia, weakness or even complete hemiplegia on the right, and dysphagia to the point where enteral nutrition can be administered only through a feeding tube. Another patient may have a large vessel stroke affecting only a small amount of one cerebellar hemisphere, and after rehabilitation, have minimal, if any, deficits at all. Ischemic lacunar strokes can be similarly variable. At times, an old lacunar stroke is found on an MRI scan, and the patient was never known to have any deficits. A lacunar stroke affecting the pons or midbrain can have persistent cranial nerve deficits such as double vision or dysarthria and hemiparesis if the motor pathways are affected.

Hemorrhagic stroke prognosis can be variable as well. These patients are often sicker in the initial phase of their illness, particularly if the hemorrhage has led to hydrocephalus or brain stem compression. But compared with patients with ischemic strokes of similar size and location, patients who survive hemorrhagic strokes can recover more. Once the blood products are absorbed, the parenchyma of the brain can recover and function again.

Patients with several comorbidities have a more difficult stroke recovery than those with fewer. Advanced age makes rehab very difficult, and there are often complications that can slow recovery or even cause regression. Infections of the urinary tract or lungs can easily worsen stroke symptoms. Older patients are also more likely to suffer from premorbid conditions, such as weakness, dysphagia, and dementia, to name a few, that can be worsened after a stroke.

Other conditions such as hypertension, hyperlipidemia, smoking history, diabetes, atherosclerosis, and cardiac abnormalities will increase the risk of recurrent stroke, which may impair recovery from the initial event.

CLINICAL SYNOPSIS

- Stroke is a major cause of death and disability throughout the world.
- Ischemic strokes are characterized by the sudden onset of focal neurological deficits and are divided into large vessel emboli and small vessel lacunar strokes.
  - Large vessel emboli often come from the heart or carotid arteries.
  - Lacunar strokes result from vascular risk factors such as hypertension, diabetes, hyperlipidemia, and smoking.
- Hemorrhagic strokes also have the sudden onset of neurological deficits and can be accompanied by headache and alterations in consciousness.
  - Hemorrhages within the brain itself often result from hypertension or vascular malformations.
  - Subarachnoid hemorrhages may be caused by aneurysms or may be spontaneous.
  - Subdural and epidural hemorrhages can be the result of trauma.
- Treatment for ischemic strokes involves thrombolysis with tissue plasminogen activator and, in some cases, retrieval of the thrombus with endovascular procedures.
- Rehabilitation with physical, occupational, and speech/language therapy is often necessary after a stroke.
- Secondary stroke prevention is highly dependent on the mechanism of the original stroke, such as anticoagulation in the setting of atrial fibrillation and blood pressure control in the setting of a lacunar stroke.

CASE STUDY

A 24-year-old law student was taking final exams when, during a break, he collapsed in the hallway. He was surrounded by friends, and they immediately called emergency medical services. About 20 minutes after the fall, he arrived in the local emergency department. On exam, he could not move the left side of his body or left lower face, his eyes were deviated to the right, he did not respond to painful stimuli to the left arm or leg, he was unaware of his deficits, and did not pay any attention to the examiners when they stood at his left side. His National Institutes of Health (NIH) stroke scale score was 19. He had no significant past medical history and was not taking any medications. His symptoms were immediately recognized as being consistent with a stroke, and a head CT without contrast was normal. A CT angiogram showed an occlusive thrombus in his proximal right middle cerebral artery territory. His blood pressure was 168/82 mmHg, and his other vital signs were within normal limits. No contraindications for IV-tPA were identified, and so it was started approximately 50 minutes after the onset of his symptoms. A CT perfusion study showed that he had minimal infarct burden in the right middle cerebral artery territory, but significantly increased mean transit time and delayed blood flow throughout that entire area. Because of this, he was immediately taken to the neuroendovascular suite, where, using a retrievable stent, a thrombectomy was performed. He was then admitted to the neurointensive care unit and monitored closely for 2 days. His symptoms began to improve within hours after the procedure, and 1 week later, he was discharged from the hospital with some very mild left arm weakness and continued problems with neglect; his NIH stroke scale had dropped to only 3.

Neuropsychological testing was performed shortly after discharge and determined that he required accommodations to continue his studies such as extended exam times and the need to sit on the left side of the lecture hall so that he would not neglect any of the presentations. He continued outpatient occupational therapy for several months and regained his baseline neurological status before 1 year, and graduated from law school with honors only one semester behind schedule. The cause of his stroke was found to be hyperhomocysteinemia, a rare genetic cause of hypercoagulability. After 6 months of anticoagulation, high doses of B vitamins reduced his homocysteine to normal levels, and anticoagulation was stopped and only a low-dose aspirin was continued.

ACKNOWLEDGMENT

Research presented in this chapter was supported by a grant from the National Institute of Neurological Disorders and Stroke (1K08NS079622).

REFERENCES

Amarenco, P., Bogousslavsky, J., Callahan, A., III, Goldstein, L. B., Hennerici, M., Rudolph, A. E., . . . Stroke Prevention by Aggressive Reduction in Cholesterol Levels (SPARCL) Investigators. (2006). High-dose atorvastatin after stroke or transient ischemic attack. *The New England Journal of Medicine, 355*(6), 549–559. doi:10.1056/NEJMoa061894

Berkhemer, O. A. (2015). A randomized trial of intraarterial for acute ischemic stroke. *The New England Journal of Medicine, 372*, 11–20.

Bullock, J. D. (1978). The blindness of Saint Paul. *Ophthalmology, 85*(10), 1044–1053.

Caplan, L. R. (2004). Cerebrovascular disease: Historical background, with an eye to the future. *Cleveland Clinic Journal of Medicine, 71*(Suppl. 1), S22–S24.

Hong, K. S., Yegiaian, S., Lee, M., Lee, J., & Saver, J. L. (2011). Declining stroke and vascular event recurrence rates in secondary prevention trials over the past 50 years and consequences for current trial design. *Circulation, 123*(19), 2111–2119. doi:10.1161/CIRCULATIONAHA.109.934786

Mathew, S. K., & Pandian, J. D. (2010). Newer insights to the neurological diseases among biblical characters of Old Testament. *Annals of the Indian Academy of Neurology, 13*(3), 164–166. doi:10.4103/0972-2327.70873

Mozaffarian, D., Benjamin, E. J., Go, A. S., Arnett, D. K., Blaha, M. J., Cushman, M., . . . American Heart Association Statistics Subcommittee, Stroke Statistics Subcommittee. (2015). Heart disease and stroke statistics—2015 update: A report from the American Heart Association. *Circulation, 131*(4), e29–e322. doi:10.1161/CIR.0000000000000152

Nilsen, M. L. (2010). A historical account of stroke and the evolution of nursing care for stroke patients. *The Journal of Neuroscience Nursing, 42*(1), 19–27.

Quest, D. O. (1990). Stroke: A selective history. *Neurosurgery, 27*(3), 440–445.

The National Institute of Neurological Disorders and Stroke rt-PA Stroke Study Group. (1995). Tissue plasminogen activator for acute ischemic stroke. *The New England Journal of Medicine, 333*(24), 1581–1587. doi:10.1056/NEJM199512143332401

CHAPTER 4

Brain Tumors

SHAROON QAISER
DONITA LIGHTNER

OVERVIEW

*And still they gazed, and still the wonder grew,
That one small head could carry all he knew.
(Oliver Goldsmith,* The Deserted Village, *1809)*

Brain tumor, like any other tumor, is an abnormal growth of cells that proliferate in a dysregulated manner (Quinn, Gonçalves, Sehovic, Bowman, & Reed, 2015). They may originate from intrinsic brain tissue, or primary brain tumors, or represent metastatic disease from cancers involving other parts of the body. Primary brain tumors can be classified on the basis of location, types of tissue involved, benign versus malignant, and other types.

Location

The calvarium is divided by a tent-like extension of dura mater called the "tentorium cerebelli." This is an important landmark as brain tumors are divided on the basis of their location in relation to tentorium cerebelli into supratentorial and infratentorial tumors. About 54% to 70% of childhood tumors are in posterior cranial fossa (infratentorial) and, owing to their anatomical location and limited space, may present as critical brain lesions capable of causing hydrocephalus and with the risk of herniation (Rorke & Schut, 1989). Additionally, tumors are further classified on the basis of which lobe of the brain is involved.

Type of Tissue Involved

Gliomas
Glial cells are nonneuronal cells of the central nervous system and generally provide support to neuronal tissue. Functions include structural support, nutritional support, and even degradation of dead neurons and clearance of infection. Tumors originating from glial cells are called "gliomas" and, on the basis of the type of glial cell involved, are further divided into subtypes:

- *Astrocytomas*: These include astrocytoma, anaplastic astrocytoma, and glioblastomas, depending on the histological characteristics and aggressiveness of the tumor. Glioblastomas and anaplastic astrocytomas are the most aggressive and malignant primary tumors.

- *Oligodendrogliomas*: These involve oligodendrocytes and are usually less aggressive than their astrocytoma counterparts. Calcifications are frequently seen histologically, and these tumors are more commonly associated with seizures.

- *Schwannomas*: Schwann cells are involved in myelin sheath formation, and therefore tumors involving Schwann cells are called "schwannomas." They are generally low-grade, benign tumors, but can cause significant local damage. Acoustic schwannomas are associated with a genetic disease, neurofibromatosis type 2, and can cause hearing loss, vertigo, and ataxia.

- *Ependymomas*: Ependymal cells compose the epithelial-like lining of the ventricular system of the brain and spinal cord. Tumors involving these cells are called "ependymomas." In the pediatric age group, these tumors are usually intracranial, in contrast to the adult population in which they are usually spinal. They can also be found supratentorially in brain parenchyma and are hypothesized to occur because of abnormal cellular migration during fetal development.

- *Meningiomas*: These tumors originate from meningeal tissue of the dura mater, the covering of the brain and spinal cord. Meningiomas are the most common primary brain tumors in the adult population and are relatively rare in children. The majority of these tumors are low-grade, benign lesions; infrequently, they are high grade and, if so, are frequently related to prior exposure to radiation. Because they irritate the surface of the brain, that is, the cortex, regardless of histological grade, they can be a focus for seizures.

Benign Versus Malignant

Brain tumors may be slowly growing tumors, with a long insidious course, and may be found as incidental findings on autopsy. This is a classic history of benign or low-grade lesions. On the other hand, they may grow aggressively over a short period of time and present as critical malignant brain tumors with quickly progressing neurological deficits and intractable headaches. This is more characteristic of malignant or high-grade tumors.

Other Tumors

The cranium has other structures and glands that also can contribute to brain tumors and present in a variety of different ways. These include the following:

- Pituitary tumors
- Pineal tumors
- Craniopharyngiomas
- CNS lymphomas

Irrespective of their origin, primary and metastatic tumors may have similar presenting features, depending on location and mass effect. Usually, the clinical course may be insidious but can present acutely depending on location, complication, and mass effect. The management of brain tumors involves a multidisciplinary approach and is challenging in terms of morbidity and mortality.

HISTORY

Early Greek physician Hippocrates mentioned "abnormal brain growths" as early as 400 BCE. In 1930, Harvey Cushing, a pioneer of neurosurgery, was probably the first to report a large series of posterior fossa tumors using a pneumoencephalogram or x-ray (Cushing, 1930). Symptom onset is frequently insidious. However, owing to complications such as hemorrhage or increased intracranial pressure, patients may present acutely. The clinical manifestations of brain tumors reflect the location of the tumor. As a result, different types of brain tumors may present similarly, if they are in the same location.

In children with brain tumors, there can be extreme variability in time from onset of symptoms to diagnoses of brain tumor, as migraines or gastrointestinal illness are much more common. According to one study from the United Kingdom, symptom onset to diagnosis for children with brain tumors was an average of 3.3 months. Headache was the most common symptom (40%) and, at the time of diagnosis, children had an average of six signs and/or symptoms (Cushing, 1930). Headache is not always consistent in characteristics and quality (McKinney, 2004).

Mental status changes, especially memory loss and decreased alertness, may be a clue of frontal lobe tumor or hydrocephalus. Likewise, emotional changes or behavioral disturbances leading to depersonalization could present temporal or frontal lobe tumors. Loss of visual fields indicates a tumor along the visual pathway. In children, posterior fossa tumors can cause obstructive hydrocephalus, leading to irritability, gait changes (i.e., ataxia), headaches, and vomiting.

PATHOPHYSIOLOGY

Limited intracranial space due to fusion of bones and compression of neurological structures and pathways play an important role in the manifestation of brain tumors. The pathogenesis includes direct invasion, infiltration and/or supplantation of normal parenchymal tissue with neoplastic and results in disruption of normal neurological function. Another critical aspect involves increased intracranial pressure by mass effect or impedance of normal cerebrospinal fluid flow, resulting in herniation or shifting of brain tissue, which can be fatal. Furthermore, new blood vessel formation (i.e., neovascularization) from tumor-secreting growth factors can disrupt the normal blood–brain barrier and result in worsening edema.

ETIOLOGY

The cause of primary tumor is not understood and is likely related to a cascade of genetic mutations. There are few factors known to increase the risk of primary brain tumors, and they include the following:

- Radiation exposure. Radiation therapy or even repetitive head computed tomographies (CTs) or skull x-rays are known to induce primary brain tumors after 20 to 30 years (Tsang, Laperrierre, & Simpson, 2007).
- There are few inherited conditions that are associated with brain tumors, including tuberous sclerosis, neurofibromatosis, Von Hippel–Lindau syndrome, Li–Fraumeni syndrome, and Turcot syndrome (Frantzen, Klasson, & Links, 2012; Gold & Cohen, 2003; Itoh, Hirata, & Ohsato, 1993).
- There is some association of infectious agents and brain tumors, specifically lymphomas, like Epstein–Barr virus and HIV in immunocompromised hosts (Delecluse, Feederle, O'Sullivan, & Taniere, 2007).
- To date, the data to support or refute cellular phone use and risk of brain tumor is lacking.

EPIDEMIOLOGY

In the United States, annual incidence of primary brain tumors range from 7 to 19 cases per 100,000 populations. According to the American Cancer Society, 22,800 cases of tumors involving the nervous system will be diagnosed by end of 2015 and the number of metastatic tumors will be even higher. Meningiomas are the most common of all primary brain tumors and comprise 34% of all primary brain tumors. Pituitary adenomas are frequent incidental findings on autopsy (Siegel, 2015).

Brain tumors are the second most common cause of cancer in children. They comprise 15% to 25% of all childhood malignancies and, unfortunately, have very high morbidity and mortality. The incidence rate of primary brain tumors is 3.6 per 100,000 children each year, higher than the international incidence rate, likely due to better registration (McCormack, 2015). In children below the age of 20 years, brain tumors are the second leading cause of cancer-related deaths (American Brain Tumor Association, 2014).

There is an age-based difference in both location and types of brain tumors. Posterior fossa tumors are more common in children. The risk of supratentorial brain tumors increases from early adolescence to adulthood. Low-grade gliomas are more common in the younger age groups as compared with high-grade gliomas, which are typically seen in the fifth decade of life.

CLINICAL PRESENTATION

Patients with brain tumors can have a wide range of signs and symptoms upon presentation owing to location of the lesion. Usually, clinical presentation depends on the pathogenesis rather than types of brain tumors. Headache may be the most common but a nonspecific symptom of brain tumor in pediatric population (Forsyth & Posner, 1993; Purdy & Kirby, 2004). The most common symptoms of brain tumors based on their location are presented in Table 4.1.

TABLE 4.1 SYMPTOMS OF BRAIN TUMOR BASED UPON LOCATION

Tumor Site	Manifestations
Childhood posterior fossa tumor	Headache (40%) Vomiting Irritability Unsteadiness Ataxia Vision difficulties Progressive obtundation
Childhood supratentorial tumor (less common)	Seizures Hemiparesis Speech difficulties Intellectual disturbance
Frontal lobe	Memory loss Decreased alertness Sleepiness or change in mental status Seizures
Temporal lobe	Depersonalization Emotional changes Behavior disturbances Seizures
Others	Visual changes Altered sense of smell Sensory disturbance Focal neurological defects involving cranial nerves

DIAGNOSTIC CONSIDERATIONS

Brain tumors are usually insidious and may present late in the course of disease, and so diagnostic considerations should be made depending on clinical picture. Pituitary tumors require specialized serum evaluations to assess the hypothalamic–pituitary hormone axis. General workup of brain tumors includes the following:

- Routine laboratory tests
    - Complete blood count
    - Comprehensive metabolic panel
    - Coagulation studies
- Imaging studies
    - CT scan with/without contrast
    - Magnetic resonance imaging (MRI) with/without contrast (better modality for posterior fossa tumors)
- Confirmation test
    - Biopsy with histopathology

TREATMENT

Treating and managing brain tumors involves a multidisciplinary approach. Management consists of treating acute symptoms caused by raised intracranial pressure, focal mass effect, and edema on the surrounding structures. Treatment for raised intracranial pressure is listed in Table 4.2. Various treatment options include the following:

TABLE 4.2 TREATMENT FOR RAISED INTRACRANIAL PRESSURE

Mannitol
3% Hypertonic saline
Dexamethasone (especially if there is peritumoral edema)
Surgical interventions: externalized ventricular drain, endoscopic third ventriculostomy, surgical decompression

Chemotherapy

There are many anticancer drug therapies that are used to achieve the following goals:

- Destroy cancer cells remaining after surgery (i.e., cytotoxic chemotherapy)
- Slow the tumor growth (i.e., cytostatic chemotherapy)
- Reduce symptoms

Radiotherapy

Depending on the type and location of tumor, radiotherapy alone or in conjunction with chemotherapy and/or surgical resection can be offered to patients with both primary and/or metastatic brain tumors.

Surgical Resection

Surgical resection is oftentimes indicated for primary brain tumors, unless the tumor is infiltrating the eloquent cortex or brainstem (e.g., the optic nerves or the language centers). Depending on the location of the lesion, whole tumor, gross total resection, part of tumor, or subtotal resection may be removed to relieve symptoms. Studies indicate that a gross total resection is better than a subtotal for prognosis.

PROGNOSIS

Over many decades, the length of survival following diagnosis of brain tumors has improved overall, but is still poor as compared with other malignancies such as leukemia or lymphoma. Different prognostic factors include age of the patient, histological types and grades of tumors, location, and presenting symptoms. Better prognostic factors include being female gender, age less than 20, extent of tumor resection, supratentorial location, certain biological markers, and less than grade 3 angiogenesis (Ma, de Pennington, Hofer, Blesing, & Stacey, 2013). The 5-year survival of adult patients with any type of brain tumors in the United States is 23% in men and 26% in women, which is 10% more than that among a similar population in the United Kingdom and 7% higher across Europe. Prognosis of brain tumors in pediatric age group has improved in the last three decades with 5-year survival rate of around 70% in the United States and 59% in the United Kingdom (Ma et al., 2013). However, improved survival rates are associated with increasing morbidity, especially in postresection cases. More recent studies are aimed toward understanding the biological and genetic bases of brain tumors, and it may open new horizons of understanding pathogenesis and may present useful prognostic indicators.

CLINICAL SYNOPSIS

Brain tumors are abnormal growths of cells in the cranial cavity. Tumor types include the following:
- Primary versus metastatic
- Benign versus malignant
- Location:
  - Supratentorial
  - Infratentorial
- Tissue type:
  - Gliomas:
    - Astrocytomas
    - Glioblastomas
    - Oligodendroglial tumors
    - Schwannomas
    - Ependymomas
  - Meningiomas
  - Others:
    - Pituitary tumors
    - Pineal gland tumors
    - Craniopharyngiomas
    - CNS lymphomas

Presentation depends on cause of symptoms, which may consist of any of the following:
- Raised intracranial pressure
- Local mass effect or normal brain tissue
- Mass shifting of intracranial contents
- Cerebral vascular events/effects due to aforementioned mechanisms

Common symptoms include the following:
- Headache

- Nausea
- Vomiting
- Altered mental status
- Gait changes
- Ataxia
- Visual changes with loss of peripheral vision or diplopia
- Seizures
- Focal weakness or deficit
- Speech deficits

Diagnosis:
- Common labs:
  - Complete blood count (CBC)/comprehensive metabolic panel (CMP)/coagulation studies
  - Specialized hormonal studies in case of pituitary tumors
- Imaging:
  - CT scan
  - MRI
- Biopsy with histopathology

Management types include acute symptomatic versus tumor load reduction strategies:
- Acute management for raised intracranial pressure (see Table 4.2)
  - Raise head of bed to 30 degrees
- Chemotherapy
- Radiotherapy
- Surgical resection

CASE STUDY

An 11-year-old previously healthy boy presented to neurology clinic with a 2- to 3-week history of headache, nausea, and early morning vomiting. Problems walking started 7 days before presentation. According to his mother, he started having diffuse headaches almost 3 weeks ago. The headaches are mild to moderate and improve as the day passes. Initially, the headaches were attributed to recent upper respiratory infection and responded to Tylenol. The headaches worsened over the next week and was associated with nausea and vomiting. His mother noticed that he complained of being sick first thing when he woke. The boy was seen by his primary care physician and was advised supportive measures. For the last week, his mother noticed his gait had become clumsy, or ataxic, and he wobbled as he walked. Frequently, he lost his balance and fell multiple times while walking in a room with a flat, even surface. Because of gait changes, he was referred to child neurology. On exam, his vital signs were within normal limits for age. He was afebrile. Positive findings included papilledema bilaterally with a broad-based gait. He was uncomfortable and could not comply to complete the cerebellar exam. However, there were no focal findings and all other systems were unremarkable. Because of concerns of raised intracranial pressure, he was admitted to neurology for further workup. An MRI was done and showed a posterior fossa mass. Neurosurgery and oncology were consulted as a multidisciplinary team, and an EVD was placed to relieve intracranial pressure. Brain biopsy later confirmed glioblastoma. He was referred to neuro-oncology for further management in conjunction with neurosurgery.

REFERENCES

American Brain Tumor Association. (2014). *Brain tumor statistics*. Retrieved from www.abta.org/privacy-policy.html

Cushing, H. (1930). *Experience with the cerebellar medulloblastoma: A critical review* (Vol. 7). Copenhagen, Denmark: Levin & Munksgaard.

Delecluse, H. J., Feederle, R., O'Sullivan, B., & Taniere, P. (2007). Epstein–Barr virus-associated tumors: An update for the attention of the working pathologist. *Journal of Clinical Pathology, 60*(12), 1358–1364. doi:10.1136/jcp.2006.044586

Forsyth, P. A., & Posner, J. B. (1993). Headaches in patients with brain tumors: A study of 111 patients. *Neurology, 43*(9), 1678–1683.

Frantzen, C., Klasson, T. D., & Links, T. P. (2012). Von Hippel-Lindau syndrome. *Gene Review*. Retrieved from www.ncbi.nlm.nih.gov/books/NBK1463

Gold, D. R., & Cohen, B. H. (2003). Brain tumors in neurofibromatosis. *Current Treatment Options in Neurology, 5*(3), 199–206.

Itoh, H., Hirata, K., & Ohsato, K. (1993). Turcot's syndrome and familial adenomatous polyposis associated with brain tumor: Review of related literature. *International Journal of Colorectal Disease, 8*(2), 87–94.

Ma, R., de Pennington, N., Hofer, M., Blesing, C., & Stacey, R. (2013). Diagnostic and prognostic markers in gliomas: An update. *British Journal of Neurosurgery, 27*(3), 311–315. doi:10.3109/02688697.2012.752432

McCormack, V. (2015). *Estimated incidence, mortality and prevalence worldwide in 2012*. Retrieved from http://globocan.iarc.fr/Pages/fact_sheets_cancer.aspx

McKinney, P. A. (2004). Brain tumors: Incidence, survival, and etiology. *Journal of Neurology, Neurosurgery, and Psychiatry, 75*(Suppl. 2), ii12–ii17.

Purdy, R. A., & Kirby, S. (2004). Headaches and brain tumors. *Neurologic Clinics, 22*(1), 39–53. doi:10.1016/S0733-8619(03)00099-9

Quinn, G. P., Gonçalves, V., Sehovic, I., Bowman, M. L., & Reed, D. R. (2015). Quality of life in adolescent and young adult cancer patients: A systemic review of literature. *Patient Related Outcome Measures, 6*, 19–51. Retrieved from www.ncbi.nlm.nih.gov/pmc/articles/PMC4337625

Rorke, L. B., & Schut, L. (1989). Introductory survey of pediatric brain tumors. In R. L. McLaurin, L. Schut, J. L. Venes, & F. Epstein (Eds.), *Pediatric neurosurgery* (pp. 335–337). Philadelphia, PA: Saunders.

Siegel, R. (2015). *Cancer facts & figures: American Cancer Society*. Retrieved from www.cancer.org/acs/groups/content/@editorial/documents/document/acspc-044552.pdf

Tsang, R. W., Laperrierre, N. J., & Simpson, W. J. (2007). Glioma arising after radiation therapy for pituitary adenoma: A report of 20 patients and estimation of risk. *Neuro-Oncology, 9*(4), 447–453.

CHAPTER 5

Neuroinfection

JULIA NOVITSKI
KATHLEEN ELVERMAN
DONNA KWAN
EVAN SCHULZE
CHRISTOPHER GROTE

OVERVIEW

Neuroinfection (or neurological infection) occurs when a virus, bacteria, parasite, fungus, or prion attack the brain and/or spinal cord, the effects of which can range from mild illness to serious impairment and even death. A neuroinfection can be a *primary* diagnosis; however, it can also be *secondary* to other conditions such as abscess elsewhere in the body. A neuroinfection can also precipitate other neurological conditions such as seizures, cerebral edema, and increased intracranial pressure (Roos & Brosch, 2012).

Infection of the nervous system can involve the brain ("encephalitis"), the meninges covering the brain ("meningitis"), or both ("meningoencephalitis"). Another type of neuroinfection is human immunodeficiency virus (HIV), which causes acquired immune deficiency syndrome (AIDS) and has a devastating effect on the body's immune system as well as the brain. A related, but distinct condition known as "HIV encephalopathy" is commonly used to describe the neural dysfunction underlying cognitive deficits associated with HIV.

Many neuroinfections are preventable or responsive to treatment. Although early diagnosis and intervention can make a major contribution to potential recovery, neuroinfections are frequently

74 ACQUIRED BRAIN INJURY

underdiagnosed or misdiagnosed and go untreated (Tan et al., 2008). The number of infectious agents that cause neuroinfection is massive, although their clinical expression is more limited. Here, we discuss some of the more common neuroinfections seen in clinical settings.

HISTORY

The study of neuroinfectious diseases is a relatively new specialty within the field of neurology. In the United States, the field of neurology as a separate specialty did not emerge from neuropsychiatry until after World War II, and the American Academy of Neurology (AAN) was established in 1948. Neuroinfectious diseases have traditionally been studied as part of the neuropathology curriculum in neurology, and it was not until 1964 that Hiram H. Merritt published a stand-alone chapter on infectious disease in his *Textbook of Neurology* (Millichap & Epstein, 2009). Nevertheless, early clinicians in the field of neurology had long been treating patients with various forms of infections of the nervous system. For instance, the first bacterial meningitis outbreak was recorded in 1805 in Geneva, Switzerland by Swiss physician Gaspard Vieusseux (Tyler, 2009), while encephalitis due to the influenza virus was first described in 1917 by Constantin von Economo. In fact, the Pasteur Institute in Paris opened in 1888 to treat patients with rabies (Millichap & Epstein, 2009). Research on, and treatment of, neuroinfectious diseases has developed partly as a result of several large-scale infectious disease epidemics that took place in the 20th century, including the influenza epidemic in 1917, the polio epidemic in the 1940s and 1950s, and the AIDS epidemic in the 1980s. In the present day, neurologists with specialization in neuroinfectious diseases care for patients in a variety of clinical settings in which patients may require management of medical complications, including seizures, increased intracranial pressure, autoimmune disorders, immunosuppression, and opportunistic infections.

PATHOPHYSIOLOGY

Different pathogens (e.g., viruses, bacteria, and other microorganisms) may invade the body and infect various organs, including the central nervous system (CNS). Neuroinfections occur when these pathogens enter the CNS (Kaneshiro, 2014). Some infections affect meningeal cells (e.g., enteroviruses), resulting in benign aseptic meningitis, whereas other viruses may affect specific classes of neurons in the brain and spinal cord, giving rise to more serious conditions, including encephalitis and poliomyelitis. Although the blood–brain barrier (BBB) protects the CNS from pathogens, once an infection has set in, the same mechanism prevents the entry of immunocompetent cells and antibodies, which can make treatment more difficult (Adams, Victor, & Ropper, 1997; Koyuncu, Hogue, & Enquist, 2013).

Encephalitis

Encephalitis is a rare but serious condition. The majority of pathogens that cause encephalitis are viruses, although other causes include bacteria, rickettsia, parasites, and fungi. After they enter the body, viruses multiply and enter the bloodstream (viremia), where they are typically cleared by the reticuloendothelial system. However, if the viremia is large enough, the virus may invade the CNS through the choroid plexus and cerebral capillaries. Despite the presence of the BBB, viruses have adapted strategies to enter the CNS through hematogenous (bloodstream) dissemination and retrograde neuronal dissemination (neuronal pathways). Once across the BBB, the viral infection disrupts normal cell functioning and may result in hemorrhage and an inflammatory response, with greater affliction of gray compared with white matter in the brain. Some viruses are thought to affect specific brain regions (e.g., herpes simplex virus targets inferior and medial temporal lobes), whereas others may result in multifocal demyelination of the white matter (e.g., measles, Epstein–Barr virus) (Adams et al., 1997; Howes & Lazoff, 2015).

Meningitis

Bacterial Meningitis

Bacteria may reach the meninges through the bloodstream or direct contact with the meninges (e.g., neurosurgery, shunting, open head wounds; National Center for Immunization and Respiratory Diseases, 2014). The common pathogenesis begins when bacteria first colonize tissue outside the CNS such as the nasopharynx. From here, the infection may enter the bloodstream and access the subarachnoid space. Similar to the infection process of encephalitis, the bacteria are thought to gain access to the cerebrospinal fluid (CSF) though the porous capillaries of the choroid plexus. Unfortunately, the CSF is a poor environment for fighting infection, and an immune response is often outpaced by bacterial growth. Eventually, cellular destruction by the bacteria and the immune response will lead to significant inflammation of the meningeal tissue (typically the arachnoid membrane), and damage to the BBB and brain tissue may occur (Dando et al., 2014).

Viral Meningitis
The pathogenesis of each family of viruses that causes meningitis varies; however, viral meningitis generally results from a complication of common infections (National Center for Immunization and Respiratory Diseases, 2014). In most cases, the viral infection originates within the respiratory or gastrointestinal tracts and progresses to the lymphatic system (Irani, 2008). The dissemination of the virus in meningitis is similar to that in encephalitis. The cellular destruction and immune response of the viral infection incites inflammation of the tissue, which is thought to give rise to clinical symptoms.

Human Immunodeficiency Virus

HIV enters the CNS through monocytes and lymphocytes that become infected before crossing the BBB. Although the virus attacks many regions of the brain, the basal ganglia, hippocampus, frontal cortex, and white matter tend to be most significantly affected (Schouten, Cinque, Gisslen, Reiss, & Portegies, 2011). CD4+ T-helper cells (commonly referred to as "CD4 cells"), which play a key role in maintaining the body's immune system, are preferentially targeted by HIV (Palmisano & Vella, 2011). Among healthy adults, CD4 count typically ranges from 500 to 1,200 cells/mm^3, whereas among individuals with HIV, CD4 count below 200 cells/mm^3 often signifies progression to AIDS (U.S. Department of Health and Human Services, 2015).

While HIV itself can cause neuronal damage, particularly because of inflammation from HIV-infected cells, opportunistic infections also result in significant neural disruption (Schouten et al., 2011). Low CD4 count, and the associated degradation of the immune system, leads to increased risk of contracting opportunistic infections such as cryptococcosis, progressive multifocal leukoencephalopathy, toxoplasmosis, tuberculosis, and neurosyphilis, to name a few (Smith, Smirniotopoulos, & Rushing, 2008). Opportunistic infections further attack the already immunosuppressed individual and are a common cause of death among patients with HIV/AIDS.

ETIOLOGY

Encephalitis

Viruses are transmitted in a variety of ways, including through direct human-to-human contact (e.g., herpes simplex virus, mumps, measles, rubella, varicella zoster viruses), dogs and wild animals (e.g., rabies virus), bats and pigs (e.g., Nipah virus), rodents (e.g., Lassa virus), mosquitos (e.g., West Nile, St. Louis encephalitis viruses), and ticks (e.g., Colorado tick fever virus). Viruses that cause encephalitis include herpes simplex virus (HSV-1, HSV-2) and other herpes viruses (e.g., varicella zoster virus, cytomegalovirus, Epstein–Barr virus), adenoviruses, arboviruses (e.g., West Nile virus, St. Louis virus, Japanese encephalitis, tick-borne viruses), arenaviruses, bunyaviruses, rabies, measles/mumps/rubella, and reoviruses (e.g., Colorado tick fever virus) (Mayo Clinic, 2014). In the United States, the most common encephalitis etiologies include herpes simplex virus, West Nile virus, and enteroviruses. Nevertheless, despite diagnostic testing, the cause remains unknown in approximately half of the cases of viral encephalitis (Kennedy, 2004; World Health Organization, 2006).

Routine vaccinations have reduced encephalitis due to certain viruses, including measles, mumps, rubella, polio, rabies, and varicella (chickenpox). The leading cause of more severe cases of encephalitis in all ages is HSV (90% caused by HSV-1 and 10% by HSV-2). It is a serious yet treatable condition and has an incidence of approximately 1 in 1 million per year, with around 2,000 cases occurring annually in the United States (Kennedy, 2004; Tunkel et al., 2008).

Meningitis

Community-acquired bacterial meningitis in adolescents and adults most commonly occurs secondary to a nasopharyngeal or inner-ear infection. The two most common bacterial agents causing meningitis (*Streptococcus pneumoniae* and *Neisseria meningitidis*) may be passed through contact with an infected person's saliva and respiratory secretions during coughing, sneezing, and kissing (National Center for Immunization and Respiratory Diseases, 2014; Thigpen et al., 2011). Bacteria may also come into contact with the meninges owing to neurosurgery, CSF shunting, traumatic brain injury, or congenital anomalies. Common microbial agents causing meningitis include *S. pneumoniae* (most common and most serious), *S. agalactiae, N. meningitidis, Listeria monocytogenes, Haemophilus influenzae,* and *Escherichia coli* (National Center for Immunization and Respiratory Diseases, 2014; van de Beek, de Gans, Tunkel, & Wijdicks, 2006).

Viral meningeal infection typically occurs following a primary infection of non-CNS tissue. Like most common viruses, those that may cause meningitis can be transmitted though contact with infected persons or objects (e.g., infected feces, saliva, mucus or sputum, blood, or blister fluid; National Center for Immunization and Respiratory Diseases, 2014). Viruses causing meningitis are similar to those that may also cause encephalitis.

Human Immunodeficiency Virus

HIV is acquired through contact with the blood and/or bodily fluids of an infected individual. Mechanisms of transmission include sexual contact (vaginal, anal, or oral), sharing intravenous drug needles, accidental needle-stick injuries, and mother-to-child transmission during pregnancy or breast-feeding.

Increased risk of HIV transmission is driven significantly by viral load, measured by the number of copies per mL of plasma HIV-1 RNA (Maartens, Celum, & Lewin, 2014). An individual in the acute state of HIV infection (i.e., approximately 2–4 weeks after the virus is acquired) has a higher chance of transmitting it to others because of a high viral load at this stage, especially through risky sexual behavior and intravenous drug use. Importantly, HIV testing during this time is likely to be negative if the body has not yet produced sufficient HIV antibodies to be detectable. Thus, an individual may be infected with HIV and transmit the virus without being aware.

Historically, blood transfusions (and organ donations) constituted another potential mechanism of HIV transmission. Infection via transfusion has become increasingly more rare since initial implementation of blood donation screenings in 1985 (Palmisano & Vella, 2011) and universal donation screening with nucleic acid testing (NAT) in 1999 (Zou et al., 2010). Recent research revealed a 1 in 2 million occurrence of NAT-positive HIV cases in a sample of 66-million blood samples taken between the years of 1999 and 2008 (Zou et al., 2010).

EPIDEMIOLOGY

Encephalitis

In the United States, encephalitis affects 7 per 100,000 people annually, with several thousand cases reported to the Centers for Disease Control and Prevention (CDC) every year. Infection is the most common cause of encephalitis, and viruses are the most common etiological agents. Although rare, HSV is the most common cause of encephalitis in Western countries, its incidence being 0.2 per 100,000. Arboviruses (transmitted through insects) are another common cause of encephalitis, with an incidence similar to HSV. However, most people who are bitten by infected insects do not go on to develop clinical illness, and of those who do, less than 10% go on to develop encephalitis. The rarest cause of encephalitis in the United States is rabies (0–3 cases annually). Risk factors for contracting encephalitis include the following (Granerod & Crowcroft, 2007; Howes & Lazoff, 2015; Mayo Clinic, 2014):

- *Age:* Certain age groups are at greater risk for some types of encephalitis, such as young children and older adults. HSV encephalitis is more common in people 20 to 40 years of age.
- *Sex:* Males are slightly more likely to be affected by encephalitis than are females.
- *Weakened immune system:* Individuals with HIV/AIDS and those with weakened immune systems or who take immunosuppressant drugs are at greater risk.
- *Geographic regions:* Encephalitis occurs worldwide. Herpesviruses tend to have a global distribution, whereas arboviruses are more geographically restricted. Mosquito or tick-borne diseases tend to be more prevalent in certain geographic regions.
- *Season of the year:* Mosquito and tick-borne diseases are more common during the warm months of the year in the United States and may be present year round in warmer areas.

Meningitis

Bacterial Meningitis
The annual incidence of bacterial meningitis is estimated to be 4 to 6 cases per 100,000 adults (van de Beek et al., 2006). In the United States, approximately 500 deaths occur annually as a result of bacterial meningitis (Thigpen et al., 2011). The most common causative bacteria of community-acquired bacterial meningitis in adults is *S. pneumoniae* followed by *N. meningitidis*, together accounting for 75% to 90% of cases.

Viral Meningitis
In temperate regions, rates of viral meningitis are highest in the summer and fall seasons, with no seasonal variability in tropical or subtropical climates (Logan & MacMahon, 2008). Viral meningitis is thought to be much more common than bacterial meningitis; however, because of frequent spontaneous recovery in mild cases, true incidence and prevalence rates are difficult to calculate. In a retrospective study of individuals aged 16 and older, the incidence of viral meningitis was 7.6 per 100,000 individuals (Kupila et al., 2006). Risk factors for contracting meningitis include the following (National Center for Immunization and Respiratory Diseases, 2014):

- *Skipping vaccinations:* If a person has not completed the recommended childhood or adult vaccination schedule, the risk of meningitis is higher.

- *Age:* Most cases occur at the extremes of age (<2 or >60 years; Thigpen et al., 2011).

- *Living in a community setting:* College students living in dormitories, personnel on military bases, and children in boarding schools and childcare facilities are at increased risk of meningococcal meningitis. This increased risk likely occurs because the bacterium is spread by the respiratory route and tends to spread quickly in large groups.

- *Compromised immune system:* Factors that may compromise a person's immune system, including AIDS, alcoholism, diabetes, and use of immunosuppressant drugs, also make the person more susceptible to meningitis. Removal of the spleen, an important part of one's immune system, may also increase the person's risk.

Human Immunodeficiency Virus

According to the CDC, approximately 915,000 people in the United States were living with an HIV diagnosis as of 2012. The annual rate of diagnosis for the overall population in 2013 was 15 per 100,000 people, with this rate having been stable since 2009. Rate of diagnosis varied by a number of factors including age, race/ethnicity, and sex. The highest rates of HIV diagnosis (per 100,000) were seen among individuals who were between the ages 25 and 29 (rate of 36.3), African American (rate of 55.9), and men (rate of 29.4). Sixty-eight percent of diagnosed cases in 2013 were attributed to male-to-male sexual contact and intravenous drug use. The rates of death due to HIV have recently decreased in the overall population. Although the incidence of HIV diagnosis has decreased in recent years, the overall prevalence has increased because of increased life expectancy with improved treatment options (Division of HIV/AIDS Prevention, National Center for HIV/AIDS, Viral Hepatitis, Sexual Transmitted Diseases and Tuberculosis Prevention, Centers for Disease Control and Prevention, 2013).

Among those with HIV, only a portion of individuals develops encephalitis or meningitis. Postmortem studies of individuals with HIV have shown a 10% to 30% incidence of HIV encephalitis (Schouten et al., 2011). Cryptococcal meningitis, the most common opportunistic infection among individuals with HIV, occurs in 5% to 7% of patients, typically following progression to AIDS, at which point the risk of contracting opportunistic infection is highest. Aseptic meningitis is the second most common form of meningitis in HIV and is frequently caused by the HIV infection itself (Singh, Thomas, & Uppal, 2013).

CLINICAL PRESENTATION

Encephalitis

Common symptoms of a viral infection include fever, headache, altered level of consciousness, confusion, seizures, and neurological deficits. In addition, nausea and vomiting, fatigue, muscle pain, neck stiffness, and photophobia may also be present. In cases of mild encephalitis, symptoms may be similar to other illnesses (e.g., low fever, mild headache, and fatigue). The diagnosis of encephalitis may be supported by analysis of spinal fluid and neuroimaging abnormalities. For HSV, abnormal brain MRI findings are typically present within 48 hours following the onset of symptoms, which include presence of hyperintensities in the frontotemporal, insular, and cingulate regions. For West Nile and St. Louis encephalitis, brain MRI abnormalities include hyperintensities in the basal ganglia and the thalamus. For varicella zoster encephalitis, brain MRI may show demyelinating lesions and hemorrhagic and ischemic infarctions. In newborns, symptoms may include irritability, increased crying, vomiting and lack of appetite, and body stiffness. Symptoms that warrant emergency care include loss of consciousness, paralysis, seizures, and sudden mental status changes (McKean, Ross, & Dressler, 2012; Tunkel et al., 2008).

Meningitis

The initial symptom presentation between bacterial and viral meningitis may be similar, with no reliable differentiation based on clinical indicators (Logan & MacMahon, 2008). *Bacterial meningitis* tends to progress rapidly and tends to be more severe, with the emergence of severe neurological symptoms (National Center for Immunization and Respiratory Diseases, 2014; Tunkel et al., 2004; van de Beek et al., 2006). Notably, pneumococcal meningitis is particularly dangerous. In a study investigating the clinical presentation of those with confirmed pneumococcal meningitis, nearly 40% had focal neurological deficits, 34% had aphasia, 17% had cranial nerve palsies, and 11% had hemiparesis upon hospital admission (Weisfelt, de Gans, van der Poll, & van de Beek, 2006). Individuals with *viral meningitis* will often experience spontaneous recovery or may require standard supportive treatment. Nevertheless, enteroviral meningitis causes considerable morbidity with high fever and severe headache despite appropriate treatment (Logan & MacMahon, 2008).

Common symptoms of meningitis in adults include fever, stiff neck, altered mental status (Glasgow Coma Scale score below 14), headache, sensitivity to bright light, fatigue and drowsiness, lethargy, nausea, and vomiting (Logan & MacMahon, 2008; National Center for Immunization and Respiratory Diseases, 2014; van de Beek et al., 2006). Common neurological complications secondary to meningitis include seizures, brain infection, cerebral edema, hydrocephalus, abscess formation, and intracranial hemorrhage (van de Beek et al., 2006).

Human Immunodeficiency Virus

In the acute stage of HIV infection, symptoms often include fatigue, fever, diarrhea, headache, rashes, mouth sores, muscle stiffness or aching, sore throat, swollen lymph glands, and yeast infections. Many HIV-positive individuals are asymptomatic for many years, up to a decade or more, despite having detectable levels of infection and being capable of transmitting the disease. Symptoms become increasingly apparent with onset of opportunistic infections. Neuroimaging findings among HIV patients frequently reveal significant atrophy, particularly in the basal ganglia, as well as white matter abnormalities in frontal regions and the corpus callosum. Such findings are commonly associated with cognitive deficits (Schouten et al., 2011).

Neuropsychological deficits occur among HIV patients in both asymptomatic and symptomatic stages of the disease. These deficits have been found to precede the onset of opportunistic infections in 12% of patients and occur in up to 50% of all patients with HIV/AIDS (Ellis, Langford, & Masliah, 2007). Consistent with the epidemiology of the HIV infection overall, the incidence of cognitive impairment among those with HIV has decreased over the years, although its prevalence has increased (because of more people living longer with the disease). HIV-associated neurocognitive disorder, commonly referred to as "HAND," can be broken down into mild and major neurocognitive disorder (NCD) due to HIV on the basis of the degree to which cognitive test performance falls below average and everyday functioning is impaired. The pattern of cognitive deficits among individuals with NCD due to HIV is typically characterized by reduced processing speed, executive functioning deficits, poor attention, and impairment in memory (Schouten et al., 2011).

DIAGNOSTIC CONSIDERATIONS

Encephalitis

Primary encephalitis (caused by a specific virus) can be distinguished from *secondary* encephalitis (caused by the body's immune reaction). Additionally, infections can either be *acute* (e.g., postinfectious encephalomyelitis, flaccid paralysis) or *chronic* (e.g., spongiform encephalopathies, retrovirus disease). "Encephalitis" should also be distinguished from "encephalopathy," which occurs secondary to factors such as metabolic disturbances, ischemia, hypoxia, intoxications, or organ and systemic infections (Adams et al., 1997). Common different diagnosis for viral encephalitis includes ruling out other etiological factors, including bacteria (Lyme disease, syphilis, tuberculosis), fungi, rickettsia, parasites, protozoa, autoimmune disease, and allergic reactions to medications (Kaneshiro, 2014). Patients with encephalitis may also exhibit acute cognitive difficulties (e.g., confusion, speech problems), focal neurologic signs (e.g., abnormal reflexes), seizures, behavioral changes, and other symptoms, including increased intracranial pressure, neck stiffness, skin rash, and signs in other organs, such as lungs and liver (Howes & Lazoff, 2015).

Meningitis

The classic triad of symptoms in those with meningitis consists of fever, neck stiffness, and altered mental status; however, the sensitivity of making a positive detection of meningitis by relying solely on these symptoms is low, with a 44% detection rate (van de Beek et al., 2006). The cornerstone in the diagnosis of *bacterial meningitis* is CSF examination. When examination of the CSF reveals no presence of a bacterial agent, the patient is said to have aseptic meningitis and workup for a viral etiology may be pursued. The usual approach to *viral meningitis* diagnosis is to test the CSF for enteroviruses, herpes simplex virus, and varicella zoster virus. Serology can also be done to test for mumps, Epstein–Barr virus, and HIV (Logan & MacMahon, 2008).

Meticulous history taking is essential in targeting risk factors and must include evaluation of exposure to infected individuals, outdoor activity in areas of endemic Lyme disease, travel history with possible exposure to tuberculosis, as well as history of medication use, intravenous drug use, and sexually transmitted disease risk. Common differential diagnoses include chemical irritation (chemical meningitis), neoplasm, granulomatous disease, acute disseminated encephalomyelitis, CNS lupus, and other inflammatory conditions.

Human Immunodeficiency Virus

A variety of CSF markers are used in the process of HIV diagnosis, as well as in monitoring disease progression and treatment response. These CSF markers provide measures of the virology of the disease, host response (e.g., inflammation and neurotoxicity), and CNS tissue damage (Schouten et al., 2011). Given the common occurrence of opportunistic infection among those with HIV/AIDS, the impact of comorbid disease processes should always be considered when working with HIV patients.

With regard to diagnosing NCD in individuals with HIV, differential diagnosis should include consideration of factors such as aging, effects of comorbid infection, and possible toxicity due to treatment (Schouten et al., 2011). Functional neuroimaging has shown some promise in aiding with early detection of NCD due to HIV. Studies of brain activation in patients with HIV have shown a pattern of compensatory recruitment (i.e., recruitment of more widespread brain regions) before the onset of cognitive deficits (Ellis et al., 2007). However, these findings are fairly nonspecific because this pattern of compensatory brain activation is common among patients with other NCDs as well, such as that due to Alzheimer's disease.

TREATMENT

Encephalitis

Antiviral drugs, including acyclovir and ganciclovir, are used to treat viral encephalitis, especially herpesviruses. Other treatments, such as antiseizure medicines, steroids (reduction of brain swelling), acetaminophen (for headaches and fever), and sedatives (for restlessness or irritability) may be used as part of supportive treatment to aid recovery. Patients are also often evaluated to determine their need for physical, occupational, speech, and cognitive rehabilitation (Kaneshiro, 2014; McKean et al., 2012).

Meningitis

Bacterial Meningitis
Research suggests a link between the severity of acute disease progression and the presence of permanent neurological damage, highlighting the importance of timely intervention. It has been recommended to initiate empirically supported antibiotic therapy before brain imaging, hospital transfer for elevated care, and lumbar puncture when disease progression is eminent (van de Beek et al., 2006). The treatment of bacterial meningitis is with targeted

or empirical antibiotic therapy. Recent studies have suggested the use of concurrent dexamethasone therapy may be of benefit by attenuating the inflammatory response in the subarachnoid space (Tunkel et al., 2004).

Viral Meningitis
Treatment for viral meningitis most often consists of supportive therapy including rest, hydration, antipyretics, and pain or anti-inflammatory medications as needed. Antiviral therapies may also be used with viral meningitis (Irani, 2008; Logan & MacMahon, 2008).

Human Immunodeficiency Virus

HIV is treated with antiretroviral therapy (ART). The first antiretroviral medication, azidothymidine (AZT; also known as "zidovudine" or "ZDV"), was approved for the treatment of HIV/AIDS in the United States in 1987. Combination antiretroviral therapy (cART; also known as "highly active antiretroviral therapy" or "HAART") was first discussed in 1995, with widespread implementation growing throughout the late 1990s (Palmisano & Vella, 2011). Six classes of antiretroviral medications are currently available (Ene, Duiculescu, & Ruta, 2011). cART treatments typically use three or more medications from at least two different classes, with the goal of reducing HIV replication and increasing CD4 count (Ellis et al., 2007). These medications are designed to attack the HIV infection that is present throughout the body. However, the degree to which HIV in the brain is effectively treated by these medications is often decreased by their inability to penetrate the BBB. Specific attention to the CSF permeability of medications within a cART regimen may have significant implications for the degree of neural damage and cognitive impairment that a patient experiences.

Consistent medication adherence is an additional treatment concern, with implications for reducing the risk of medication resistance (Maartens et al., 2014). This topic is particularly important among patients with complicated treatment regimens and significant negative side effects. It is important to consider the potentially reciprocal relationship between neurocognitive deficits and treatment adherence. Also, the degree to which cognitive impairment may contribute to poor adherence should be assessed in all HIV patients, particularly given the executive functioning and memory deficits commonly seen among these patients.

PROGNOSIS

Encephalitis

Prognosis for viral encephalitis varies depending on the type of virus and the patient's overall health. In general, patients at the extremes of the age range and those who are immune compromised tend to have poorer outcomes. The acute phase typically lasts between 1 and 2 weeks, though recovery can take up to several months. Permanent brain dysfunction may result from cases of severe encephalitis, affecting various functions such as memory, speech, vision, hearing, and muscle control (Kaneshiro, 2014).

The most common cause of encephalitis, HSV, has a mortality rate of 50% to 75% if left untreated (20% when treated), and the majority of survivors experience persisting mental and motor disabilities in addition to seizures and impaired memory functioning. Mortality rate for West Nile and St. Louis encephalitis may be up to 30%, with potential for neurologic sequelae after treatment, including memory loss and movement disorders. Prevention recommendations include avoiding contact with an infected individual, minimizing exposure to mosquitos, and obtaining routine vaccinations (Howes & Lazoff, 2015).

Meningitis

Bacterial Meningitis
Mortality for bacterial meningitis is highest in the first year of life, decreases in midlife, and increases again in old age. Bacterial meningitis is fatal in 1 in 10 cases, and 1 of every 7 survivors is left with a severe neurological impairment. In 50% of patients, several complications may develop in the days to weeks following infection. Even with effective antibiotic therapy, long-term sequelae are seen in as many as 30% of survivors (van de Beek et al., 2006). Among the bacterial pathogens, *S. pneumoniae* causes the highest mortality (20%–30%) and morbidity (15%) in adults and children with meningitis (Kastenbauer & Pfister, 2003; Thigpen et al., 2011). Serious complications impacting outcome include seizures, hearing or vision loss, cranial nerve dysfunction, hydrocephalus, ataxia, focal paralysis, and cognitive impairment (van de Beek et al., 2006).

Viral Meningitis
The prognosis for viral meningitis is usually excellent, with most cases resolving without complication within 7 to 10 days. Of note, children and older adults and those with significant medical co-morbidities and immunodeficiency may have a poorer outcome (Logan & MacMahon, 2008). The mortality rate for viral meningitis without encephalitis is less than 1%.

Human Immunodeficiency Virus

Despite advances in treatment, HIV continues to be a disease without a cure. However, the advent of cART in the late 1990s dramatically shifted the prognostic landscape for HIV. Having historically been an intensely progressive and fatal disease, HIV has since shifted to being a disease with a chronic, yet considerably more manageable course (Maartens et al., 2014). This is evidenced by the decreased incidence and increased prevalence (due to extended life expectancy) noted previously. A decrease in the occurrence of opportunistic infections has been shown among patients on antiretroviral medications (Ellis et al., 2007). Additionally, better cognitive prognoses are also associated with cART, and treatment regimens including antiretroviral medications with high CSF penetration are associated with improved neuropsychological performance (Schouten et al., 2011).

CLINICAL SYNOPSIS

Overview

- Neuroinfection occurs when a virus, bacteria, parasite, fungus, or prion attacks the brain and/or spinal cord.
- Infection of the CNS can involve the brain (encephalitis), the meninges covering the brain (meningitis), or both (meningoencephalitis).
- HIV/AIDS is a viral infection that compromises the body's immune system and can cause both encephalitis and meningitis, as well as HIV encephalopathy.
- Early diagnosis and treatment is imperative for recovery from neuroinfection.
- Neuroinfections may lead to diffuse myelin damage, neuronal tissue loss or damage, or vascular damage

Etiology

- Common viruses that cause neuroinfection are herpesviruses, enteroviruses, West Nile, and Lyme disease and can be transmitted through contact with infected humans, animals, or insects, though the etiology is unclear in about 50% of cases.
- Bacterial neuroinfections are commonly secondary to nasopharyngeal or inner-ear infections.
- The risk of contracting a neuroinfection may depend on various factors, such as age, sex, immune system status, vaccinations, sexually risky behaviors, exposure to unsanitary conditions, geographic locations, international travel, and recent medical surgery or an infection in another part of the body.

Symptoms

- Symptoms of neuroinfection may be similar to flulike illness, which can lead to misdiagnosis.
- Classic triad of symptoms for meningitis includes neck stiffness, fever, and altered mental status, though it may be present in less than 50% of cases.
- Other symptoms may include double vision, photophobia, speech difficulties, muscle weakness, gait disturbance, rash, personality changes, behavioral changes, and seizures.

Diagnosis and Treatment

- Diagnostic procedures include obtaining patient's history, neurological examination, CSF and blood tests, and brain imaging.
- Treatment depends on the etiological agent and severity of infection:
    - Antiviral agents for viral etiologies
    - Antibacterial therapy for bacterial etiologies
    - Skull puncture and shunting to relieve intracranial pressure

Rehabilitation and other follow-up treatment may include the following:
- Physical and occupational therapy to improve strength and balance and establish independence with activities of daily living
- Speech therapy to relearn muscle control and coordination to produce speech
- Neuropsychological assessment to measure postinfection cognitive functioning
- Psychotherapy to learn coping strategies and behavioral skills to improve mood

CASE STUDY

Five days after a 59-year-old woman returns from a camping trip, she developed body aches, worsening pain when rotating her neck, and sluggishness. Symptoms persisted for several more days, and on arrival to the ER, she was confused and had a high-grade fever. Laboratory workup showed normal head CT and blood composition; however, CSF analysis showed elevated protein and IgM antibody. EEG showed diffuse bilateral focal abnormalities and global slowing. She was diagnosed with West Nile virus encephalitis and hospitalized for 10 days, during which she received supportive therapy (i.e., hydration, prevention of secondary infection) because no specific antiviral treatment was available.

Ten weeks after discharge, the patient continued to have physical symptoms of severe muscle weakness, headaches, fatigue, and decreased psychomotor speed. In addition, cognitive symptoms included difficulty concentrating and memory loss. She was irritable with family members, withdrawn from friends, and was increasingly anxious about her absence from work.

Physical rehabilitation included restoring muscle tone, building strength, and increasing balance. Functional rehabilitation included modifying the home environment to reduce fall risk, assessing fitness to drive, developing guidelines for return to work, and developing compensatory strategies to aid memory and concentration.

Psychological services can aid in addressing the patient's anxiety, helping her to process the effects of the sudden illness, and reducing potential for depression. Although progress is very gradual, the patient can expect a high chance of complete recovery within a year.

REFERENCES

Adams, R. D., Victor, M., & Ropper, A. H. (1997). Infections of the nervous system (bacterial, fungal, spirochetal, parasitic, and sarcoid). In M. Navrozov (Ed.), *Principles of neurology.* New York, NY: McGraw-Hill.

Dando, S. J., Mackay-Sim, A., Norton, R., Currie, J., St. John, J. A., Ekberg, J. A. K., . . . Beaham, I. R. (2014). Pathogens penetrating the central nervous system: Infection pathways and the cellular and molecular mechanisms of invasion. *Clinical Microbiology Reviews, 27*(4), 691–726.

Division of HIV/AIDS Prevention, National Center for HIV/AIDS, Viral Hepatitis, Sexual Transmitted Diseases and Tuberculosis Prevention, Centers for Disease Control and Prevention. (2013). *HIV surveillance report.* Retrieved from www.cdc.gov/hiv/library/reports/surveillance

Ellis, R., Langford, D., & Masliah, E. (2007). HIV and antiretroviral therapy in the brain: Neuronal injury and repair. *Nature Reviews: Neuroscience, 8*(1), 33–44. doi:10.1038/nrn2040

Ene, L., Duiculescu, D., & Ruta, S. M. (2011). How much do antiretroviral drugs penetrate into the central nervous system? *Journal of Medicine and Life, 4*(4), 432–439.

Granerod, J., & Crowcroft, N. S. (2007). The epidemiology of acute encephalitis. *Neuropsychological Rehabilitation, 17*(4/5), 406–428. doi:10.1080/09602010600989620

Howes, D. S., & Lazoff, M. (2015). *Encephalitis.* Retrieved from http://emedicine.medscape.com/article/791896-overview

Irani, D. N. (2008). Aseptic meningitis and viral myelitis. *Neurology Clinics, 26*(3), 635–viii.

Kaneshiro, N. K. (2014). *Encephalitis.* Baltimore: University of Maryland Medical Center. Retrieved from http://umm.edu/health/medical/ency/articles/encephalitis

Kastenbauer, S., & Pfister, H. W. (2003). Pneumococcal meningitis in adults: Spectrum of complications and prognostic factors in a series of 87 cases. *Brain, 126,* 1015–1025.

Kennedy, P. G. (2004). Viral encephalitis: Causes, differential diagnosis, and management. *Journal of Neurology, Neurosurgery and Psychiatry, 75*(Suppl. 1), i10–i15.

Koyuncu, O. O., Hogue, I. B., & Enquist, L. W. (2013). Virus infections in the nervous system. *Cell Host Microbe, 13*(4), 379–393. doi:10.1016/j.chom.2013.03.010

Kupila, L., Vuorinen, T., Vainiopaa, R., Hukkanen, V., Marttila, R. J., & Kotilainen, P. (2006). Etiology of aseptic meningitis and encephalitis in an adult population. *Neurology, 66*, 75–80.

Logan, S. A., & MacMahon, E. (2008). Viral meningitis. *British Medical Journal, 336*(7634), 36–40. doi:10.1136/bmj.39409.673657.AE

Maartens, G., Celum, C., & Lewin, S. R. (2014). HIV infection: Epidemiology, pathogenesis, treatment, and prevention. *Lancet, 384*(9939), 258–271. doi:10.1016/S0140-6736(14)60164-1

Mayo Clinic. (2014). *Encephalitis.* Scottsdale, AZ: Author. Retrieved from www.mayoclinic.org/diseases-conditions/encephalitis/basics/definition/con-20021917

McKean, S. C., Ross, J. J., Dressler, D. D., Brotman, D. J., & Ginsberg, J. S. (2012). *Principles and practice of hospital medicine.* New York, NY: McGraw-Hill Medical.

Millichap, J. J., & Epstein, L. G. (2009). Emerging subspecialties in neurology: Neuroinfectious diseases. *Neurology, 73*(4), e14–e15. doi:10.1212/WNL.0b013e3181af7a46

National Center for Immunization and Respiratory Diseases. (2014). *Bacterial meningitis.* Atlanta, GA: Centers for Disease Control and Prevention. Retrieved from www.cdc.gov/meningitis/bacterial.html

Palmisano, L., & Vella, S. (2011). A brief history of antiretroviral therapy of HIV infection: Success and challenges. *Annali dell'Istituto Superiore di Sanità, 47*(1), 44–48. doi:10.4415/ANN_11_01_10

Roos, K. L., & Brosch, J. R. (2012). Meningitis and encephalitis. In S. C. McKean, J. J. Ross, D. D. Dressler, D. J. Brotman, & J. S. Ginsberg (Eds.), *Principles and practice of hospital medicine.* New York, NY: McGraw-Hill Medical.

Schouten, J., Cinque, P., Gisslen, M., Reiss, P., & Portegies, P. (2011). HIV-1 infection and cognitive impairment in the cART era: A review. *AIDS, 25*(5), 561–575. doi:10.1097/QAD.0b013e3283437f9a

Singh, N. N., Thomas, F. P., & Uppal, G. (2013). *Meningitis in HIV.* Retrieved from http://emedicine.medscape.com/article/1952165-overview

Smith, A. B., Smirniotopoulos, J. G., & Rushing, E. J. (2008). From the archives of the AFIP: Central nervous system infections associated with human immunodeficiency virus infection: Radiologic-pathologic correlation. *Radiographics, 28*(7), 2033–2058. doi:10.1148/rg.287085135

Tan, K., Patel, S., Gandhi, N., Chow, F., Rumbaugh, J., & Nath, A. (2008). Burden of neuroinfectious diseases on the neurology service in a tertiary care center. *Neurology, 71*(15), 1160–1166. doi:10.1212/01.wnl.0000327526.71683.b7

Thigpen, M. C., Whitney, C. G., Messonnier, N. E., Zell, E. R., Lynfield, R., Hadler, J. L., . . . Schuchat, A.; Emerging Infections Programs Network. (2011). Bacterial meningitis in the United States, 1998–2007. *The New England Journal of Medicine, 364*(21), 2016–2025. doi:10.1056/NEJMoa1005384

Tunkel, A. R., Glaser, C. A., Bloch, K. C., Sejvar, J. J., Marra, C. M., Roos, K. L., . . . Whitley, R. J; Infectious Diseases Society of America. (2008). The management of encephalitis: Clinical practice guidelines by the Infectious Diseases Society of America. *Clinical Infectious Diseases, 47*(3), 303–327. doi:10.1086/589747

Tunkel, A. R., Hartman, B. J., Kaplan, S. L., Kaufman, B. A., Roos, K. L., Scheld, W. M., & Whitley, R. J. (2004). Practice guidelines for the management of bacterial meningitis. *Clinical Infectious Diseases, 39*(9), 1267–1284. doi:10.1086/425368

Tyler, K. L. (2009). Chapter 28: A history of bacterial meningitis. *Handbook of Clinical Neurology, 95*, 417–433. doi:10.1016/S0072-9752(08)02128-3

U.S. Department of Health and Human Services. (2015). *CD4 count*. Washington, DC: Author. Retrieved from www.aids.gov/hiv-aids-basics/just-diagnosed-with-hiv-aids/understand-your-test-results/cd4-count

van de Beek, D., de Gans, J., Tunkel, A. R., & Wijdicks, E. F. (2006). Community-acquired bacterial meningitis in adults. *The New England Journal of Medicine, 354*(1), 44–53. doi:10.1056/NEJMra052116

Weisfelt, M., de Gans, J., van der Poll, T., & van de Beek, D. (2006). Pneumococcal meningitis in adults: New approaches to management and prevention. *Lancet Neurology, 5*(4), 332–342. doi:10.1016/S1474-4422(06)70409-4

World Health Organization. (2006). *Neurological disorders: Public health challenges* (pp. 95–111). Geneva, Switzerland: Author.

Zou, S., Dorsey, K. A., Notari, E. P., Foster, G. A., Krysztof, D. E., Musavi, F., . . . Stramer, S. L. (2010). Prevalence, incidence, and residual risk of human immunodeficiency virus and hepatitis C virus infections among United States blood donors since the introduction of nucleic acid testing. *Transfusion, 50*(7), 1495–1504. doi:10.1111/j.1537-2995.2010.02622.x

CHAPTER 6

Neurotoxic and Metabolic Injuries

BRUCE J. DIAMOND
JOSEPH E. MOSLEY
KATHERINE MAKAREC
KRISTA DETTLE

OVERVIEW

In this chapter, we briefly examine brain injuries manifested as acute and chronic impairments and disturbances across a variety of cognitive, motor, neuropsychiatric, perceptual-motor, visuospatial, emotional, tissue, systemic, and electro-chemical domains secondary to neurotoxic and metabolic injuries.

Chronic Hepatic Encephalopathy

Chronic hepatic encephalopathy (CHE) is a reversible metabolic neuropsychiatric syndrome (Hilsabeck & Webb, 2013). Mild CHE (M-CHE) requires neuropsychological testing to reveal cognitive impairments. M-CHE is associated with poor quality of life and a high risk for accidents (Bajaj & Mullen, 2010).

Uremic Encephalopathy

Uremic encephalopathy (UE), a potentially debilitating disorder, can be experienced in both acute and chronic renal failure (Seifter & Samuels, 2011). It involves subtle decline in mentation, emotional changes, and progression into full-blown delirium, seizures, coma, cognitive, motor, and neuropsychiatric impairments.

Hyperhomocysteinemia and Alzheimer's Disease

Homocysteine (Hcy) is a nonessential, nonproteinogenic amino acid synthesized from dietary methionine (Petras et al., 2014). Elevation of total plasma Hcy, known as "hyperhomocysteinemia" (HHcy), is associated with neurodegenerative diseases of the central nervous system (CNS) such as epilepsy, stroke, and dementia, including Alzheimer's disease (AD) (Petras et al., 2014). HHcy is theorized to be a risk factor that, if properly managed, may help postpone the onset of AD (Van Dam & Van Gool, 2009), although causal links are tenuous and controversial (Farkas et al., 2013).

Metabolic Risk Factors of Sporadic Alzheimer's Disease

Approximately 95% of AD cases are of the sporadic type in which multifactorial genetic, lifestyle, and environmental influences contribute to pathogenesis (Chakrabarti et al., 2015). This type of AD usually becomes fully symptomatic after age 60, termed "late-onset AD" (LOAD) (Lim , Martins, & Martins, 2014). However, distinct and measurable changes may begin in affected individuals' brains years before onset (Liu et al., 2014). Accordingly, research has focused on identifying pathogenic mechanisms and early biomarkers of metabolic origin (Chakrabarti et al., 2015).

Organophosphates and Pesticides

Pesticide chemicals are used throughout the United States and the developing world to manage insects, birds, weeds, plant pathogens, mollusks, and biological agents (United States Environmental Protection Agency, 2007).

Wernicke's Encephalopathy

Wernicke's encephalopathy (WE) is an acute neuropsychiatric disorder caused by thiamine (B_1) deficiency; left untreated, it can result in Korsakoff's syndrome (Galvin et al., 2010).

Toxic Metabolic Encephalopathy

The term "encephalopathy" derives from the Greek *encephalos* (brain) and *pathos* (suffering or experience). Toxic metabolic encephalopathy (TME) characteristically involves delirium and an acute confusional state accompanied by global cerebral dysfunction in the absence of primary structural brain disease (Chen & Young, 1996).

Lead Poisoning

Lead (Pb) poisoning is insidious but treatable and is now more commonly seen in developing countries, in those living in older homes, or environments with lead contamination in the soil. It can be an acute (less commonly seen and typically due to occupational exposure) (Flora, Gupta, & Tiwari, 2012) or a chronic condition. Lead can be ingested (e.g., recently in a popular noodle brand in India) (Bhullar, Thind, & Singla, 2015), inhaled (e.g., lead dust from deteriorating paints), or absorbed through the skin. The impact on children under 6 years of age can be devastating (developmental delay or, in severe cases, death) if not treated.

HISTORY

Chronic Hepatic Encephalopathy

Associations between hepatic disease and mental disorders were first recorded by Hippocrates. Galen later developed a model of liver functioning that recognized its importance to brain functioning, hypothesizing that the liver used food in the stomach to prepare blood for systemic distribution (Davidson & Summerskill, 1956).

Uremic Encephalopathy

Metabolic encephalopathy was a diagnostic term first used in 1927 to define the clinical presentation of brain dysfunction caused by systemic factors (Varelas & Graffagnino, 2013). UE is one of the most debilitating disorders associated with renal failure.

Hyperhomocysteinemia and Alzheimer's Disease

In 1992, it was suggested that B vitamin deficiencies might contribute to cognitive decline in patients with dementia. During the same year, three independent groups suggested that because metabolism of Hcy depends on normal levels of B vitamins, Hcy levels might be elevated in patients with AD (McCaddon, 2006), known as the "homocysteine hypothesis of AD" (McCaddon, 2006). Using data from the Framingham Heart Study, Seshadri and colleagues (2002) published the first sufficiently powered epidemiological study investigating relationships between Hcy levels and AD.

Metabolic Risk Factors of Sporadic Alzheimer's Disease

At the turn of the 20th century, Alois Alzheimer, psychiatrist and neuroanatomist, discovered and characterized the histological alterations that we recognize today as the hallmark features of AD, plaques and neurofibrillary tangles. Although the response in the medical community was not enthusiastic, these histopathological findings and the accompanying symptom profile and illness course described by Alzheimer had not previously been seen or recognized as a disease profile (Hippius & Neundörfer, 2003).

Organophosphates and Pesticides

While many organophosphates and pesticides are known neurotoxins, research is only beginning to characterize the neuropsychological sequelae following exposure (Schultz & Ferraro, 2013). Organophosphates and carbamates contribute to the majority of the available data (National Research Council, 1993).

Wernicke's Encephalopathy

Wernicke first described WE in 1881 with a characteristic triad of symptoms: confusion, ataxia, and oculomotor abnormality. It was recognized in China over 1,000 years ago as wet beriberi, a disease caused by malnutrition brought on by a limited diet consisting of polished white rice (Fan, 2004).

Toxic Metabolic Encephalopathy

In 1912, Kinnier Wilson coined the term "metabolic encephalopathy" to describe a global cerebral dysfunction induced by systemic factors (Varelas & Graffagnino, 2013).

Lead Poisoning

Lead poisoning is thought to have played a role in the fall of the Roman Empire and has been mined by humans for 6,000 years (Hernberg, 2000). Although lead poisoning was known in the ancient world, it was forgotten until 1772 when Sir George Backer made the connection between lead ingestion and the Devonshire colic (Hernberg, 2000). Tanquerel des Planches provided the first modern description of lead poisoning in 1839 (Hernberg, 2000). Since 1978, lead-based paints stopped being sold in the United States. Most of the developed world stopped producing lead-based gasoline in the 1920s; it was not until the 1990s, after a period of decline, that it was virtually eliminated (Hernberg, 2000).

PATHOPHYSIOLOGY

Chronic Hepatic Encephalopathy

Ammonia neurotoxicity largely mediates observed neuropathology (Hilsabeck & Webb, 2013). When ammonia in the blood reaches the brain, astrocytes attempt to eliminate it by synthesizing glutamine from molecules of ammonia and glutamate (Bajaj & Mullen, 2010). As glutamine accumulates, its osmotic effect causes perivascular astrocytes to absorb water and swell, causing a cascade of events, for example, brain edema, increased intracranial pressure (ICP), alterations in neurotransmission, oxidative stress, and release of proinflammatory cytokines.

Uremic Encephalopathy

The pathogenesis is thought to be complex with accumulation of metabolites, imbalance in excitatory and inhibitory neurotransmitters, elevated parathyroid hormone, and abnormal calcium control (Lacerda, Krummel, & Hirsch, 2010). Buildup of dialyzable uremic toxins such as urea, guanidine compounds, hippuric acid, polyamines, phenols, indolic acids, and myo-inositol are thought to play a role in the pathophysiology (Varelas & Graffagnino, 2013).

Hyperhomocysteinemia and Alzheimer's Disease

Hcy is considered a potent neurotoxin, and elevated levels are risk factors for AD (Seshadri et al., 2002). Although exact mechanism(s) are unknown, there is evidence that HHcy may promote dementia via multiple pathways, including cerebral microangiopathy, endothelial dysfunction, oxidative stress, neuronal DNA damage, excitotoxicity, and apoptosis (Sachdev, 2005). HHcy may influence pathophysiological processes of AD, such as potentiating the neurotoxicity of amyloid β-peptide, disrupting microtubules by promoting tau phosphorylation, disturbing proteins controlling cell division in the cerebral cortex, and contributing to vascular pathology of AD (Chakrabarti et al., 2015; Sachdev, 2005). The pathogenesis of HHcy in AD in particular remains unclear (Zhuo, Wang, & Praticò, 2011). The increase in Hcy with AD appears to be associated with biochemical damage resulting from oxidative stress (Köseoglu & Karaman, 2007). Other theories have suggested that HHcy damages DNA repair mechanisms, leading to apoptosis and vulnerability to further injury (Kruman et al., 2002). As such, HHcy is linked with hippocampal or cortical atrophy in healthy older adults (den Heijer et al., 2003) and white-matter changes in AD patients (Kim et al., 2009). Still others suggest factors such as inhibition of adult neurogenesis (Kruman, Mouton, Emokpae, Cutler, & Mattson, 2005), immune activation (Schroecksnadel, Leblhuber, Frick, Wirleitner, & Fuchs, 2004), and blockage of the nitric oxide signaling pathway (Selley, 2004).

Metabolic Risk Factors of Sporadic Alzheimer's Disease

Histopathological study of the AD brain reveals two characteristic findings: (a) extracellular neuritic plaques (NPs) and (b) cytoplasmic neurofibrillary tangles (NFTs) (Chakrabarti et al., 2015). The central cores of NPs contain amyloid beta (Aβ) peptide in oligomerized states, surrounded by detritus composed of degenerating neurons, microglia, and macrophages (Bird & Miller, 2008). By contrast, NFTs are composed of twisted neurofilaments of abnormally phosphorylated tau (τ) protein (Chakrabarti et al., 2015). Concomitant findings include neuronal loss, synaptic degeneration, dendrites, and axons, as well as destruction of cholinergic neurons and the neurotransmitter (NT) acetylcholine (Bird & Miller, 2008; Chakrabarti et al., 2015).

Organophosphates and Pesticides

Given the prevalence of organophosphates and pesticides and the fact that the chronic neurotoxic effects of these substances are not yet clearly established, issues related to neurotoxicity have seen increasing scrutiny in recent years (McElgunn, 2010). Existing evidence suggests that acute, high-level exposure results in complex systemic dysfunction, brought about by biochemical mechanisms directly affecting the nervous system (National Research Council, 1993). More specifically, confusion, agitation, coma, and respiratory failure are triggered by overstimulation of nicotinic and muscarinic acetylcholine receptors in the CNS (Eddleston, Buckley, Eyer, & Dawson, 2008). Data also indicate that lower-level chronic exposure may lead to subtle, but measurable, long-term neurological dysfunction (National Research Council, 1993).

Wernicke's Encephalopathy

Thiamine is a water-soluble B vitamin, the active form of which is thiamine pyrophosphate that is integral to three major enzymes required for glucose metabolism (Spector, 1982). It is commonly derived from food sources, notably flour-based products (e.g., bread) that have been enriched with B_1 and other vitamins and minerals since WWII in the United States (Isenberg-Grzeda, Kutner, & Nicolson, 2012). Thiamine is found throughout the body, with higher concentrations in skeletal muscle, liver, heart, and brain (Spector & Johanson, 2007).

Toxic Metabolic Encephalopathy

Underlying mechanisms may include disturbances in neurotransmission along with disruption of energy metabolism, cellular depolarization, secretion of cytokines, and changes in blood flow (Campbell et al., 2009; Surtees & Leonard, 1989).

Lead Poisoning

There is no known safe level of lead (Flora et al., 2012) and it impacts almost all major organ systems including blood (binding to red blood cells), renal, cardiovascular, and peripheral and central nervous systems. Lead in the blood is excreted in urine and bile at a rate of 1 to 3 mL/min and has a half-life of 30 days (Mason, Harp, & Han, 2014). Residual lead binds to red blood cells and is stored in bone with a half-life of 20 to 30 years. Lead is known to interfere with developmental aspects of CNS (neuronal migration, neuronal and glial differentiation, and synapse formation) (Mason et al., 2014).

ETIOLOGY

Chronic Hepatic Encephalopathy

Intestinal flora and protein metabolism by deamination of amino acids produce ammonia. Gut-derived ammonia is absorbed into the hepatic portal system, the major source of blood flow from the gut to the liver. A normal liver would rapidly convert ammonia to urea for excretion by the kidneys. However, a cirrhotic (diseased) liver synthesizes ammonia into urea more slowly, or not at all, allowing ammonia to accumulate in the blood.

Uremic Encephalopathy

UE severity tends to be higher with acute renal failure, but can be experienced with chronic renal failure as well (Varelas & Graffagnino, 2013).

Hyperhomocysteinemia and Alzheimer's Disease

While the direct cause of AD remains unknown, various theories have been explored. A majority of cases are sporadic, with environmental and genetic factors contributing in varying degrees (Zhuo et al., 2011). Determining whether HHcy is an independent causal risk factor, or is secondary to neurodegeneration, remains a significant issue (Farkas et al., 2013). Increased levels of homocysteine are often the result of disturbed methionine metabolism. The amino acid methionine is converted to Hcy, which is then normally

(a) converted back to methionine or (b) converted to the amino acid cystathionine (Petras et al., 2014). However, genetically inherited enzyme mutations, end-stage renal disease, hypothyroidism, and dietary vitamin deficiencies can negatively influence the metabolism of methionine, causing hyperhomocysteinemia. Adequate stores of folic acid, vitamin B_{12}, and vitamin B_6 are critical for normal Hcy metabolism (Maron & Loscalzo, 2009).

Metabolic Risk Factors of Sporadic Alzheimer's Disease

- *Hyperinsulinemia*: In a hyperinsulinemic brain, insulin competes with Aβ for enzymatic degradation, resulting in a state of Aβ accrual. However, evidence suggests that hyperinsulinemia of type 2 diabetes is associated with lower brain and CSF insulin levels (Chakrabarti et al., 2015). Type 2 diabetes would thus involve both insulin deficiency and insulin resistance (Chakrabarti et al., 2015).
- *Insulin resistance*: Although the mechanism is unclear, insulin resistance may directly contribute to the development of AD pathology by potentiating Aβ accumulation and tau phosphorylation (Chakrabarti et al., 2015; Kim & Feldman, 2015). Defective insulin signaling and glucose metabolism may be characteristic of the AD brain (Kim & Feldman, 2015).
- *Hypercholesterolemia*: Cellular cholesterol levels may play a role in both the generation of Aβ and the amyloid cascade (Frisardi et al., 2010). That is, cholesterol-influenced increases in Aβ oligomer levels result in reduced intracellular cholesterol, in turn inducing hyperphosphorylation of tau (Michikawa, 2003). This cascade might ultimately lead to NFTs, decreased synaptic plasticity, and neurodegeneration (Frisardi et al., 2010).
- *Inadequate vitamin D levels*: Vitamin D_3 insufficiency has been associated with CSF Aβ levels, cognitive decline, and increased risk of AD. Patients with AD show decreased phagocytosis of soluble Aβ by macrophages, thereby delaying clearance of Aβ from the brain. Vitamin D_3 alone or combined with curcuminoids may activate macrophages to phagocytize Aβ, increasing its clearance in AD patients (Chakrabarti et al., 2015; Masoumi et al., 2009).

- *Increased proinflammatory cytokines*: AD patients' brains evidence inflammation activated by microglial release of proinflammatory cytokines. Moreover, increased proinflammatory cytokine levels might promote the phosphorylation of tau or production of Aβ, which contribute to the AD neurodegeneration process (Chakrabarti et al., 2015).

Organophosphates and Pesticides

Pesticide chemicals are used across the country, with the greatest usage in the midwestern states (United States Department of the Interior, 2007). A pertinent clinical issue is that in rural, developing countries, organophosphate self-poisoning claims approximately 200,000 lives each year. Unintentional poisoning has a lesser case fatality of about 15%, but continues to be problematic due to difficulties in medical management (Eddleston et al., 2008).

Wernicke's Encephalopathy

Neuropsychiatric symptoms appear when levels of thiamine are reduced below 20% of normal limits (Spector & Johanson, 2007).

- WE is reported to average 1.3% of consecutive autopsy studies (Galvin et al., 2010).
- Among alcoholics, WE is estimated to occur in 9.3% of consecutive autopsy studies (Galvin et al., 2010).
- In nonalcoholic patients, the most prevalent contributing factor to the development of WE is digestive abnormalities of various etiologies (e.g., due to treatment of cancer, gastrointestinal surgery, hyperemesis gravidarum, starvation/fasting, gastrointestinal tract disease, AIDS, and malnutrition) (Galvin et al., 2010).
- Incidence is higher in developing countries due to higher prevalence of poor nutrition (Neki, 2015).

Toxic Metabolic Encephalopathy

Metabolic encephalopathies are chemical disorders that adversely impact consciousness, cognition and alertness; they are primarily attributable to systemic septic, toxic, or metabolic derangements, but not structural lesions (Krishnan, Leung, & Caplan, 2014; McCandless, 2009; Young & DeRubeis, 1998).

Lead Poisoning

The etiology of lead poisoning is artificial. Lead ingestion can occur through inhalation of dust and particulate matter (e.g., leaded gasoline, phased out in the United States after 1986), orally (lead in plumbing of older homes), in the canning process (eliminated in the United States in 1995), as leaded glazes (in older pottery pieces, etc.), or through the skin (e.g., lead dust in older homes with lead paint, leaded gas). For children, environmental factors are predominant, whereas for adults, the workplace is the more likely source of exposure (Mason et al., 2014). Developing fetuses are at risk beyond external environmental exposure, as lead stored over the lifetime in the maternal bone can cross the placenta, affecting the fetus (Rothenberg et al., 1994). The impact of lead poisoning is greater on children than on adults (Bhullar et al., 2015) due to the impact of developmental processes.

EPIDEMIOLOGY

Chronic Hepatic Encephalopathy

CHE is diagnosable in 60% to 80% of individuals with cirrhosis (Bajaj & Mullen, 2010). CHE is considered a preclinical stage of Overt Hepatic Encephalopathy (Bajaj & Mullen, 2010).

Uremic Encephalopathy

As UE may present in any patient with renal disease, prevalence is difficult to establish. The extent of the problem is evidenced from the perspective that an estimated 1.3 patients per 10,000 develop end-stage renal disease (ESRD). The overall incidence of ESRD is experiencing the fastest growth in patients over 65 and is four times greater in African Americans than in Whites, although men and women are equally affected (Bucurescu, 2014).

Hyperhomocysteinemia and Alzheimer's Disease

- A number of studies have demonstrated HHcy in Alzheimer's patients (Sachdev, 2005).
- Various studies have reported a positive correlation between Hcy levels and AD symptom severity, as well as rate of disease progression (McCaddon, 2006).

- In a study of individuals without AD ($n = 1,092$) followed for 8 or more years, a 5 µmol/L increase in Hcy from baseline levels elevated the risk of developing AD by 40% (Seshadri et al., 2002).

The importance of the link between HHcy and AD is based on the fact that AD is the leading cause of neurodegenerative disease, with over 26 million people affected worldwide (Cummings, 2004) and the prevalence of AD expected to exceed 100 million by 2050 (Brookmeyer, Johnson, Ziegler-Graham, & Arrighi, 2007). HHcy is observed in 5% to 12% of the general population. Individuals with alcoholism, chronic kidney disease, and inadequate vitamin intake have a higher incidence (Davis, 2014). Despite associations between HHcy and cognitive disorders, the clinical benefit of Hcy reduction has yet to translate into palpable gains (Maron, & Loscalzo, 2009), with some theorizing that there may be methodological problems in the research and/or application (Andrieu et al., 2009).

Metabolic Risk Factors of Sporadic Alzheimer's Disease

- An estimated 5.2 million older Americans have AD, the majority of whom are women.
- AD is the sixth leading cause of all deaths in the United States.
- Older African Americans are twice as likely to develop AD as older European Americans.

Organophosphates and Pesticides

Statistics show that as many as 25 million U.S. workers are at risk for severe intoxication by pesticide (Miller, 2004) and that merely residing in or near a place where pesticides are used appears to have health effects (Eckerman et al., 2007).

Wernicke's Encephalopathy

- WE is found in 1.3% of consecutive autopsy studies (Galvin et al., 2010).
- Alcoholics: WE occurs in approximately 9.3% of consecutive autopsy (Galvin et al., 2010).

- In nonalcoholic patients, the most prevalent contributing factor to the development of WE is digestive abnormalities of various etiologies (e.g., due to treatment of cancer, gastrointestinal surgery, hyperemesis gravidarum, starvation/fasting, gastrointestinal tract disease, AIDS, and malnutrition) (Galvin et al., 2010).
- Incidence is higher in developing countries due to poor nutrition (Neki, 2015).

Toxic Metabolic Encephalopathy

The incidence of delirium has been estimated to be between 5% and 40% for hospitalized patients in general, and between 11% and 80% for critically ill patients (Varelas & Graffagnino, 2013).

Lead Poisoning

- National Health and Nutrition Examination Survey estimated blood lead levels of greater than 10 μg/dL among U.S. children (1988–1991) and prevalence at 8.6% but dropping to 1.4% during 1999–2004 (Mason et al., 2014). Lead poisoning is still considered a common health threat in developing countries (Bhullar et al., 2015).
- A 2015 review of the literature by White, Bonilha, and Ellis (2015) found the incidence of blood lead levels to be highest among African American, followed by Mexican American, and lowest in White children under the age of 6 years.
- In adults, higher lead levels are associated with individuals working in industrial settings (e.g., battery plants), in contrast to children who are exposed to lead in the immediate home environment (e.g., lead paint and in the soil) (Mason et al., 2014).

CLINICAL PRESENTATION

Chronic Hepatic Encephalopathy

Patients with cirrhosis and a clinical neurological exam negative for obvious abnormalities should undergo neuropsychological testing for M-CHE (Bajaj & Mullen, 2010). A typical M-CHE symptom profile includes impairments in attention, executive functions, processing speed, visuo-motor coordination, and visuospatial construction speed (Hilsabeck & Webb, 2013).

Uremic Encephalopathy

Symptom presentation is insidious, with family and caregivers typically noticing changes before patients. Subtle decline in mentation along with emotional changes can progress into delirium, seizures, and coma. Symptoms may include loss of memory, impaired concentration, lethargy, fatigue, insomnia, irritability, depressed mood, delusions, psychosis, slurred speech, muscle twitches, and restless legs (Bucurescu, 2014). Additionally, action tremors, asterixis, hyperreflexia, myoclonus, anorexia, and, in long-term cases, peripheral neuropathy may be part of the clinical progression (Varelas & Graffagnino, 2013).

Hyperhomocysteinemia and Alzheimer's Disease

Elevated plasma homocysteine levels do not cause acute, overt symptoms. Rather, increased homocysteine levels are expressed as a variety of progressive vascular and neurological disorders, including AD (Maron & Loscalzo, 2009).

Metabolic Risk Factors of Sporadic Alzheimer's Disease

Sporadic AD often begins insidiously with relatively subtle symptoms: recent memory loss and word-finding difficulties. With disease progression, symptoms may include memory deficits, apraxia, and impairments in language and executive functions. In the final stages of AD, symptoms include severe confusion, disorientation, and wandering. Psychiatric symptoms may develop at this point, along with behavioral problems, hypophagia, and incontinence (Chakrabarti et al., 2015; Lim et al., 2014).

Organophosphates and Pesticides

Research on the neuropsychological impact of pesticide exposure has shown mixed results. It is still not clear whether some pesticides have a greater impact than do others (Schultz & Ferraro, 2013); however, cholinesterase inhibitors such as organophosphates typically lead to cognitive deficits (Roldan-Tapia et al., 2006). Both acute poisoning and chronic exposure (>10 years) have been shown to result in similar disturbances of perception and visuo-motor processing (Riccio, Avila, & Ash, 2010). Acute poisoning patients exhibit impairment in verbal and perceptual learning, recall, and constructive abilities, along with disturbed mood states (Roldan-Tapia et al., 2006). Symptoms may also include dizziness, headaches, nausea, skin and eye problems, long-term respiratory problems, cancer, diabetes, and birth defects (Arcury, Quandt, & Mellen, 2003; Daniels, Olshan, & Savitz, 1997; Garcia, 2003).

Wernicke's Encephalopathy

Although WE is characterized by a triad of symptoms, namely, confusion, ataxia, and oculomotor abnormality, the likelihood of any one patient displaying all three is low, with estimated co-occurrence among alcoholics being as low as 16% (Caine, Halliday, Kril, & Harper, 1997).

Toxic Metabolic Encephalopathy

The primary clinical feature of TME is delirium and is manifested as disordered cognitive function, impaired behavior, dysregulation of the sleep–awake cycle (Earnest & Parker, 1993), bilateral asterixis, paratonia, tremor, and multifocal myoclonus (Krishnan et al., 2014; Young & DeRubeis, 1998). Acute confusional states present as disruptions in attention, concentration, memory, intellectual function, visuospatial and perceptual function, language abilities, abstract thinking, problem-solving, and mood/emotion (Parks, Zec, & Wilson, 1993).

Lead Poisoning

Neuropsychological and behavioral impairments span multiple domains: intelligence, memory, executive functioning, attention, processing speed, language comprehension, visual spatial skill, motor skills, and affect (e.g., depression, anxiety, aggression, and antisocial behavior) and are correlated with lead levels in adults and children (Mason et al., 2014). Prenatal and early postnatal exposure appears to be associated with higher lead levels and global developmental delays (Spreen, Tupper, Risser, Tukko, & Edgell, 1984).

DIAGNOSTIC CONSIDERATIONS

Chronic Hepatic Encephalopathy

The International Society for Hepatic Encephalopathy and Nitrogen Metabolism (ISHEN) recommends the use of the Repeated Battery for Assessment of Neuropsychological Status (RBANS) or the Psychometric Hepatic Encephalopathy Score (PHES) for identifying CHE (Hilsabeck & Webb, 2013). Two of the following four tests may also be used: Parts A and B of the trail making test, the digit symbol test, and the block design test (Bajaj & Mullen, 2010; Hilsabeck & Webb, 2010).

Uremic Encephalopathy

When acute change in mental status is first observed, computed tomography (CT) and magnetic resonance imaging (MRI) scans are useful in eliminating the possibility of intracranial hemorrhage and subdural hematoma (Bucurescu, 2014). Due to acute renal failure further complicating sepsis, it may be challenging to differentiate UE from septic encephalopathy (Varelas & Graffagnino, 2013). Blood tests can confirm electrolyte and renal function abnormalities, whereas the electroencephalogram (EEG) can help monitor progress (Bucurescu, 2014).

Hyperhomocysteinemia and Alzheimer's Disease

In addition to the relationship between HHcy and AD, mildly elevated Hcy levels may also raise the risk of developing non-AD dementia including vascular dementia, Parkinson's disease–associated dementia, and multiple sclerosis–related cognitive decline (Maron & Loscalzo, 2009). Severity of HHcy is based on total plasma concentration of Hcy (Petras et al., 2014):

- Normal Hcy = 4 to 14.99 µmol/L
- Mild HHcy = 15 to 29.99 µmol/L
- Moderate HHcy = 30 to 99.99 µmol/L
- Severe HHcy ≥ 100 µmol/L

Blood tests for deficiencies in folate, B_{12}, B_6, methionine, and betaine may reveal a nutritional cause of abnormal metabolism. Clinicians should inquire about current medications that affect folate and B_{12} levels, as well as use of alcohol, coffee, and cigarettes (Miller, 2003).

Metabolic Risk Factors of Sporadic Alzheimer's Disease

Unequivocal diagnosis of AD is not possible until autopsy. In patients 65 years or older, the aforementioned symptoms, in conjunction with impairments in multiple cognitive domains (i.e., as assessed by the Mini Mental State Exam), are considered diagnostic of probable AD (Chakrabarti et al., 2015). MRI may be used to characterize diffuse brain atrophy, as well as to rule out other neurological, vascular, neoplastic, and dementing pathology.

Organophosphates and Pesticides

Major and subtle effects on the peripheral nervous system are typically assessed using nerve conduction tests, stimulus–response times, reflex arcs, vibratory sensitivity measures (sensory function), evoked brain responses, electroencephalogram (EEG), and biochemical markers of neurotransmitter and neuroendocrine levels. Cognitive-behavioral processes are assessed using psychological testing but may be confounded by nonpesticide factors. Furthermore, developmental evaluations are needed to identify age-related vulnerabilities to neurotoxins in both children and adults (National Research Council, 1993).

Wernicke's Encephalopathy

The classic triad of symptoms of WE are narrow and do not capture the full range of possible presenting symptoms. Thus confusion can include many states including, but not limited to, disorientation, apathy, incoherence, disorders of memory, anxiety, and fearfulness (Isenberg-Grzeda et al., 2012). Ocular signs can also include many abnormalities (e.g., ophthalmoplegia, nystagmus, conjugate gaze oasis, retinal hemorrhages, scotomas). Ataxia is just one of several possible cerebellar signs often seen in WE. These diagnostic considerations are likely the reason for the underdiagnosis of WE; estimates of 80% not diagnosed in life with estimates as high as 80% of missed diagnoses (Isenberg-Grzeda et al., 2012)

Toxic Metabolic Encephalopathy

TME is an underrecognized and undertreated condition, generally resulting from systemic disease (Ely, Shintani, Truman, et al., 2004; Ely, Stephens, Jackson, et al., 2004; Milbrandt et al., 2004; Teodorczuk, Reynish, & Milisen, 2012). The presentation is frequently confused with dementia (Teodorczuk, Reynish, & Milisen, 2012); suspected delirium should be verified with a mental status and neurological examination. Assessment should include brain MRI for arriving at an accurate diagnosis (Sharma, Eesa, & Scott, 2009), chest x-ray, noncontrast CT scan of the head, examination of blood sugar, blood gases, plasma ammonia, blood lactate, plasma electrolytes, plasma ketones and amino acids, liver function, cortisol levels, and urinary organic acids during the acute illness to identify possible metabolic disorders (Krishnan et al., 2014; Surtees & Leonard, 1989). Current medications should be reviewed to identify those with anticholinergic and sedative effects, which may confound the differential diagnosis (Krishnan et al., 2014).

Lead Poisoning

If lead exposure is suspected, a careful screening history including neuropsychological assessment as well as blood analysis should be undertaken.

TREATMENT

Chronic Hepatic Encephalopathy

Treatment strategies target the gut, focusing on reducing or eliminating ammonia. Lactulose reduces plasma ammonia levels by increasing fecal nitrogen excretion and inhibiting bacterial ammonia production (Hilsabeck & Webb, 2010). Rifaximin inhibits growth of ammonia-producing bacteria and is a second line of treatment (Stinton & Jayakumar, 2013).

Uremic Encephalopathy

Interventions include hemodialysis, peritoneal dialysis, renal transplant, and neurosurgical procedures for intracranial bleeding. Potential complications include dialysis equilibrium syndrome and rejection encephalopathy (Bucurescu, 2014). Use of medication to correct anemia and thiamine deficiency may improve cognitive functioning (Angel & Young, 2011; Seifter & Samuels, 2011). Medication should be administered with caution because toxicity increases with impaired renal function. A low-sodium, low-protein diet is also recommended (Bucurescu, 2014).

Hyperhomocysteinemia and Alzheimer's Disease

Patients with known cerebrovascular and neurological disease may be treated with folic acid 1 to 5 mg/d, B_{12} 0.4 to 2 mg/d, and B_6 10 mg/d, with the goal of decreasing Hcy levels below 15 µmol/L. A diet low in protein and methionine is also recommended. As there is no known cure for AD, a better understanding of modifiable risk factors is vital. Hypotheses linking B-group–vitamin deficiency and cognitive impairment were present in the literature before homocysteine theories gained popularity in the 1990s (Morris, 2003). Although HHcy is treatable with vitamins B_6, B_{12}, and folic acid (Selhub, 1999), trials have not demonstrated cognitive improvement in AD patients. Vitamin therapy shows promise in decreasing brain atrophy in individuals with mild cognitive impairment (Smith et al., 2010).

Metabolic Risk Factors of Sporadic Alzheimer's Disease

There are currently no well-established pharmacologic or lifestyle choices known to decrease the risk of developing AD or to cease its progression, and thus treatment should focus on controlling symptoms and prevention. Metabolic risk factors for sporadic AD may be especially important as they might serve as early markers of AD and be amenable to treatment.

Early treatment of metabolic anomalies may prevent or slow AD onset.

- Controlling type 2 diabetes may require insulin, metformin, or sulfonylureas.
- Metabolic syndrome hypercholesterolemia and dyslipidemia might be treated with statins, fibrates, or high-dose niacin, in addition to other lifestyle changes.
- Disordered methionine–homocysteine metabolism may be corrected with administration of vitamins B_6, B_{12}, and folic acid.

- Vitamin D insufficiency may be treated by administration of vitamin D_3.

Organophosphates and Pesticides

Decades after the beginning of organophosphate use, the effectiveness of implementing the core treatments (atropine, oximes, and diazepam) is still uncertain. Poisoned patients frequently develop agitated delirium of complex etiology. Contributing factors are not only the pesticide, but also atropine toxicity, hypoxia, and medical complications. Although prevention is the best treatment, pharmacological interventions are often initiated. Acutely agitated patients show improvement following treatment with diazepam. Animal research suggests that diazepam reduces neural damage and can further prevent respiratory failure and death; however, this remains unsubstantiated in human patients (Eddleston et al., 2008).

Wernicke's Encephalopathy

Immediate treatment with intravenously or intramuscularly administered thiamine is the recommended treatment (Neki, 2015).

Toxic Metabolic Encephalopathy

The treatment of TME is largely supportive, focusing on the management of cerebral perfusion pressure and restoration of the brain's normal metabolic environment (Earnest & Parker, 1993; Surtees & Leonard, 1989). Many TMEs can be reversed with the timely diagnosis and treatment of infectious, traumatic, or surgically related causes of the acute underlying illness (Campbell et al., 2009). However, some metabolic encephalopathies caused by sustained hypoglycemia and thiamine deficiency (e.g., WE) often result in permanent structural brain damage with significant functional impairments (e.g., memory disorders, executive dysfunction, motor involvement) (Mayes, 1988).

Lead Poisoning

Removal of lead from the home or work environment and chelation therapy has shown efficacy.

PROGNOSIS

Chronic Hepatic Encephalopathy

M-CHE is a preclinical stage of the more severe overt hepatic encephalitis. Although cognitive deficits associated with M-CHE may improve, a significant number of patients show little or no improvement (Stinton & Jayakumar, 2013).

Uremic Encephalopathy

Prognosis is more favorable with early recognition. Reversal of signs and symptoms can occur as soon as days or weeks. If left untreated, UE may lead to coma and death (Bucurescu, 2014). Appropriately tailored therapies to minimize complications of renal disease and treatment risks require close collaboration between nephrologists and neurologists (Lacerda et al., 2010).

Hyperhomocysteinemia and Alzheimer's Disease

Although an effective treatment for AD has yet to be discovered, strategies to manage risk factors (e.g., lowering of high blood pressure) can help decrease incidence and cost. A 1-year delay in onset could mean 9.2 million less cases by 2050 and billions of dollars in savings (Brookmeyer et al., 2007). While vitamin B therapy decreases Hcy levels, lower Hcy levels generally do not slow AD progression or reverse cognitive symptoms (Maron & Loscalzo, 2009). Future research should focus on early detection of AD in order to improve chances of favorable prognosis.

Metabolic Risk Factors of Sporadic Alzheimer's Disease

Given that there are currently no pharmacologic treatments known to decrease the risk of developing AD or to cease its progression, the prognosis at this point is challenging for patients, family members, and friends. However, a symptom-focused approach in combination with a supportive social network could favorably modify the day-to-day quality of life.

Organophosphates and Pesticides

Chronic pesticide exposure negatively affects cognitive ability and contributes to the likelihood of developing neurodegenerative brain conditions such as Alzheimer's and Parkinson's diseases (Schultz & Ferraro, 2013). The greater the quantity and exposure time, the greater the likelihood of these consequences (Roldan-Tapia, Parron, & Sanchez-Santed, 2005). Future studies are needed to determine specific mechanisms that are affected, as well as prevention strategies for minimizing long-term effects.

Wernicke's Encephalopathy

If left untreated, WE is likely to develop into the more permanent and debilitating Korsakoff's syndrome (Isenberg-Grzeda et al., 2012). With thiamine treatment, the prognosis is generally good (Galvin et al., 2010; Neki, 2015).

Toxic Metabolic Encephalopathy

The prognosis depends on the initial causes, severity, and the time to reverse and stabilize the patient. Prognosis varies from complete recovery to a poor outcome that often includes permanent brain damage or even death (Varelas & Graffagnino, 2013).

Lead Poisoning

Neonatal and early postnatal exposure to high levels of lead yields a poor prognosis. CNS damage may be permanent. Later acute exposure and even chronic exposure has a better prognosis with some return of function reported, although progressive cognitive deficits can be found years afterwards (Mason et al., 2014).

CLINICAL SYNOPSIS

Chronic Hepatic Encephalopathy

- *Symptoms*: Poor quality of life, high risk of traffic violations and accidents. Impairments in attention, executive functions, processing speed, visuo-motor coordination, and visuospatial construction speed.

- *Diagnostics*: Repeated Battery for Assessment of Neuropsychological (RBANS) or Psychometric Hepatic Encephalopathy Score (PHES).
- *Treatment*: Targets the gut, reducing or eliminating ammonia. Lactulose reduces plasma ammonia; Rifaximin inhibits bacteria that produce ammonia.

Uremic Encephalopathy

- *Symptoms*: Memory loss, progressing into delirium, seizures, and coma; impaired concentration; lethargy; fatigue; insomnia; irritability; depressed mood; delusions; psychosis; slurred speech; muscle twitches and restless legs; action tremors; asterixis; hyperreflexia; myoclonus; anorexia; and peripheral neuropathy.
- *Diagnostics*: Blood tests for electrolyte and renal function. Electroencephalogram (EEG) to monitor progress. CT and MRI scans for possible intracranial hemorrhage and subdural hematoma.
- *Treatment*: Hemodialysis, peritoneal dialysis, renal transplant, and neurosurgery for intracranial bleeding.

Hyperhomocysteinemia and Alzheimer's Disease

- *Symptoms*: A variety of progressive vascular and neurological disorders, including AD.
- *Diagnostics*: Determine current medications that affect folate and B_{12} levels, as well as evaluate use of alcohol, coffee, and cigarettes.
- *Treatment*: Patients with known cerebrovascular and neurological disease may be treated with folic acid 1 to 5 mg/d, B_{12} 0.4 to 2 mg/d, and B_6 10 mg/d to decrease Hcy levels below 15 μmol/L. A diet low in protein and methionine is recommended.

Metabolic Risk Factors of Sporadic Alzheimer's Disease

- *Symptoms*: Anterograde memory loss, word-finding difficulties, apraxia, and impairments in language and executive functions, and in final stages, confusion, disorientation, wandering, behavioral problems, hypophagia, and incontinence.

- *Diagnostics*: Unequivocal diagnosis on autopsy. Probable AD: based on aforementioned symptoms and impairments in multiple cognitive domains.
- *Treatment*: Should focus on controlling symptoms and prevention.

Organophosphates and Pesticides

- *Symptoms*: Cholinesterase inhibitors (organophosphates) typically lead to cognitive deficits; acute poisoning and chronic exposure associated with disturbances in perception, visuo-motor processing, verbal and perceptual learning, recall, constructive abilities, mood states, dizziness, headaches, nausea, skin and eye problems, respiratory problems, cancer, diabetes, and birth defects.
- *Diagnostics*: Nerve conduction tests, stimulus–response times, reflex arcs, vibratory sensitivity measures (sensory function), evoked brain responses, electroencephalogram (EEG), and biochemical markers of neurotransmitter and neuroendocrine levels. Cognitive-behavioral processes are assessed via psychological testing.
- *Treatment*: Management is based on prevention. Acutely agitated patients show improvement following treatment with diazepam.

Wernicke's Encephalopathy

- *Symptoms*: Triad of symptoms = confusion, ataxia, and oculomotor abnormality. Confusion includes disorientation, apathy, incoherence, disorders of memory, anxiety, and fearfulness. Ocular signs can include ophthalmoplegia, nystagmus, conjugate gaze oasis, retinal hemorrhage, and scotomas. Ataxia is just one of several possible cerebellar signs.
- *Diagnostics*: Clinicians should consider the full range of possible presenting symptoms in this underdiagnosed disorder.
- *Treatment*: Immediate intravenous or intramuscular thiamine administration.

Toxic Metabolic Encephalopathy

- *Symptoms*: Delirium, disordered cognitive function, impaired behavior, dysregulation of the sleep–awake cycle, bilateral asterixis, paratonia, tremor, and multifocal myoclonus. Acute confusional: Disruptions in attention/concentration, memory, intellectual function, visuospatial and perceptual function, language abilities, abstract thinking, problem-solving, and mood/emotion.

- *Diagnostics*: Suspected delirium: Verify with a mental status and neurological examination, chest x-ray, MRI, and non-contrast CT of the brain. Assessment of blood sugar, gases and lactate, plasma ammonia, plasma electrolytes, plasma ketones, plasma amino acids, liver function, cortisol levels, and urinary organic acids during the acute illness to identify patients at risk for metabolic disorder.

- *Treatment*: Largely supportive, focusing on the management of cerebral perfusion pressure and restoration of the brain's normal metabolic environment.

Lead Poisoning

- *Symptoms*: Neuropsychological and behavioral impairments can affect intelligence, memory, executive functioning, attention, processing speed, language comprehension, visual spatial skill, motor skills, and affect.

- *Diagnostics*: If lead exposure is suspected, a careful screening history, neuropsychological assessment as well as blood analysis should be undertaken.

- *Treatment*: Removal of lead from the home or work environment is needed. Chelation therapy is the standard treatment.

ACKNOWLEDGMENT

The authors wish to acknowledge the editorial support of Christina Angelo.

REFERENCES

Andrieu, S., Coley, N., Aisen, P., Carrillo, M. C., DeKosky, S., Durga, J., . . . Vellas, B. (2009). Methodological issues in primary prevention trials for neurodegenerative dementia. *Journal of Alzheimer's Disease, 16*(2), 235–270. doi:10.3233/JAD-2009-0971

Angel, M. J., & Young, G. B. (2011). Metabolic encephalopathies. *Neurologic Clinics, 29*(4), 837–882. doi:10.1016/j.ncl.2011.08.002

Arcury, T. A., Quandt, S. A., & Mellen, B. G. (2003). An exploratory analysis of occupational skin disease among Latino migrant and seasonal farmworkers in North Carolina. *Journal of Agricultural Safety and Health, 9*(3), 221–232.

Bajaj, J., & Mullen, K. (2010). Hepatic encephalopathy. In C. Armstrong & L. Morrow (Eds.), *Handbook of medical neuropsychology* (pp. 469–477). New York, NY: Springer.

Bhullar, D. S., Thind, A. S., & Singla, A. (2015). Childhood lead poisoning: A review. *Journal of Punjab Academy of Forensic Medicine and Toxicology, 15*(1), 43–49.

Bird, T. D., & Miller, B. L. (2008). Alzheimer's disease and primary dementias. In A. S. Fauci, E. Braunwald, D. L. Kasper, S. L. Hauser, D. L. Longo, J. L. Jameson, & J. Loscalzo (Eds.), *Harrison's principles of internal medicine* (17th ed., pp. 2393–2406). New York, NY: McGraw-Hill.

Brookmeyer, R., Johnson, E., Ziegler-Graham, K., & Arrighi, H. M. (2007). Forecasting the global burden of Alzheimer's disease. *Alzheimer's and Dementia, 3*(3), 186–191. doi:10.1016/j.jalz.2007.04.381

Bucurescu, G. (2014, February 13). *Neurological manifestations of uremic encephalopathy.* Retrieved from http://emedicine.medscape.com/article/1135651-overview

Caine, D., Halliday, G. M., Kril, J. J., & Harper, C. G. (1997). Operational criteria for the classification of chronic alcoholics: Identification of Wernicke's encephalopathy. *Journal of Neurology, Neurosurgery and Psychiatry, 62*(1), 51–60.

Campbell, N., Boustani, M. A., Ayub, A., Fox, G. C., Munger, S. L., Ott, C., . . . Singh, R. (2009). Pharmacological management of delirium in hospitalized adults: A systematic evidence review. *Journal of General Internal Medicine, 24*(7), 848–853. doi:10.1007/s11606-009-0996-7

Chakrabarti, S., Khemka, V. K., Banerjee, A., Chatterjee, G., Ganguly, A., & Biswas, A. (2015). Metabolic risk factors of sporadic Alzheimer's disease: Implications in the pathology, pathogenesis and treatment. *Aging and Disease, 6*(4), 282–299. doi:10.14336/AD.2014.002

Chen, R., & Young, G. B. (1996). Metabolic encephalopathies. *Bailliere's Clinical Neurology, 5*(3), 577–598.

Cummings, J. L. (2004). Alzheimer's disease. *The New England Journal of Medicine, 351*(1), 56–67. doi:10.1056/NEJMra040223

Daniels, J. L., Olshan, A. F., & Savitz, D. A. (1997). Pesticide and childhood cancers. *Environmental Health Perspectives, 105*(10), 1068–1077.

Davidson, E., & Summerskill, W. (1956). Psychiatric aspects of liver disease. *Postgraduate Medical Journal, 32*, 487–494. doi:10.1136/pgmj.32.372.487

Davis, C. P. (2014). *Homocysteine (elevated homocysteine, homocystinuria, hyperhomocysteinemia)*. Retrieved from www.medicinenet.com/homocysteine/article.htm

den Heijer, T., Vermeer, S. E., Clarke, R., Oudkerk, M., Koudstaal, P. J., Hofman, A., & Breteler, M. M. (2003). Homocysteine and brain atrophy on MRI of non-demented elderly. *Brain, 126*(Pt. 1), 170–175.

Earnest, M. P., & Parker, W. D. (1993). Metabolic encephalopathies and coma from medical causes. In J. Grotta (Ed.), *Management of the acutely ill neurological patient* (p. 1). New York, NY: Churchill Livingstone.

Eckerman, D. A., Gimenes, L. S., de Souza, R. C., Galvao, P. R., Sarcinelli, P. N., & Chrisman, J. R. (2007). Age related effects of pesticide exposure on neurobehavioral performance of adolescent farm workers in Brazil. *Neurotoxicology and Teratology, 29*(1), 164–175. doi:10.1016/j.ntt.2006.09.028

Eddleston, M., Buckley, N. A., Eyer, P., & Dawson, A. H. (2008). Management of acute organophosphorus pesticide poisoning. *Lancet, 371*(9612), 597–607. doi:10.1016/S0140-6736(07)61202-1

Ely, E. W., Shintani, A., Truman, B., Speroff, T., Gordon, S. M., Harrell, F. E., . . . Dittus, R. S. (2004). Delirium as a predictor of mortality in mechanically ventilated patients in the intensive care unit. *JAMA, 291*, 1753–1762.

Ely, E. W., Stephens, R. K., Jackson, J. C., Thomason, J. W., Truman, B., Gordon, S., . . . Bernard, G. (2004). Current opinions regarding the importance, diagnosis, and management of delirium in the intensive care unit: A survey of 912 healthcare professionals. *Critical Care Medicine, 32*(1), 106–112.

Fan, K. W. (2004). Jiao Qi disease in medieval China. *The American Journal of Chinese Medicine, 32*(6), 999–1011. doi:10.1142/S0192415X04002594

Farkas, M., Keskitalo, S., Smith, D. E., Bain, N., Semmler, A., Ineichen, B., . . . Linnebank, M. (2013). Hyperhomocysteinemia in Alzheimer's disease: The hen and the egg? *Journal of Alzheimer's Disease, 33*(4), 1097–1104. doi:10.3233/JAD-2012-121378

Flora, G., Gupta, D., & Tiwari, A. (2012). Toxicity of lead: A review with recent updates. *Interdisciplinary Toxicology, 5*(2), 47–58. doi:10.2478/v10102-012-0009-2

Frisardi, V., Solfrizzi, V., Seripa, D., Capurso, C., Santamato, A., Sancarlo, D., ... Panza, F. (2010). Metabolic-cognitive syndrome: A cross-talk between metabolic syndrome and Alzheimer's disease. *Ageing Research Reviews, 9*, 399–417.

Galvin, R., Brathen, G., Ivashynka, A., Hillbom, M., Tanasescu, R., Leone, M. A., & EFNS. (2010). EFNS guidelines for diagnosis, therapy and prevention of Wernicke encephalopathy. *European Journal of Neurology, 17*(12), 1408–1418. doi:10.1111/j.1468-1331.2010.03153.x

Garcia, A. M. (2003). Pesticide exposure and women's health. *American Journal of Industrial Medicine, 44*(6), 584–594. doi:10.1002/ajim.10256

Hernberg, S. (2000). Lead poisoning in a historical perspective. *American Journal of Industrial Medicine, 38*(3), 244–254.

Hilsabeck, R. & Webb, A. (2013). Hepatic encephalopathy. In L. Ravdin & H. Katzen (Eds.), *Handbook on the neuropsychology of aging and dementia*. New York, NY: Springer.

Hippius, H., & Neundörfer, G. (2003). The discovery of Alzheimer's disease. *Dialogues in Clinical Neuroscience, 5*(1), 101–108.

Isenberg-Grzeda, E., Kutner, H. E., & Nicolson, S. E. (2012). Wernicke-Korsakoff-syndrome: Under-recognized and under-treated. *Psychosomatics, 53*(6), 507–516. doi:10.1016/j.psym.2012.04.008

Kim, B., & Feldman, E. (2015). Insulin resistance as a key link for the increased risk of cognitive impairment in the metabolic syndrome. *Experimental & Molecular Medicine, 47*, 1–10.

Kim, S. R., Choi, S. H., Ha, C. K., Park, S. G., Pyun, H. W., & Yoon, D. H. (2009). Plasma total homocysteine levels are not associated with medial temporal lobe atrophy, but with white matter changes in Alzheimer's disease. *Journal of Clinical Neurology (Seoul, Korea), 5*, 85–90.

Köseoglu, E., & Karaman, Y. (2007). Relations between homocysteine, folate and vitamin B12 in vascular dementia and in Alzheimer disease. *Clinical Biochemistry, 40*(12), 859–863. doi:10.1016/j.clinbiochem.2007.04.007

Krishnan, V., Leung, L. Y., & Caplan, L. R. (2014). A neurologist's approach to delirium: Diagnosis and management of toxic metabolic encephalopathies. *European Journal of Internal Medicine, 25*(2), 112–116. doi:10.1016/j.ejim.2013.11.010

Kruman, I. I., Kumaravel, T. S., Lohani, A., Pedersen, W. A., Cutler, R. G., Kruman, Y., ... Mattson, M. P. (2002). Folic acid deficiency and homocysteine impair DNA repair in hippocampal neurons and sensitize them to amyloid toxicity in experimental models of Alzheimer's disease. *Journal of Neuroscience, 22*(5), 1752–1762.

Kruman, I. I., Mouton, P. R., Emokpae, R., Jr., Cutler, R. G., & Mattson, M. P. (2005). Folate deficiency inhibits proliferation of adult hippocampal progenitors. *Neuroreport, 16*(10), 1055–1059.

Lacerda, G., Krummel, T., & Hirsch, E. (2010). Neurologic presentations of renal diseases. *Neurologic Clinics, 28*(1), 45–59. doi:10.1016/j.ncl.2009.09.003

Lim, W., Martins, I., & Martins, R. (2014). The involvement of lipids in Alzheimer's disease. *Journal of Genetics and Genomics, 41,* 261–274.

Liu, Y., Yu, J., Wang, H., Han, P., Tan, C., & Wang, C., . . . Tan, L. (2014). APOE genotype and neuroimaging markers of Alzheimer's disease: Systematic review and meta-analysis. *Journal of Neurology, Neurosurgery, and Psychiatry, 86*(2), 127–134.

Maron, B. A., & Loscalzo, J. (2009). The treatment of hyperhomocysteinemia. *Annual Review of Medicine, 60,* 39–54. doi:10.1146/annurev.med.60.041807.123308

Mason, L. H., Harp, J. P., & Han, D. Y. (2014). Pb neurotoxicity: Neuropsychological effects of lead toxicity. *BioMed Research International, 2014,* 1–8. (Article ID 840547). doi:10.1155/2014/840547

Masoumi, A., Goldenson, B., Ghirmai, S., Avagyan, H., Zaghi, J., Abel, K., . . . Fiala, M. (2009). 1 alpha, 25-dihydroxy vitamin D3 interacts with curcuminoids to stimulate amyloid-beta clearance by macrophages of Alzheimer's disease patients. *Journal of Alzheimer's Disease, 17,* 703–717.

Mayes, A. R. (1988). *Human organic memory disorders.* Cambridge, United Kingdom: Cambridge University Press.

McCaddon, A. (2006). Homocysteine and cognition: A historical perspective. *Journal of Alzheimer's Disease, 9*(4), 361–380.

McCandless, D. W. (2009). *Metabolic encephalopathy.* New York, NY: Springer.

McElgunn, B. (2010). The developing brain: A largely overlooked health endpoint in risk assessments for synthetic chemical substances. *International Journal of Disability, Development and Education, 57*(3), 315–330. doi:0.1080/1034912X.2010.501234

Michikawa, M. (2003). Cholesterol paradox: Is high total or low HDL cholesterol level a risk factor for Alzheimer's disease? *Journal of Neuroscience Research, 72,* 141–146.

Milbrandt, E. B., Deppen, S., Harrison, P. L., Shintani, A. K., Speroff, T., Stiles, R. A., . . . Ely, E. W. (2004). Costs associated with delirium in mechanically ventilated patients. *Critical Care Medicine, 32*(4), 955–962.

Miller, A. L. (2003). The methionine-homocysteine cycle and its effects on cognitive diseases. *Alternative Medicine Review, 8*(1), 7–19.

Miller, G. T. (2004). *Sustaining the earth* (6th ed.). Pacific Grove, CA: Thompson Learning.

Morris, M. S. (2003). Homocysteine and Alzheimer's disease. *Lancet Neurology, 2*(7), 425–428.

National Research Council. (1993). *Pesticides in the diets of infants and children*. Washington, DC: National Academies Press.

Neki, N. S. (2015). Wernicke's encephalopathy. *Journal of Pioneering Medical Science, 5*(3), 107–112.

Parks, R. W., Zec, R. F., & Wilson, R. S. (1993). *Neuropsychology of Alzheimer's disease and other dementias*. New York, NY: Oxford University Press.

Petras, M., Tatarkova, Z., Kovalska, M., Mokra, D., Dobrota, D., Lehotsky, J., & Drgova, A. (2014). Hyperhomocysteinemia as a risk factor for the neuronal system disorders. *Journal of Physiology and Pharmacology, 65*(1), 15–23.

Riccio, C. A., Avila, L., & Ash, M. J. (2010). Pesticide poisoning in a preschool child: A case study examining neurocognitive and neurobehavioral effects. *Applied Neuropsychology, 17*(2), 153–159. doi:10.1080/09084281003715618.

Roldan-Tapia, L., Nieto-Escamez, F. A., del Aguila, E. M., Laynez, F., Parron, T., & Sanchez-Santed, F. (2006). Neuropsychological sequelae from acute poisoning and long-term exposure to carbamate and organophosphate pesticides. *Neurotoxicology and Teratology, 28*(6), 694–703. doi:10.1016/j.ntt.2006.07.004

Roldan-Tapia, L., Parron, T., & Sanchez-Santed, F. (2005). Neuropsychological effects of long-term exposure to organophosphate pesticides. *Neurotoxicology and Teratology, 27*(2), 259–266. doi:10.1016/j.ntt.2004.12.002

Rothenberg, S. J., Karchmer, S., Schnaas, L., Perroni, E., Zea, F., & Fernandez Alba, J. (1994). Changes in serial blood lead levels during pregnancy. *Environmental Health Perspectives, 102*(10), 876–880.

Sachdev, P. S. (2005). Homocysteine and brain atrophy. *Progress in Neuro-Psychopharmacology and Biological Psychiatry, 29*(7), 1152–1161. doi:10.1016/j.pnpbp.2005.06.026

Schroecksnadel, K., Leblhuber, F., Frick, B., Wirleitner, B., & Fuchs, D. (2004). Association of hyperhomocysteinemia in Alzheimer's disease with elevated neopterin levels. *Alzheimer Disease and Associated Disorders, 18*(3), 129–133.

Schultz, C. G., & Ferraro, F. R. (2013). The impact of chronic pesticide exposure on neuropsychological functioning. *The Psychological Record, 63*(1), 175–184. doi:10.11133/j.tpr.2013.63.1.013

Seifter, J. L., & Samuels, M. A. (2011). Uremic encephalopathy and other brain disorders associated with renal failure. *Seminars in Neurology, 31*(2), 139–143. doi:10.1055/s-0031-1277984

Selhub, J. (1999). Homocysteine metabolism. *Annual Review of Nutrition, 19*, 217–246. doi:10.1146/annurev.nutr.19.1.217

Selley, M. L. (2004). Homocysteine increases the production of asymmetric dimethylarginine in cultured neurons. *Journal of Neuroscience Research, 77*(1), 90–93. doi:10.1002/jnr.20070

Seshadri, S., Beiser, A., Selhub, J., Jacques, P., Rosenberg, I., D'Agostino, R., . . . Wolf, P. (2002). Plasma homocysteine as a risk factor for dementia and Alzheimer's disease. *The New England Journal of Medicine, 346*(7), 476–483.

Sharma, P., Eesa, M., & Scott, J. N. (2009). Toxic and acquired metabolic encephalopathies: MRI appearance. *AJR: American Journal of Roentgenology, 193*(3), 879–886. doi:10.2214/AJR.08.2257

Smith, A. D., Smith, S. M., de Jager, C. A., Whitbread, P., Johnston, C., Agacinski, G., . . . Refsum, H. (2010). Homocysteine-lowering by B vitamins slows the rate of accelerated brain atrophy in mild cognitive impairment: A randomized controlled trial. *PLOS ONE, 5*(9), e12244. doi:10.1371/journal.pone.0012244

Spector, R. (1982). Thiamine homeostasis in the central nervous system. *Annals of the New York Academy of Science, 378*, 344–354.

Spector, R., & Johanson, C. E. (2007). Vitamin transport and homeostasis in mammalian brain: Focus on vitamins B and E. *Journal of Neurochemistry, 103*(2), 425–438. doi:10.1111/j.1471-4159.2007.04773.x

Spreen, O., Tupper, D., Risser, A., Tukko, H., & Edgell, D. (1984). *Human developmental neuropsychology.* New York, NY: Oxford University Press.

Surtees, R., & Leonard, J. V. (1989). Acute metabolic encephalopathy: A review of causes, mechanisms and treatment. *Journal of Inherited Metabolic Disease, 12*(Suppl. 1), 42–54.

Stinton, L., & Jayakumar, S. (2013). Minimal hepatic encephalopathy. *Canadian Journal of Gastroenterology, 27*(10), 572–574.

Teodorczuk, A., Reynish, E., & Milisen, K. (2012). Improving recognition of delirium in clinical practice: A call for action. *BMC Geriatrics, 12*, 55. doi:10.1186/1471-2318-12-55

United States Department of the Interior. (2007). *Pesticide use: Pesticide National Synthesis Project*. Retrieved from https://water.usgs.gov/nawqa/pnsp/usage/maps

United States Environmental Protection Agency. (2007). *What are pesticides?* Retrieved from www.epa.gov/pesticides/about/index.htm

Van Dam, F., & Van Gool, W. A. (2009). Hyperhomocysteinemia and Alzheimer's disease: A systematic review. *Archives of Gerontology and Geriatrics, 48*(3), 425–430. doi:10.1016/j.archger.2008.03.009

Varelas, P. N., & Graffagnino, C. (2013). Metabolic encephalopathies and delirium. *Neurocritical Care Society Practice Update Manual*, 521–535.

White, B. M., Bonilha, H. S., & Ellis, C., Jr. (2016). Racial/ethnic differences in childhood blood lead levels among children <72 months of age in the United States: A systematic review of the literature. *Journal of Racial and Ethnic Health Disparities, 3*(1), 145–153. doi:10.1007/s40615-015-0124-9

Young, G. B., & DeRubeis, D. A. (1998). Metabolic encephalopathies. In G. B. Young, A. H. Ropper, & C. F. Bolton (Eds.), *Coma and impaired consciousness* (p. 307). New York, NY: McGraw-Hill.

Zhuo, J. M., Wang, H., & Praticò, D. (2011). Is hyperhomocysteinemia an Alzheimer's disease (AD) risk factor, an AD marker, or neither? *Trends in Pharmacological Sciences, 32*(9), 562–571. doi:10.1013/j.tips.2011.05.003

CHAPTER 7

Hypoxia / Anoxia

JILL Z. STUART
THOMAS J. FARRER
ALEX L. HEINTZELMAN

OVERVIEW

Hypoxic and anoxic brain injuries can damage many different organ systems, and some organs are particularly vulnerable due to their high oxygen consumption. For example, although the brain constitutes only a mere 2% of the total body mass, it uses 20% of the body's total oxygen consumption (Hopkins & Bigler, 2008). Hypoxic brain injury refers to a reduction of oxygen to the brain tissue, and anoxia refers to total absence of oxygen. Isolated hypoxia/anoxia refers strictly to lack of oxygen, whereas ischemia refers to a restriction of blood supply to tissues, which causes not only a shortage of oxygen, but also a shortage of essential cellular metabolites (i.e., glucose) (Howard, Holmes, & Koutroumanidis, 2011). Neurons in particular are sensitive to oxygen deprivation because they are not capable of storing oxygen and glucose for later use (Hopkins & Bigler, 2008). In fact, brain cells can begin to die within 5 minutes after oxygen supply has been cut off.

Advances in medicine make it increasingly likely that a significant number of individuals will have a hypoxic or anoxic event. For example, cardiac or pulmonary crises are no longer the death sentence they used to be, but surviving these events can lead to other medical and/or psychosocial complications. A large percentage of patients who have had hypoxic or anoxic brain injuries are unable to return to their premorbid level of functioning and many will be unable to return to work. Therefore, hypoxic/anoxic brain injuries have the potential to become a significant public health concern.

This chapter will describe the pathophysiology behind anoxic and hypoxic brain injuries, common etiologies, and the epidemiology of such events. We will also discuss clinical presentations, diagnostic considerations, and treatment recommendations for neurotrauma and neurorehabilitation professionals. Finally, a clinical case of anoxic brain injury following an episode of cardiac arrest will be presented with a brief discussion highlighting the relevant medical, cognitive, and treatment needs of the patient.

HISTORY

Both research and clinical examination of hypoxic and anoxic injury have evolved with time. In fact, a PubMed search of "anoxic brain injury" indicates that the number of indexed publications has increased from 599 in 2000 to 783 in 2005, 936 in 2010, and 1,014 in 2015 (National Library of Medicine [pubmed.gov]). This increase in research related to hypoxic and anoxic injury is likely related to multiple factors, including diet, obesity, environmental pollutants, and increasing rates of chronic obstructive pulmonary disease (COPD) and asthma. Cardiovascular and pulmonary diseases continue to be common public health concerns. There are also increased incidence rates of obstructive sleep apnea (OSA), COPD, and acute respiratory distress syndrome (ARDS), all of which correlate with lifestyle factors such as alcohol consumption, sedentary living, and tobacco use (Franklin & Lindberg, 2015; Raherison & Girodet, 2009). This is especially true among older adults. Specifically, the elderly are particularly vulnerable to lifestyle risks and other injuries, which is a significant public health concern given people are more likely to live to an older age and due to the fact that the average age of the adult population is increasing. In addition, the increased rates of obesity in the United States correlate in a rise in rates of COPD and OSA (Franklin & Lindberg, 2015; Raherison & Girodet, 2009). Second, as critical care medicine has advanced, mortality rates have declined following such emergencies as cardiac arrest, stroke, and carbon monoxide poisoning (Rab et al., 2015; Wilson, Staniforth, Till, das Nair, & Vesey, 2014). With high survival rates, more individuals experience long-term deficits from oxygen deprivation to the brain.

PATHOPHYSIOLOGY

Overall, the extent of brain damage is directly linked to the length of time without oxygen (Busl & Greer, 2010). Once circulation is interrupted, cell death occurs in several ways: necrosis, apoptosis, autophagy, excitotoxicity, decreased ATP production, and calcium influx (Hopkins & Bigler, 2008; Northington, Chavez-Valdez, & Martin, 2011). In purely hypoxic brain injuries, with sustained circulation, glucose is still supplied to the brain and toxic metabolites are able to be washed away (Busl & Greer, 2010). During hypoxia or anoxia, there is a decrease of adenosine triphosphate (ATP) production, which ultimately results in a pathophysiological cascade that leads to neuronal death (Hopkins & Haaland, 2004). One of the first results is anoxic depolarization, which leads to changes in electrolyte composition both inside and outside of cells and a decrease in ATP (Busl & Greer, 2010). This change in electrolyte composition causes a decrease in cell membrane function and ultimately an approximate 25% increase in total cell calcium (Busl & Greer, 2010). This high intracellular calcium results in mitochondrial damage that causes further ATP depletion (Busl & Greer, 2010). Ultimately, the cytoskeleton is damaged and therefore cells cannot maintain their structure, which is a crucial factor in the process of cell death (Busl & Greer, 2010). This mechanism is referred to as "death by calcium" and can cause protein degradation (Biagas, 1999). In addition to the aforementioned processes, which occur from the initial oxygen deprivation, ischemic reperfusion injury can also cause neuronal damage (Hopkins & Bigler, 2008).

Although neuroanatomical damage can often be widespread (Hopkins, Kesner, & Goldstein, 1995), the hippocampus, a structure that plays a crucial role in memory and storage of semantic knowledge, is one of the most vulnerable structures and widely known structures to be damaged by hypoxic/anoxic injury. In addition, the cerebral cortex neurons, cerebellum, deep white matter, corpus callosum, fornix, mammillary bodies, and basal ganglia are particularly susceptible to the drop in cerebral blood flow and therefore are less resistant to oxygen deprivation (Garcia-Molina et al., 2006; Hopkins & Bigler, 2012). Deficits in memory due to hippocampal damage is perhaps one of the most common neuropathological outcomes of hypoxic injury; however, some researchers have suggested that changes in watershed areas and the basal ganglia are even more common (Caine & Watson, 2000). A study comparing the effects of hypoxia on the brain due to either carbon monoxide poisoning or OSA revealed hippocampal atrophy in both groups, whereas generalized brain atrophy was more prevalent in the carbon monoxide group (Gale & Hopkins, 2004). The amount of neuronal tissue loss has been suggested as an important factor in neuropsychological outcome in the absence of focal lesions (Hopkins, Tate, & Bigler, 2005).

ETIOLOGY

The most common cause of hypoxic–ischemic brain injury is cardiac arrest. Other causes of hypoxic (not necessarily ischemic) injuries include profound hypotension (associated with pulmonary embolism, surgery, shock, sepsis, metabolic encephalopathy, and drug overdose), as well as hypovolemia due to blood loss, drowning, stroke, and neonatal injuries (Howard et al., 2011). Isolated hypoxic brain injuries include any situation that results in decreased oxygen flow, such as suffocation, airway obstruction, strangulation, drowning, or poisoning. According to the National Institutes of Health (NIH), common causes of hypoxia include smoke inhalation, carbon monoxide poisoning, choking, high altitudes, compression of the trachea, and suffocation or strangulation, including as a result of attempted suicide. Other causes include asthma, OSA, and COPD (Hopkins & Bigler, 2008; Howard et al., 2011). Isolated hypoxia is more common in children as they are more likely to suffer from asphyxia, whereas adults are more likely to have cardiac arrest and suffer from ischemia (Biagas, 1999). Children who survive asphyxia at birth often develop problems such as cerebral palsy, mental retardation, and learning difficulties (Bryce, Boschi-Pinto, Shibuya, Black, & WHO Child Health Epidemiology Reference Group, 2005).

EPIDEMIOLOGY

Cardiac death is the leading cause of mortality in the United States (Chiota, Freeman, & Barrett, 2011), with only a 10% survival rate if occurring outside the hospital setting (Hinduja, Gupta, Yang, & Onteddu, 2014). The survival rate of an in-hospital cardiac arrest is between 2.4% and 18.1% (Hinduja et al., 2014). An autopsy study of patients with cardiopulmonary arrest revealed 21% with hypoxic brain damage (Hinduja et al., 2014). One study of anoxic brain injury revealed interesting age/sex differences, with incidents of anoxic injury in men peaking around age 60 related to cardiac causes, whereas for women there was a peak in the 20- to 30-year-old age group related to a higher prevalence of suicide or parasuicide (Fitzgerald, Aditya, Prior, McNeill, & Pentland, 2010). According to Franklin and Lindberg (2015), the prevalence of OSA, a condition causing intermittent hypoxia, in general population–based studies is roughly 22% in men and 17% in women. Carbon monoxide poisoning in the United States has resulted in extremely large numbers of patients diagnosed but a relatively low death rate. Specifically, carbon monoxide poisoning accounts for 50,000 emergency department visits and 2,700 deaths annually in the United States (Ruth-Sahd, Zulkosky, & Fetter, 2011). Hypoxia due to carbon monoxide poisoning has an increased incidence in colder months, when use of furnaces and fireplaces increases.

As the incidence of hypoxic and anoxic injuries rise, more information is needed on the public health impact of hypoxia/anoxia, including the financial burden as a result of the functional impact of these brain injuries. Cullen and Weisz (2011) note that research on patients with anoxic brain injuries pales in comparison to the research on patients with traumatic brain injury (TBI); however, there is a trend in the literature showing worse functional outcomes in patients with anoxic brain injuries compared with TBI. Of the studies that do exist, most studies do not include older adults with nontraumatic brain injuries such as anoxia. Certainly, the variability in etiology, age ranges, and severity of brain injury can make it difficult to set up direct comparisons between groups.

CLINICAL PRESENTATION

Pure hypoxic brain injury does not always cause severe brain injury if systemic circulation is maintained (Busl & Greer, 2010); however, hypoxic/anoxic brain injuries often result in neurocognitive deficits. In their review, Caine and Watson (2000) found that hypoxic brain injury resulted in amnestic memory impairment in over half (54%) of the individual case reports they analyzed; executive deficits or personality changes (i.e., frontal symptoms) were the second most commonly reported neuropsychological sequela, followed by visuospatial deficits. A similar pattern emerged in their review of group studies. Garcia-Molina et al. (2006) investigated cognitive outcomes across two different groups of patients with cerebral anoxic injuries. Although deficits in multiple domains of cognition were reported, the authors found more significant verbal memory deficits with episodes of ischemic anoxia than in patients with hypoxemic anoxia. In general, the degree of neurocognitive impairment tends to mirror the degree of neuropathological damage (Hopkins & Bigler, 2008).

Brain imaging for anoxic/hypoxic injuries often reveals both focal and diffuse neuropathologic lesions and atrophy (Hopkins & Bigler, 2008). Hopkins and Bigler (2008) note that commonly ordered scans (e.g., CT and MR) may appear to be normal or show only subtle changes during the acute period; however, newer imaging techniques (e.g., diffusion-weighted magnetic resonance imaging [MRI]), can reveal more extensive changes even in the acute phase. Damage is commonly reported in the hippocampus, white matter, cerebellum, and corpus callosum, as noted previously in this chapter. For example, using voxel-based morphometry, Di Paola et al. (2008) found a bilateral reduction of hippocampal gray matter in persons who had anoxic/hypoxic injuries as compared with healthy subjects. In terms of diffuse damage, common findings may include generalized cerebral atrophy and enlargement of the ventricles, with enlarged ventricle to brain ratios (Hopkins & Bigler, 2008). Diffuse damage is likely to appear over time, not acutely following hypoxic injury.

Psychosocial impairments are important considerations in overall quality of life post hypoxic brain injury. Not surprisingly, quality of life may vary significantly depending on the extent of the hypoxic/anoxic injury, particularly with greater cognitive impairments that affect one's ability to work, independence for ADLs, or interpersonal relationships. Psychological and behavioral changes often occur following hypoxic/anoxic brain injuries. Symptoms can vary widely and may include symptoms of euphoria, irritability, hostility, emotional lability, apathy, depression, anxiety, and occasionally mania (Hopkins & Bigler, 2008). Emotional and personality changes can be difficult for the patient, as well as for loved ones or caregivers. In a study of psychosocial outcomes of anoxic brain injury following cardiac arrest, Wilson et al. (2014) found that patients who had anoxia following cardiac arrest demonstrated more significant psychosocial difficulties, including anxiety, depression, PTSD, and social problems. Social difficulties were associated with subjective ratings of memory and executive dysfunction.

DIAGNOSTIC CONSIDERATIONS

The following tips are provided for consideration in diagnosing hypoxic/anoxic brain injuries and clinical management:

- The main method of detecting hypoxic/anoxic brain injury is clinical examination, including level of consciousness (e.g., Glasgow Coma Scale [GCS]), as well as vestibular and brain stem reflexes.
- Take a meticulous history. This is important not only to gain clarity about the nature and the extent of the hypoxic/anoxic brain injury itself, but also to gain information about a patient's medical history, including comorbid risk factors and any prior brain insults. Often the patient may be unable to provide a good history; therefore, it is important to try to obtain this information from family members or a caregiver who knows the patient well.
- Treatment of comorbid conditions, especially cardiovascular and cerebrovascular risk factors, is important when caring for the patient's immediate medical needs, as well as in reducing the risk for repeat or additional brain insults. Additionally, as discussed in the prognosis section, hypoxic/anoxic injuries may result in new medical consequences that also warrant evaluation and treatment, such as movement disorders or seizures.
- It is important to consider whether the patient may be "locked-in," a condition in which the patient is conscious and aware of what is happening, but unable to move or communicate. Repeated examination and electroencephalogram (EEG) can be helpful if this is of concern.
- MRI, EEG, and somatosensory evoked potentials (SSEPs) can provide helpful information about the nature and severity of hypoxic–ischemic injuries.
- Refrain from the urge to provide a definite prognosis too early. Often patients or family members will press providers for such a response. Instead, it would be helpful to state that it is difficult, if not impossible, to predict an individual patient's recovery in the acute phase of hypoxic/anoxic brain injury. You can also encourage repeat clinical assessment over time to monitor the patient's progress.

- If you are working as part of a medical team, it may be helpful to designate one person to be responsible for communicating information about the patient's condition, or at least defer such communications until after the patient has been staffed by the multidisciplinary team. This will help reduce giving of misinformation or conflicting information across providers.

- As noted previously in this chapter, cognitive/neuropsychological outcomes following hypoxic/anoxic injury are highly variable, not unlike the injury itself. A neurocognitive evaluation during the subacute phase may be helpful in determining the patient's treatment needs, particularly in planning for discharge and determining whether the patient has decision-making capacity. Serial evaluations can be used to track response to treatment interventions and recovery over time.

TREATMENT

Resuscitation is typically the first step in treatment (Howard et al., 2011). Medication options may be most beneficial in sub- or postacute stages to facilitate recovery and function (Anderson & Arciniegas, 2010). For example, stimulant medication may boost processing speed, arousal, and possibly attention and memory. Additionally, cholinesterase inhibitors may help memory impairment. Howard et al. (2011) reported that induced hypothermia has been shown to help minimize neurological damage in patients with prolonged cardiac arrest. Although somewhat controversial, hyperbaric oxygen has been investigated as a possible treatment for patients with hypoxic injuries due to carbon monoxide poisoning and other types of brain injury; however, benefits beyond improving initial Glasgow Coma Scale scores are inconclusive (Bennett, Trytko, & Jonker, 2012).

In addition to medical interventions, behavioral strategies are particularly effective. In particular, compensatory tools, or external memory aides, including calendars, notes, and cell phone alarm reminders, are useful in helping patients become more functionally independent. Patients should be encouraged to keep all vital information, such as appointments, important names and phone numbers, and medication instructions in one place, ideally a calendar or day–date book. Centralizing this information reduces the organizational demands and prevents the patient from having to search for information in multiple places. This is particularly important in this population given the prevalence of memory and executive impairment. Environmental modifications are also useful for reducing distraction or limiting competing demands. For example, creating distraction-free work spaces in quiet areas may be helpful for patients with attention problems. Providing clear and written instructions can minimize executive demands for persons with difficulty planning and organizing tasks. Certainly many of these strategies can be taught in formal rehabilitation programs, but unfortunately, as Hopkins and Bigler (2012) note, unlike TBI or stroke, there has not been a systematic approach to rehabilitation for persons who have had hypoxic/anoxic injuries.

Beyond direct intervention, psychoeducation for the patient and his or her family members is a beneficial form of treatment in its own right. This includes providing information about the nature of hypoxic/anoxic injuries, as well as the impact of the injury on the patient's cognitive and psychosocial functioning. Understanding changes in memory (e.g., difficulty learning new information), as well as reduced attention or executive functioning is important in helping family members adjust their expectations and set the patient up for success. For example, it can be frustrating for family to tolerate longer latencies in the patient's response time or slowed processing speed. As such, it can be tempting to speak for the patient or to complete a task in order to minimize their own frustration or prevent the patient from experiencing difficulty. However, this is not beneficial to the patient and negates his or her opportunity for practice. Instead, family members are encouraged to give the patient extra time to respond. It is also helpful for others to be mindful that they are not giving the patient too much information at once. In cases with more significant cognitive impact, family members may also need to plan how they can supervise or assist patients with activities of daily living. A sudden change in a person's level of independence can be quite a shock for the individual and/or their families, but education can go a long way in helping families cope and support the patient.

PROGNOSIS

Several factors affect the prognosis following cardiac arrest, including the duration of arrest, age of the patient, timing and effectiveness of resuscitation efforts, and fever in the first 48 hours (Howard et al.,

2011). The best outcomes are seen in patients with only mild cerebral hypoxia with only short periods of impaired consciousness, and worse outcomes following more severe hypoxia. Out-of-hospital cardiac arrest carries worse prognosis, likely due to a longer latency in receiving intervention as compared with in-hospital arrest. Poor prognosis is also associated with older age and having comorbid risk factors, such as cerebrovascular disease, diabetes, and obesity. The effects of certain kinds of hypoxias may take time to develop. For example, the long-term effects of serious carbon monoxide poisoning usually may take several weeks to appear. Similarly, the effects of intermittent hypoxemia associated with OSA develop over time. Seizures, although uncommon in the initial stages following hypoxic–ischemic brain injury, may occur during the recovery period (Howard et al., 2011). Movement disorders or parkinsonian symptoms can also occur because the basal ganglia are vulnerable to oxygen deprivation. In fact, the onset of movement disorder may not develop until months later, particularly for younger patients (Howard et al., 2011). Dystonia can occur from damage to the putamen, and akinetic syndromes can occur when there is damage to the global pallidus. Watershed or boundary-zone infarctions can also occur after hypoxic–ischemic brain injuries. Rarely, delayed posthypoxic leukoencephalopathy can occur, a condition in which patients seem to have made a complete recovery from hypoxic injury only to relapse with cognitive deterioration, frontal lobe signs, and parkinsonian features (Howard et al., 2011).

A study comparing 93 patients with anoxic brain injury to patients with TBI found that patients with anoxic injuries had poorer prognosis, with more severe cognitive impairments than the TBI group (Fitzgerald et al., 2010). Similar findings were reported by Cullen and Weisz (2011), who reported that patients with TBI scored better than patients with anoxic brain injury on measures of motor and cognitive tasks.

CLINICAL SYNOPSIS

- Hypoxic brain injury refers to a reduction of oxygen to the brain tissue and anoxia refers to total absence of oxygen.
- Isolated hypoxia/anoxia refers strictly to lack of oxygen, whereas ischemia refers to a restriction of blood supply to

- tissues, which causes not only a shortage of oxygen, but also of essential cellular metabolites.
- Advances in medicine will likely increase the incidence of hypoxic and anoxic brain injuries in an aging population in the coming years.
- Cardiovascular and pulmonary diseases are the leading causes of hypoxic/anoxic brain injuries in adults, particularly following cardiac arrest.
- The brain is vulnerable to oxygen deprivation because it cannot store oxygen.
- Certain brain structures, including the hippocampus, cerebellum, white matter, basal ganglia, and corpus callosum are especially vulnerable to damage following hypoxic/anoxic brain injury.
- Diagnosis of hypoxic and anoxic injury is done through thorough clinical exam, history, and imaging.
- The neuropsychological effects often include impairments in memory (anterograde amnesia), executive functions, and visuospatial skills.
- Brain imaging of hypoxic and anoxic injuries using advanced MRI techniques often show both focal and diffuse pathological changes, although diffuse changes are not always present in the acute phase.
- Hypoxic and anoxic brain injuries can cause psychosocial difficulties both as a pathological result of the injury or because of difficulty coping with functional changes postinjury. Depression, anxiety, and social and functional changes are commonly reported.
- Treatment of hypoxic/anoxic brain injuries should include resuscitation, medical stabilization, psychoeducation about neuropsychological effects, and provision of behavioral and compensatory strategies to offset neurocognitive difficulties.
- Several factors affect the prognosis following cardiac arrest, including the duration of arrest, age of the patient, timing and effectiveness of resuscitation efforts, and fever in the first 48 hours.

Outcomes following hypoxic and anoxic brain injuries can be quite variable, reflecting the wide spectrum of injury severity. Therefore, it is important to remember that the effects of hypoxic/anoxic brain injuries may develop or change over time, including cognitive and psychiatric symptoms, as well as additional medical concerns such as seizures and movement disorders.

CASE STUDY

A 63-year-old man with 20 years of education was admitted and intubated for respiratory failure after being found at home, by his wife, in respiratory distress. He was admitted to the intensive care unit (ICU) with respiratory, kidney, and liver failure, and hypoperfusion due to accidental overdose of opioid pain medication he was taking for a kidney stone. Brain MRI revealed mild, age-appropriate diffuse cerebral atrophy with associated prominence of the cerebral sulci and ventricles, as well as scattered white matter FLAIR hyperintensities attributed to chronic small vessel ischemic disease. Per medical records, the patient was initially admitted to the neuro-ICU intubated and sedated, was transitioned to dexmedetomidine hydrochloride for sedation, and, over the next 24 hours, neurologic examination improved significantly and patient was extubated. Upon extubation, patient was noted to be alert and oriented ×4 with clear speech and no focal deficits. He was discharged home after 4 days.

Patient presented for a neuropsychological evaluation approximately 3 months following hospitalization with complaints of memory problems. He was able to recall the days before the aforementioned hospitalization, but he was unable to remember most of his hospitalization, except for a vague memory of waking with tubes in his mouth. Although he had some improvement in the months following the hypoxic event, he continued to have memory problems. His wife reported that he forgets conversations. For example, he and his wife always discuss a plan for the day, but he must write it down or else he will forget it. His attention span is limited and he has trouble multitasking. His wife sets out his medications as he cannot recall if he had already taken them. His wife has also been managing their finances since the hospitalization. Results of his neuropsychological evaluation noted some areas of relative weakness in this previously high-functioning man. Specifically, he demonstrated rather circumscribed deficits in learning new information, as well as reduced semantic fluency and slowed processing speed. Overall, his profile was most notable for anterograde amnesia (difficulty learning and retaining new information) suggestive of medial temporal dysfunction. Such memory difficulty is often seen following an anoxic injury as described previously in this chapter.

Maximal cognitive recovery from acute hypoxic/anoxic injury would be expected within 6 to 12 months, but it is unlikely that this patient will return to his cognitive baseline. As such, he would not be able to successfully return to work at his previously high-level job. Since the time of his neuropsychological evaluation, he has been participating in weekly cognitive remediation using spaced retrieval. Spaced retrieval is a technique that has been shown to be useful in helping patients with memory impairment to acquire new information (Schacter, Rich, & Stampp, 1985). Specifically, the patient is given a relatively circumscribed piece of information and prompted to retrieve it at increasingly longer intervals. The theory posits that people better remember information when they are successful the first time (i.e., almost immediately) and information is more likely to be lasting if the information is retrieved frequently over extended periods of time. This technique is particularly helpful with adaptive living skills as it can be used to help patients remember to do a task. It can also be used to help patients remember someone's name or associate a name and face.

REFERENCES

Anderson, C. A., & Arciniegas, D. B. (2010). Cognitive sequelae of hypoxic-ischemic brain injury: A review. *NeuroRehabilitation, 26*(1), 47–63. doi:10.3233/NRE-2010-0535

Bennett, M. H., Trytko, B., & Jonker, B. (2012). Hyperbaric oxygen therapy for the adjunctive treatment of traumatic brain injury. *Cochrane Database of Systematic Reviews, 12*, CD004609. doi:10.1002/14651858.CD004609.pub3

Biagas, K. (1999). Hypoxic-ischemic brain injury: Advancements in the understanding of mechanisms and potential avenues for therapy. *Current Opinion in Pediatrics, 11*(3), 223–228.

Bryce, J., Boschi-Pinto, C., Shibuya, K., Black, R. E., & WHO Child Health Epidemiology Reference Group. (2005). WHO estimates of the causes of death in children. *Lancet, 365*(9465), 1147–1152. doi:10.1016/ S0140-6736(05)71877-8

Busl, K. M., & Greer, D. M. (2010). Hypoxic-ischemic brain injury: Pathophysiology, neuropathology and mechanisms. *NeuroRehabilitation, 26*(1), 5–13. doi:10.3233/NRE-2010-0531

Caine, D., & Watson, J. D. (2000). Neuropsychological and neuropathological sequelae of cerebral anoxia: A critical review. *Journal of the International Neuropsychological Society, 6*(1), 86–99.

Chiota, N. A., Freeman, W. D., & Barrett, K. M. (2011). Hypoxic-ischemic brain injury and prognosis after cardiac arrest. *Continuum, 17*(5), 1094–1118. doi:10.1212/01.CON.0000407062.25284.f3

Cullen, N. K., & Weisz, K. (2011). Cognitive correlates with functional outcomes after anoxic brain injury: A case-controlled comparison with traumatic brain injury. *Brain Injury, 25*(1), 35–43. doi:10.3109/ 02699052.2010.531691

Di Paola, M., Caltagirone, C., Fadda, L., Sabatini, U., Serra., L., & Carlesimo, G. A. (2008). Hippocampal atrophy is the critical brain change in patients with hypoxic amnesia. *Hippocampus, 18*(7), 719–728. doi:10.1002/hipo.20432

Fitzgerald, A., Aditya, H., Prior, A., McNeill, E., & Pentland, B. (2010). Anoxic brain injury: Clinical patterns and functional outcomes: A study of 93 cases. *Brain Injury, 24*(11), 1311–1323. doi:10.3109/02 699052.2010.506864

Franklin, K. A., & Lindberg, E. (2015). Obstructive sleep apnea is a common disorder in the population: A review on the epidemiology of sleep apnea. *Journal of Thoracic Disease, 7*(8), 1311–1323. doi:10.3039 78.j.issn.2072-1439.2015.06.11

Gale, S. D., & Hopkins, R. O. (2004). Effects of hypoxia on the brain: Neuroimaging and neuropsychological findings following carbon monoxide poisoning and obstructive sleep apnea. *Journal of the International Neuropsychological Society, 10*(1), 60–71. doi:10.1017/ S1355617704101082

Garcia-Molina, A., Roig-Rovira, T., Ensenat-Cantallops, A., Sanchez-Carrion, R., Pico-Azanza, N., Bernabeu, M., & Tormos, J. M. (2006). Neuropsychological profile of persons with anoxic brain injury: Differences regarding physiopathological mechanism. *Brain Injury, 20*(11), 1139–1145. doi:10.1080/02699050600983248

Hinduja, A., Gupta, H., Yang, J. D., & Onteddu, S. (2014). Hypoxic ischemic brain injury following in hospital cardiac arrest: Lessons from autopsy. *Journal of Forensic and Legal Medicine, 23,* 84–86. doi:10.1016/j.jflm.2014.02.003

Hopkins, R. O., & Bigler, E. D. (2008). Hypoxic and anoxic conditions of the CNS. In J. E. Morgan & J. H. Ricker (Eds.), *Textbook of clinical neuropsychology.* New York, NY: Taylor & Francis.

Hopkins, R. O., & Bigler, E. D. (2012). Neuroimaging of anoxic injury: Implications for neurorehabilitation. *NeuroRehabilitation, 31*(3), 319–329. doi:10.3233/NRE-2012-0799

Hopkins, R. O., & Haaland, K. Y. (2004). Neuropsychological and neuropathological effects of anoxic or ischemic induced brain injury. *Journal of the International Neuropsychological Society, 10*(7), 957–961.

Hopkins, R. O., Kesner, R. P., & Goldstein, M. (1995). Item and order recognition memory in subjects with hypoxic brain injury. *Brain and Cognition, 27*(2), 180–201. doi:10.1006/brcg.1995.1016

Hopkins, R. O., Tate, D. F., & Bigler, E. D. (2005). Anoxic versus traumatic brain injury: Amount of tissue loss, not etiology, alters cognitive and emotional function. *Neuropsychology, 19*(2), 233–242. doi:10.1037/0894-4105.19.2.233

Howard, R. S., Holmes, P. A., & Koutroumanidis, M. A. (2011). Hypoxic-ischemic brain injury. *Practical Neurology, 11*(1), 4–18. doi:10.0036/jnnp.2010.235218

Kurinczuk, J. J., White-Koning, M., & Badawi, N. (2010). Epidemiology of neonatal encephalopathy and hypoxic-ischaemic encephalopathy. *Early Human Development, 86*(6), 329–338. doi:10.1016/j.earlhumdev.2010.05.010

Northington, F. J., Chavez-Valdez, R., & Martin, L. J. (2011). Neuronal cell death in neonatal hypoxia-ischemia. *Annals of Neurology, 69*(5), 743–758. doi:10.1002/ana.22419

Rab, T., Kern, K. B., Tamis-Holland, J. E., Henry, T. D., McDaniel, M., & Dickert, N. W. (2015). Cardiac arrest: A treatment algorithm for emergent invasive cardiac procedures in the resuscitated comatose patient. *Journal of the American College of Cardiology, 66*(1), 62–73. doi:10.1016/j.jacc.2015.05.009

Raherison, C., & Girodet, P. O. (2009). Epidemiology of COPD. *European Respiratory Review: An Official Journal of the European Respiratory Society, 18*(114), 213–221. doi:10.1183/09059180.00003609

Ruth-Sahd, L. A., Zulkosky, K., & Fetter, M. E. (2011). Carbon monoxide poisoning: Case studies and review. *Dimensions of Critical Care Nursing, 30*(6), 303–314. doi:10.1097/DCC.0b013e31822fb017

Schacter, D. L., Rich, S. A., & Stampp, M. S. (1985). Remediation of memory disorders: Experimental evaluation of the spaced-retrieval technique. *Journal of Clinical and Experimental Neuropsychology, 7*(1), 79–96. doi:10.1080/01688638508401243

Wilson, M., Staniforth, A., Till, R., das Nair, R., & Vesey, P. (2014). The psychosocial outcomes of anoxic brain injury following cardiac arrest. *Resuscitation, 85*(6), 795–800. doi:10.1016/j.resuscitation.2014.02.008

CHAPTER 8

Electrical and Lightning Brain Injuries

SHRAVAN PARIKH
JOSEPH FINK
MAIA FEIGON
NEIL PLISKIN

OVERVIEW

Electricity pervades modern society; it is often taken for granted, in terms of the utility, power, and ease with which it provides consumers innumerable benefits. Although electrical power is virtually ubiquitous in everyday life, injuries associated with accidental contact are relatively rare in the general population. However, electric shock is a common type of trauma in the workplace, where significant electrical injuries (EIs) disproportionately affect younger men (Martinez & Nguyen, 2000). Similarly, EI caused by lightning strikes is a relatively uncommon weather event that causes even fewer fatalities. However, the impact of electricity-related injuries and the significant amount of short- and long-term medical, social, and personal consequences deserve unique consideration.

EIs are sometimes poorly understood by neuropsychologists, as well as by physicians, clinicians, and allied health professionals. Because of the relatively low incidence rate of EI, neuropsychologists may have little or no experience with injury dynamics and issues when they first encounter a patient with such an injury. Moreover, EIs are often compared to traumatic brain injuries. However, neuropsychological sequelae of EI do not typically follow the symptom and recovery path as seen in cases of traumatic brain injury (TBI; Barrash, Kealey, & Janus, 1996; Heilbronner, 1994). In particular, perceived neuropsychological changes following a mild TBI typically resolve within 8 months to 1 year postinjury, whereas the neuropsychological sequelae found in EI may emerge after some time has elapsed and last much longer.

EI survivors may see numerous clinicians from various disciplines and specialties depending on the nature of their injuries and complaints, but it is often difficult for patients to obtain a comprehensive and integrated assessment that takes into account the physical, cognitive, and emotional changes that can occur after EI, especially when brain involvement is not evident on neuroimaging or standard neurological exam. The role of neuropsychological assessment can be particularly crucial for situations in which overt physiologic manifestations of injury are minimal or lacking, in order to help guide clinical care and medical–legal decisions.

In this chapter, we review the epidemiology of electrical and lightning injuries and consider some of both the known and poorly understood aspects of the pathophysiology of these injuries. We review the patterns of symptom presentation, diagnostic considerations, treatment, and prognosis. Finally, we conclude with two case studies that highlight the intricate details of assessing and treating individuals who have experienced a trauma due to electrical and lightning injuries.

HISTORY

EI from sources other than lightning is a relatively new phenomenon in the history of humankind. With the advent of the light bulb and industrialized electricity, the incidence of EI increased significantly in the 19th and 20th centuries. The first recorded death caused by electrical current from an artificial source was reported in 1879 when a carpenter in Lyons, France came in contact with a 250-V alternating current (AC) generator. In the United States, the first reported fatality occurred in 1881 when an intoxicated man passed out on a similar type of generator in front of a crowd in Buffalo, New York (Price & Cooper, 2013).

Lightning-related injury has presumably always been a rare part of humankind's experience. From a historical perspective, the incidence of lightning-related fatalities in the United States decreased from an average of 94 over the period from 1891 to

1894, to only 26 in 2014 (Holle, López, & Navarro, 2005; National Weather Service, 2015). Despite this, the sheer amount of lightning strikes per day, the propensity to cause significant injury or death when an individual is struck, and the magnitude of the economic, social, and personal costs deserve in-depth exploration in order to better assist health professionals in understanding the unique injury characteristics.

PATHOPHYSIOLOGY

The exact pathophysiologic mechanisms of electrical and lightning injury are not well understood because of the numerous variables that cannot be measured or controlled when an electrical current passes through tissue. However, the nature and severity of these injuries is thought to depend on the following factors (Kouwenhoven, 1949):

- Direct current (DC) versus alternating current (AC)
- Duration of exposure
- Voltage and amperage
- Body resistance
- Pathway of current

Type of Current

High-voltage DC contact tends to cause a single muscle spasm, often throwing the victim from the source, resulting in shorter duration of exposure compared with AC exposures. However, the likelihood of secondary blunt trauma due to falls, blast trauma, and trauma from flying debris is increased. Generally, the longer the duration of contact with a high-voltage current, the greater the electrothermal heating and tissue damage. However, even brief contact with a DC source can still result in cardiac arrhythmias, depending on the phase of the cardiac cycle affected (Price & Cooper, 2013; Wesner & Hickie, 2013).

The electric current involved in lightning strikes is also via DC. The amount of DC delivered by a lightning strike is far greater than that produced by typical AC domestic electricity sources. The duration of exposure, however, is generally much shorter, lasting approximately 10 to 100 ms. This current causes the release of a significant amount of heat, raising temperatures of the lightning-strike channel to approximately 30,000 K (Ritenour, Morton, McManus, Barillo, & Cancio, 2008).

AC, which is the standard form of electrical transmission, may be more dangerous than non–lightning-associated DC of the same voltage (Koumbourlis, 2002). EI from AC can cause repetitive muscle contraction, or tetany, wherein the muscle fibers are stimulated between 40 and 110 times per second by the AC cycles (Price & Cooper, 2013). The hand is the most common contact point, such as with a tool, appliance, or machinery, which results in contact with an AC electrical source. The upper extremity flexors are much stronger than the extensors, often causing the hand grasping the current source to both grip and pull the source even closer to the body. Currents greater than the "let-go threshold" (6–9 mA) can prevent the victim from releasing the current source, resulting in the "no let-go" phenomena, which extends the duration of exposure to the electrical current (Price & Cooper, 2013).

Voltage

Voltage is a measure of the difference in electrical potential between two points and is determined by the electrical source. In the scientific literature, EIs are typically divided into low (<1,000 V) or high voltage (>1,000 V). Although both can cause significant morbidity and mortality, high voltage tends to have a greater potential for tissue damage and major amputation (Bryan, Andrews, Hurley, & Taber, 2009a; Price & Cooper, 2013).

Current, expressed in amperes, is a measure of the amount of energy that flows through an object. The heat generated, as defined by Joule's law, is proportional to the amperage squared. Amperage depends on the source voltage and the resistance of the conductor. Although the voltage of the source is often known, the resistance varies according to the affected tissues and may change markedly during the exposure, making predictions of actual amperage difficult for any given EI (Price & Cooper, 2013).

Resistance

Resistance is the tendency of a material to resist the flow of electrical current. It varies for a given tissue, depending on its moisture content, temperature, and other physical properties. The higher the resistance of a tissue to the flow of current, the greater the potential for transformation of electrical energy to thermal energy. The least amount of resistance involves nerves, blood, mucous membranes, and muscle. Dry skin represents an intermediate amount of resistance, and bone, fat, and tendon yield the most resistance (Bryan et al., 2009a).

Path of Current Flow

Electric current enters a victim at contact points on the body (i.e., usually an extremity). In the case of DC, electricity enters at an "entrance" point and, after traveling along a pathway through the body, leaves through an "exit" point (Bryan et al., 2009a). In the case of AC current, which repeatedly alternates its directional flow, there are technically only contact points, none of which is solely an entrance or an exit point because of the bidirectional current flow. Contact wounds are only an indication that the body has conducted a significant amount of electrical energy to cause injury. However, the mere presence or absence of contact wounds is not sufficient to accurately predict the severity of EI. A close examination of the direct and indirect effects of the electric shock is necessary to determine the severity of the injury, course, and prognosis (Koumbourlis, 2002; Price & Cooper, 2013).

When lightning strikes an individual, the primary current arc typically travels outside the body, a phenomenon known as "flashover" (Ritenour et al., 2008). The immense current generates large magnetic fields perpendicular to the body's surface, which in turn transiently create secondary electrical currents within the body itself.

When lightning hits the ground, current spreads out from the ground contact point such that if a victim is standing nearby with feet apart, the potential difference between the feet may be in the range of 1,500 V (Pfortmueller et al., 2012). Thus, lightning injuries are more severe when a person's feet are apart in line with the ground contact point than when they are close together. When lightning directly strikes a victim's upper body, a very large potential difference between the upper and lower body is created, resulting in a brief but large current flow. Although the duration is generally not sufficient to cause Joule heating, as in high-voltage nonlightning injuries, it is sufficient to damage muscle and nerve cells (Ritenour et al., 2008).

ETIOLOGY

The causes of electrical and lightning-related injury are varied; however, research suggests that young men working in the construction or utility industry are at higher risk (American Burn Association, 2015). Subsequent injuries, such as electrical or thermal burns, deep-tissue and organ damage, brain injury, and secondary systemic disorders require prompt, comprehensive, and multidisciplinary care. The primary cause of death in these cases is typically cardiac or respiratory arrest (Price & Cooper, 2013). The following areas have been identified as high risk, in which EI is often the primary mechanism for injury and fatality (Electrical Safety Authority, 2012):

- Powerline contact
- Electrical/construction workers
- Misuse of electrical products and unapproved or counterfeit products
- Electrical infrastructure fires in buildings

In cases of lightning-related injury, the risk of being struck is contingent on regional, seasonal, and temporal factors. The following is a list of mechanisms that can occur in lightning-related injury (Ritenour et al., 2008):

- *Direct strike:* Most of the current flows through the body.
- *Contact voltage:* Occurs when lightning strikes an object that the victim is touching.
- *Ground current:* Ground current passes from the strike point through the ground and into the victim.
- *Side flash:* Splashing of current from a nearby object or person onto the victim.
- *Upward streamer:* Passage of lightning from the victim upwards.
- *Blast injury:* Sudden expansive explosion of the air around the lightning channel causing blunt trauma.

EPIDEMIOLOGY

Electrical and lightning injuries are relatively uncommon; however, their impact on victims and families is often significant. The prototypic electrical accident victim is a young man shocked while working in the electrical or construction trade, bringing significant risks for death and morbidity. Epidemiological rates of lightning-related EIs are less reliable and difficult to discern because state and federal agencies do not require they be reported (Ritenour et al., 2008). However, some studies have suggested that lightning-related injuries disproportionately affect young adult men, with low rates of fatal injuries (Jensenius, 2015; Price & Cooper, 2013; Ritenour et al., 2008).

Information on rates of burn admissions related to EI in the United States between 2005 and 2014 showed an overwhelming decline of incidents and complicating injuries sustained per year (American Burn Association, 2015). Over this period, burns related to EIs represented only 3.6% of all burn admissions that were reported. The majority of these cases was work related (60.8%) and occurred within an industry setting (38.9%). The highest rates of EIs occurred at several age peaks, including in the 20- to 29.9-year-old age group (13%) and among the 60-and-over age group (13.5%; American Burn Association, 2015).

Between 1992 and 2010, fatal EIs in the United States have declined significantly by more than 50% on an annual basis (Electrical Safety Foundation International, 2011). The dramatic reduction of EIs, especially within an industrial setting, has been attributed to better training, electrical safety standards, and even a slowdown in economic activity (Electrical Safety Foundation International, 2011). Victims who came in contact with overhead power lines comprised the largest fatal-accident category, representing 44% of all electrical fatalities between 1992 and 2010. From 2003 to 2010, the construction industry experienced the highest rates of fatal EIs (52%) compared with other industries such as professional and business services; trade, transportation, and utilities; natural resources and mining; and manufacturing. Nonfatal EIs have shown similar declining trends as well. In 2010, nonfatal EIs were down by more than 60% when compared with rates in 1992. Victims who came in contact with electric current from a machine, tool, appliance, or light fixture represented the largest group (Electrical Safety Foundation International, 2011).

From 2006 to 2014, 287 people were struck and killed by lightning in the United States (Jensenius, 2015). Men accounted for 81% of all fatalities, and more than 90% of these deaths were related to fishing and sports accidents. Ages of the victims predominantly ranged from 10 to 60 years, with somewhat fewer in the 30- to 39-year-old age group. In general, the summer months (June–August) represent a peak in lightning activity across the country. For instance, over 70% of lightning fatalities recorded between 2006 and 2014 were during the summer months (Jensenius, 2015). Some estimates on the global prevalence of lightning-related fatalities are estimated to be around 24,000 per year, while nonfatal lightning-related injuries are estimated to be approximately 240,000 per year (Holle, 2008).

CLINICAL PRESENTATION

Symptom presentation in victims of electrical and lightning injury can include a variety of physical, neurological, cognitive, and emotional changes that manifest in the acute, postacute (1 month to 5 years postinjury), and long-term phase (5 or more years postinjury). The severity of injuries can range widely from minimal (e.g., minor burns, transient confusion) to very severe (e.g., paraplegia, permanent memory loss, death; Duff & McCaffery, 2001; Fink, Rog, Bush, & Pliskin, 2010; Silversides, 1964).

Although immediate effects of EI can be quite obvious like burns and cardiac abnormalities, frequent and often clinically significant central and peripheral nervous system dysfunction is sometimes less evident in the immediate aftermath of electrical shock. Additionally, the degree of neuropsychological impairment and emotional disturbance can persist for months and years, unlike cases of uncomplicated mild TBI, in which symptoms typically dissipate in the weeks or months following the injury (Aase, Fink, Lee, Kelley, & Pliskin, 2014; Barrash et al., 1996; Hahn-Ketter et al., 2015; Pliskin et al., 1994; Wesner & Hickie, 2013).

Physical

Clinical manifestations of dermal and subcutaneous burns are among the most common acute symptoms in EI, and often lead to pain, scarring, fibrosis, and joint stiffness (Price & Cooper, 2013). Low-voltage EI burns tend to create small, well-defined burns at the sites of skin contact (Czuczman & Zane, 2009). In high-voltage injuries, the burns are typically more significant and may appear as painless, depressed, yellow-gray, charred craters with central necrosis (Czuczman & Zane, 2009; Price & Cooper, 2013). Although high-voltage injuries may spare the skin surface, they can cause significant damage to underlying soft tissues and bones. In cases of lightning-related EI, the prevalence of significant burns or soft tissue destruction is rather low due to the brief duration of the actual strike itself. However, four main types of superficial burns are typically seen: linear, puncture, feathering, and thermal (Price & Cooper, 2013; Ritenour et al., 2008).

When severe flash and flame burns are present, the patient is expected to develop severe hemodynamic, autonomic, cardiopulmonary, renal, metabolic, and neuroendocrine responses that may have devastating effects on long-term recovery (Koumbourlis, 2002).

In the case of electrical arc events, injuries may include perforated eardrums; blast effects affecting lung, abdomen, and/or head, plus acceleration–deceleration head injury; and blunt head trauma from falling or being hit by explosion shrapnel (Capelli-Schellpfeffer, Miller, & Humilier, 1999; Fink et al., 2010).

The skeletal system may have fractures or joint dislocations either from severe tetanic muscle contractions or from injury due to falls. Fractures are more common in the long bones of the upper limb and in vertebrae and increase the risk of spinal cord injury (Bryan et al., 2009b). In cases of lightning injury, skull fractures and cervical spine injury from either direct strikes or associated trauma are often seen (Pfortmueller et al., 2012). In high-voltage EI, direct electrothermal energy leading to coagulation and necrosis is the main cause of muscle injury (Czuczman & Zane, 2009).

Ocular injuries (e.g., cataracts, keratitis) and auditory sequelae (e.g., hearing loss, tinnitus, vertigo) are also common. Cardiac complications (e.g., sinus tachycardia, supraventricular tachycardia, atrial fibrillation, cardiac arrest) may occur, particularly when AC and/or high voltages are involved (Price & Cooper, 2013; Spies & Trohman, 2006).

In the postacute and long-term phases, common physical complaints include pain, fatigue, reduced range of motion, joint stiffness, headache, motor weakness, coordination problems, blurred vision, dizziness, insomnia, contracture, and paresthesia (Daniel, Haban, Hutcherson, Bolter, & Long, 1985; Hooshmand, Radfar, & Beckner, 1989; Ramati et al., 2009; Theman, Singerman, Gomez, & Fish, 2008; Wesner & Hickie, 2013).

Neurological

Although central and peripheral nervous system injury are common clinical sequelae of EI, there are no specific histologic or clinical findings that are considered pathognomonic for victims of EI. However, loss of consciousness, confusion, and cognitive impairment tend to be common among victims (Wesner & Hickie, 2013). Victims of EI have been reported to experience isolated seizures following shortly after the accident, as well as recurring seizures that may last for years after injury (Bryan et al., 2009b; Daniel et al., 1985; Hooshmand et al., 1989; Wesner & Hickie, 2013). Acute dysfunction of peripheral motor and sensory nerves is also relatively common and may cause a variety of motor and sensory deficits. This is largely in part due to the process of electroporation, which results in the formation of pores in the lipid bilayers that form cell membranes and eventually lead to rapid and diffuse necrosis (Bryan et al., 2009b).

Keraunoparalysis is a transient type of neurological paralysis that is considered to be a pathognomonic sign of lightning-related EI (Czuczman & Zane, 2009; Pfortmueller et al., 2012; Ritenour et al., 2008). Immediate and persistent neurologic syndromes associated with lightning injury include hypoxic encephalopathy and intracranial hemorrhage, usually occurring in the basal ganglia and brain stem. Delayed neurologic sequelae may include motor neuron disease and movement disorders, traumatic falls resulting in spinal cord injury, and epidural and subdural hematomas (Czuczman & Zane, 2009; Pfortmueller et al., 2012; Ritenour et al., 2008).

Cognitive and Emotional Disturbances

A large body of research suggests that a variety of cognitive deficits are frequently observed, including impairments of attention, processing speed, and memory, as well as disruptions in emotional well-being that could adversely affect cognition (Aase et al., 2014; Grigorovich, Gomez, Leach, & Fish, 2013; Pliskin et al., 2006; Wesner & Hickie, 2013). Despite the heterogeneity of neuropsychological symptom presentation, a controlled investigation concerning neuropsychological symptom constellation in EI victims highlights specific impairments. In particular, cognitive deficits in attention/concentration, mental processing speed, and motor skills were more pronounced when compared with demographically and occupationally matched samples (Pliskin et al., 2006). Furthermore, these symptoms were not directly related to the severity of the physical injury as measured by surgery and hospitalization statistics, voltage exposure, litigation, or return-to-work status (Pliskin et al., 2006).

Emotional disturbance and problems with emotion regulation are very common symptoms reported by patients following EI. Although the victims of EI are sometimes mistakenly compared with patients who have experienced uncomplicated mild TBI, symptoms observed in EI may, in contrast, persist and in some cases, worsen over time (Bianchini, Love, Greve, & Adams, 2005; Chico, Capelli-Schellpfeffer, Kelly, & Lee, 1999; Hahn-Ketter et al., 2015; Pliskin et al., 2006). The following symptoms are commonly reported and may contribute to poorer cognitive ability and affect return-to-work status (Hahn-Ketter et al., 2015). Additionally, the significance of these emotional and cognitive symptoms may be more evident postacute injury and long-term (Aase et al., 2014; Pliskin et al., 2006; Ramati et al., 2009):

- Depression
- Anxiety
- Posttraumatic stress disorder (PTSD)
- Adjustment disorders
- Irritability and attitude change
- Decreased frustration tolerance

DIAGNOSTIC CONSIDERATIONS

The injury characteristics of electrical and lightning injury are multifaceted and heterogeneous; as a result, there are many diagnostic tools that various health care professionals can use to better understand symptom severity and prognosis. Arnold and Purdue's review of the literature suggests that all patients should undergo an electrocardiogram (ECG), regardless of the type of EI. Ongoing cardiac monitoring after EI is also recommended for patients who have the following history (Arnoldo & Purdue, 2009; Czuczman & Zane, 2009):

- Documented arrhythmia or evidence of ischemia
- Loss of consciousness
- Exposure to high-voltage (>1,000 V) EI

Laboratory Tests

Specific laboratory tests are recommended for patients with EIs beyond minor cutaneous burns (Arnoldo & Purdue, 2009; Czuczman & Zane, 2009) including:

- Complete blood count (CBC)
- Electrolytes
- Blood urea nitrogen (BUN) and creatine

To test for myoglobinuria, a urinalysis should be ordered. A serum myoglobin should be drawn as well. If intra-abdominal injury is suspected and/or surgery course is projected, authors suggest the following labs should also be ordered (Arnoldo & Purdue, 2009; Czuczman & Zane, 2009):

- Liver function tests/amylase/lipase
- Coagulation profile
- Blood type and screen/cross-match

Neurodiagnostic Imaging

Czuczman and Zane (2009) recommend a head computed tomography (CT) scan to evaluate for fractures or intracranial abnormalities (e.g., hemorrhage) in patients whose EI is associated with a fall, altered level of consciousness, or abnormal findings on neurologic examination. Similarly, plain films and CT scans of the spinal cord should be ordered if spinal cord injury is suspected. Additionally, radiography should be obtained in any area where the patient has pain, clear deformity, or decreased range of motion.

Evaluation of tissue perfusion and occult muscle damage prior to surgical exploration can be done with technetium-99 pyrophosphate scintigraphy. Magnetic resonance imaging (MRI) with gadolinium can also be a helpful adjunct to better localize areas of muscle necrosis (Czuczman & Zane, 2009).

Neuropsychological Assessment

Neuropsychological evaluation, as part of an overall comprehensive assessment, can be helpful in determining the presence and severity of possible neurocognitive deficits and psychological symptoms, while appreciating key issues like effort and motivation in mixed medico-legal contexts. Although briefer assessments or screening evaluations may be sufficient in acute inpatient settings or in other contexts with severely impaired patients, the breadth and depth of assessment afforded by a comprehensive neuropsychological evaluation is usually needed to address most outpatient referral questions. A comprehensive evaluation can also help determine on which areas rehabilitative treatment should focus, while also measuring improvement, decline, or stability over time. A comprehensive neuropsychological evaluation can be particularly useful in guiding medical–legal decisions in cases where clear physiological or neurological etiologies are minimal or lacking.

TREATMENT

Individuals who sustain electrical and lightning injuries may experience a host of wounds and other injuries as the direct or indirect effects of the electrical current. The nature and extent of treatment will depend on the nature of the injuries.

High-voltage EI causes significant tissue and organ damage along the path between contact wounds. The initial phase of treatment typically relies on acute clinical issues, such as restoring and maintaining cardiopulmonary stability. Treatment involves aggressive management of wounds and other injuries, including brain injuries that require surgical intervention, and control of pain. When indicated, especially in the case of high-voltage EI, individuals may be transferred to a regional burn center for burn care and extensive occupational and physical rehabilitation.

Victims of lighting injury may appear to have significant injuries, including transient symptoms (headaches, loss of consciousness, numbness, and weakness), encephalopathy and myelopathy, delayed neurological syndromes, and secondary complications resulting from falls, blast effects, or trauma from flying debris (Cherington, 2004). After spinal cord and intracranial injuries are excluded, observation and supportive care are the mainstays of treatment. Similarly, patients with low-voltage EI who have minor cutaneous burns or persistent minor symptoms may be discharged safely if they have a normal ECG and no urinary heme pigment that would be indicative of myoglobinuria (Czuczman & Zane, 2009).

Brain injuries associated with electrical or lightning injuries can manifest with different expectations for recovery, and different treatment needs are typically characterized by (Yarnell & Lammertse, 1995):

- Global dysfunction following cardiac arrest
- Focal brain injuries from direct electrical contact to the head or from falls

- Behavioral-cognitive sequelae without gross physical signs

With the goal of maximizing functioning, neurorehabilitation efforts should begin as soon as possible and, to the extent needed, involve multiple health care disciplines (Cherington, 2004). Clinicians typically begin to turn their attention toward cognitive, emotional, and behavioral symptoms only after the acute effects of the injury have been addressed. Neuropsychological treatment on an outpatient basis can address chronic pain, cognitive, emotional, and behavioral problems, long after the acute effects of the injury have dissipated. More often than not, the approach to rehabilitation is similar to that taken with TBIs and stroke (Barrash et al., 1996; Brenner, Vanderploeg, & Terrio, 2009; Primeau, 2005).

A hierarchically arranged approach to the treatment of neuropsychological problems following polytrauma that includes TBI and PTSD has been proposed (Brenner et al., 2009; Terrio et al., 2009). The steps consist of the following:

- Education: Pattern of recovery
- Behavioral health issues
- Somatic complaints/self-care routines
- Irritability/impulsivity
- Cognitive issues

PROGNOSIS

EI produces a variety of physical, cognitive, and emotional consequences. Prognosis ultimately depends on the severity of the initial injury and the development and severity of subsequent complications. Typically, the extent of burn injuries, as opposed to the voltage, is the main prognostic indicator earlier in the recovery period (Spies & Trohman, 2006). Deeper and more extensive burns may require emergent fasciotomy, debridement, and wound exploration (Spies & Trohman, 2006).

Price and Cooper (2013) summarize the primary complications and causes of death in EI, in temporal order of occurrence:

- Cardiopulmonary arrest
- Overwhelming traumatic injuries
- Cardiac arrhythmias

- Hypoxia and electrolytes
- Intracranial injuries
- Myoglobinuric renal failure
- Abdominal injuries
- Sepsis
- Tetanus
- Iatrogenic
- Suicide

Psychiatric and neurocognitive symptoms may complicate the survivor's psychosocial adjustment even 10 or more years postinjury (Aase et al., 2014; Hahn-Ketter et al., 2015). Acute presentation of psychiatric symptomatology, specifically depression, following EI can have a more significant impact on the course of recovery as well as psychosocial adjustment even years after the injury occurred (Hahn-Ketter et al., 2015). Other studies have also shown that the presence of acute stress disorder shortly following an EI can predict a more chronic course of PTSD at least 6 months to 2 years postinjury (Difede et al., 2002; McKibben, Bresnick, Askay, & Fauerbach, 2008). Diffuse EIs can occur in some individuals even in the absence of gross external injury or in the total absence of an obvious current path that affects the central nervous system, resulting in widespread physical, neurological, and neuropsychological symptoms that can persist for years after the injury (Berg & Morse, 2004; Primeau, 2005).

CLINICAL SYNOPSIS

Burns

- Low-voltage injuries tend to create small, well-defined burns at contact sites.
- High-voltage injuries tend to create severe burns that affect deep tissues and bones.
- In lightning injury, four types of minor burns are seen: linear, puncture, feathering, and thermal.
- Extensive flash and flame burns can result in severe hemodynamic, autonomic, cardiopulmonary, renal, metabolic, and neuroendocrine responses.

Musculoskeletal

- Severe tetanic muscle contractions or injuries sustained from falls can result in joint dislocations, fractures, and TBIs.
- Fractures are more common in the long bones of the upper limb and in vertebrae, the latter of which may cause spinal cord injuries. In cases of lightning-related injury, skull fractures and cervical spine injury from associated trauma may be seen.
- In high-voltage EI, direct electrothermal energy leading to coagulation necrosis may be the main cause of muscle injury.

Ocular, Auditory, and Cardiac Complications

- Cataracts and keratitis are often seen in victims, though symptoms may not appear immediately after injury.
- Auditory complications include hearing loss, tinnitus, and vertigo.
- Cardiac complications, including sinus tachycardia, supraventricular tachycardia, atrial fibrillation, and cardiac arrest may also occur, particularly when AC and/or high voltages are involved.

Neurological

- Loss of consciousness, confusion, and cognitive impairment can occur.
- Acute dysfunction of peripheral motor and sensory nerves may result.
- Seizures include both postacute and delayed onset.
- In cases of lightning injury, keraunoparalysis may occur, along with hypoxic encephalopathy and intracranial hemorrhage commonly affecting the basal ganglia and brain stem.
- Delayed neurological sequelae may include motor neuron disease and movement disorders, traumatic falls resulting in spinal cord injury, and epidural and subdural hematomas.

Cognitive and Emotional Disturbances

- Impairments in memory, attention, language, problem-solving ability, and executive dysfunction may occur during the acute, postacute, and postinjury recovery phase.
- Emotional disturbance is one of the most commonly reported symptoms by patients. Depression, anxiety, PTSD, adjustment disorder, irritability, attitude change, and decreased frustration tolerance may be observed and contribute to poorer cognitive ability.
- Physical symptoms with or without a clear pathophysiology may continue to persist for months and years postinjury. These may include pain, fatigue, reduced range of motion, headache, joint stiffness, motor weakness, blurred vision, coordination problems, dizziness, insomnia, and paresthesia.
- A wide range of cognitive and emotional difficulties may continue to persist as well, with depression and other mood disturbances often being cited as a predictor of psychosocial outcome.

CASE STUDIES

Lightning Injury

The patient was a right-handed, 36-year-old, divorced, Caucasian male who sustained injuries in a work-related lightning-strike accident 7 years before the date of the neuropsychological evaluation. While loading a large object (possibly an industrial machine) into the back of his semitruck at a wet-dock facility, lightning reportedly struck the object (which was housed in a metal skid), injuring the patient and two other workers, and causing the death of a fourth man due to heart attack secondary to electric shock. The patient described being "dazed" immediately after the lightning strike and described his memory of the event as "skipping sections." He reported feeling "numb" at the scene of the accident and focusing on helping one of his coworkers who had apparently suffered a heart attack secondary to the electrical trauma. The patient reported that he was discharged from the hospital after being evaluated and received no medical treatment that day. MRI of the brain with and without contrast 2 months postinjury was unremarkable. The patient reported a variety of cognitive, emotional, and physical problems that he attributed to the lightning accident.

On the neuropsychological examination, he performed adequately on most of the measures of effort that were included in the battery, though his performance on one subsection of a test administered late in the day suggested that his effort may have fluctuated toward the end of testing. His general intellectual ability was low average and somewhat lower than his estimated premorbid intelligence based on sight-reading/word recognition skills. In broad terms, the patient had a variable neuropsychological profile with noted inefficiencies in the areas of learning and memory, attention, and executive functioning. In the domain of memory, he showed particular impairment in the area of visual working memory and verbal memory. In the attentional domain, he also demonstrated impaired abilities on various tasks, including an index of working memory. His executive function abilities also varied, with several of his performances below average. His visuospatial abilities were largely intact. Motor function was within normal limits for his nondominant hand and mildly impaired for his dominant hand.

Overall, the patient's impairments were consistent with sequelae often observed following EI, with both cognitive and mood disruption. Factors such as pain, subjective mood disruption, and possible medication side effects were thought to have exacerbated his cognitive dysfunction, but were thought to be unlikely to entirely explain it. It was recommended that the patient participate in a pain-management program as well as individual psychotherapy.

Electrical Injury

The patient was a right-handed, 46-year-old, married, Caucasian male who was in good health when he sustained a work-related EI approximately 5 years before the neuropsychological evaluation. He was reportedly exposed to a primary voltage of over 12,000 V, reportedly resulting in a combination of direct electrical shock plus an arc shock and a fall. He had no direct memory of the injury event nor of anything that occurred for several hours after, but reported being told of the incident by coworkers. The patient reported that he and some coworkers were "cutting" a switch into a line, and diverted the current, allowing the contractor to safely install the switch. Following the installation, he was reading several meters when he clamped onto the third phase and the meter blew up, becoming engulfed in flames. Due to the force of the current, the patient then flew backwards an estimated 15 to 20 feet, hitting his partner, who then flew back further still. The patient reported that his face was approximately 2 feet away from the explosion when it occurred and that he was wearing a cotton shirt that was wet from perspiration and rubber gloves. He was told that following the explosion, he was lying on the ground foaming from the mouth and thrashing, and that it took eight football players from the local high school to hold him down. He was unsure if there was a loss of consciousness at that time. The patient reported that paramedics then arrived and later told him that his blood was black and coagulated, with his primary visible injuries being on his legs. Within the last 5 years, since the injury, he has had many physical, cognitive, and emotional complaints. He reported experiencing physical pain and paresthesia, which were his primary concern. He also reported experiencing cognitive symptoms within the last 2 to 3 years, especially having difficulty concentrating, problems with short-term memory, and difficulty planning and organizing information. Emotionally, the patient reported that he had been much more sensitive and moody and that he has troubling, intrusive thoughts about the accident. His wife also affirmed the reported cognitive and emotional changes since the accident.

On his cognitive exam, he was found to be functioning in the borderline impaired range of general intellectual ability, which was somewhat lower than would be expected on the basis of occupational attainment. However, his reported history of academic difficulties may have indicated an undiagnosed learning disability, affecting performance on academic skill measures. A more focused neurocognitive assessment indicated some difficulty with attention, specifically with sustained attention. He also showed variable but mild to moderately impaired memory performance on encoding and retrieving both verbal and visual information. Additionally, he had difficulty with complex problem solving, organization, and abstract reasoning. He showed largely intact language, visuospatial, and motor functions. On measures of personality/emotional functioning, the patient presented defensively, but indicated that he was experiencing a significant amount of psychological turmoil including feeling misunderstood, alienated, depressed, and lacking self-confidence. He also indicated that he was bothered by intrusive thoughts about the accident and sought to avoid concomitant unpleasant emotions.

Overall, the neurocognitive findings indicated that the patient was experiencing deficits in his attentional abilities, immediate and delayed memory, and executive functioning. He was also found to be experiencing significant symptoms that were consistent with PTSD. Cognitive deficits of this sort have been documented as potential sequelae of EI, as have some of the changes in personality and emotional functioning similar to that experienced by the patient. As part of his recovery, the patient was thought to be likely to benefit from engaging in cognitive behavioral therapy and cognitive rehabilitation.

REFERENCES

Aase, D. M., Fink, J. W., Lee, R. C., Kelley, K. M., & Pliskin, N. H. (2014). Mood and cognition after electrical injury: A follow-up study. *Archives of Clinical Neuropsychology, 29*(2), 125–130. doi:10.1093/arclin/act117

American Burn Association. (2015). *2015 National Burn Repository: Report of data from 2005–2014* (pp. 1–141). Retrieved from www.ameriburn.org/2015NBRAnnualReport.pdf

Arnoldo, B. D., & Purdue, G. F. (2009). The diagnosis and management of electrical injuries. *Hand Clinics, 25*(4), 469–479. doi:10.1016/j.hcl.2009.06.001

Barrash, J., Kealey, G. P., & Janus, T. J. (1996). Neurobehavioral sequelae of high voltage electrical injuries: Comparison with traumatic brain injury. *Applied Neuropsychology, 3*(2), 75–81.

Berg, J. S., & Morse, M. S. (2004). Diffuse electrical injury. *Practical Neurology, 4*(4), 222–227.

Bianchini, K., Love, J. M., Greve, K. W., & Adams, D. (2005). Detection and diagnosis of malingering in electrical injury. *Archives of Clinical Neuropsychology, 20*(3), 365–373. doi:10.1016/j.acn.2004.09.003

Brenner, L. A., Vanderploeg, R. D., & Terrio, H. (2009). Assessment and diagnosis of mild traumatic brain injury, posttraumatic stress disorder, and other polytrauma conditions: Burden of adversity hypothesis. *Rehabilitation Psychology, 54*(3), 239–246.

Bryan, B. C., Andrews, C. J., Hurley, R. A., & Taber, K. H. (2009a). Electrical injury: Part I: Mechanisms. *The Journal of Neuropsychiatry and Clinical Neurosciences, 21*(3), iv–244. doi:10.1176/appi.neuropsych.21.3.iv

Bryan, B. C., Andrews, C. J., Hurley, R. A., & Taber, K. H. (2009b). Electrical injury: Part II: Consequences. *The Journal of Neuropsychiatry and Clinical Neurosciences, 21*(4), iv. doi:10.1176/appi.neuropsych.21.4.iv

Capellie-Schellpfeffer, M., Miller, G. H., & Humilier, M. (1999). Thermoacoustic energy effects in electrical arcs. *Annals of the New York Academy of Sciences, 888*(1), 19–32.

Cherington, M. (2004). Spectrum of neurologic complications of lightning injuries. *NeuroRehabilitation, 20*(1), 3–8.

Chico, M. S., Capelli-Schellpfeffer, M., Kelley, K. M., & Lee, R. C. (1999). Management and coordination of postacute medical care for electrical trauma survivors. *Annals of the New York Academy of Sciences, 888*(1), 334–342.

Czuczman, A. D., & Zane, R. D. (2009). Electrical injuries: A review for the emergency clinician. *Emergency Medicine Practice, 11*(10), 1–20. Retrieved from www.ebmedicine.net/topics.php?paction=dLoadTopic&topic_id=201

Daniel, M., Haban, G. F., Hutcherson, W. L., Bolter, J., & Long, C. (1985). Neuropsychological and emotional consequences of accidental, high-voltage electrical shock. *International Journal of Clinical Neuropsychology, 7*(2), 102-106.

Difede, J., Ptacek, J. T., Roberts, J., Barocas, D., Rives, W., Apfeldorf, W., & Yurt, R. (2002). Acute stress disorder after burn injury: A predictor of posttraumatic stress disorder? *Psychosomatic Medicine, 64*(5), 826–834.

Duff, K., & McCaffrey, R. J. (2001). Electrical injury and lightning injury: A review of their mechanisms and neuropsychological, psychiaric, and neurological sequelae. *Neuropsychology Review, 11*(2), 101–116.

Electrical Safety Authority. (2012). *2012 Ontario electrical safety report: Electrical safety authority.* Mississauga, ON: Author.

Electrical Safety Foundation International. (2011). *20 Years of EI data show substantial electrical safety improvement.* Rosslyn, VA: Author.

Fink, J., Rog, L., Bush, S., & Pliskin, N. (2010). Electrical injury in the workplace. In S. S. Bush & G. L. Iverson (Eds.), *Neuropsychological assessment of work-related injuries.* New York, NY: Guilford Press.

Grigorovich, A., Gomez, M., Leach, L., & Fish, J. (2013). Impact of post-traumatic stress disorder and depression on neuropsychological functioning in electrical injury survivors. *Journal of Burn Care & Research, 34*(6), 659–665.

Hahn-Ketter, A., Aase, D. M., Paxton, J., Fink, J. W., Kelley, K. M., Lee, R. C., & Pliskin, N. H. (2015). Psychiatric outcome over a decade after electrical injury: Depression as a predictor of long-term adjustment. *Journal of Burn Care and Research, 36,* 509–512.

Heilbronner, R. L. (1994). Rehabilitation of the neuropsychological sequelae associated with electrical trauma. *Annals of the New York Academy of Sciences, 720,* 224–229.

Holle, R. L. (2008, April). Annual rates of lightning fatalities by country. In *Preprints of the International Lightning Detection Conference* (pp. 21–23).

Holle, R. L., López, R. E., & Navarro, B. C. (2005). Deaths, injuries, and damages from lightning in the United States in the 1890s in comparison with the 1990s. *Journal of Applied Meteorology, 44*(10), 1563–1573.

Hooshmand, H., Radfar, F., & Beckner, E. (1989). The neurophysiological aspects of electrical injuries. *Clinical EEG and Neuroscience, 20*(2), 111–120.

Jensenius, J. S., Jr. (2015). A detailed analysis of lightning deaths in the United States from 2006 through 2014. In *National Weather Service executive summary.* Fort Worth, TX: National Weather Service. Retireved from www.srh.weather.gov

Koumbourlis, A. C. (2002). Electrical injuries. *Critical Care Medicine, 30*(11, Suppl.), S424–S430.

Kouwenhoven, W. B. (1949). Effects of electricity on the human body. *Electrical Engineering, 68*(3), 199–203.

Martinez, J. A., & Nguyen, T. (2000). Electrical injuries. *Southern Medical Journal, 93*(12), 1165–1168.

McKibben, J. B., Bresnick, M. G., Askay, S. A. W., & Fauerbach, J. A. (2008). Acute stress disorder and posttraumatic stress disorder: A prospective study of prevalence, course, and predictors in a sample with major burn injuries. *Journal of Burn Care & Research, 29*(1), 22–35.

National Weather Service. (2015). *Weather fatalitieis.* Fort Worth, TX: Author. Retrived from www.nws.noaa.gov

Pfortmueller, C. A., Yikun, Y., Haberkern, M., Wuest, E., Zimmermann, H., & Exadaktylos, A. K. (2012). Injuries, sequelae, and treatment of lightning-induced injuries: 10 Years of experience at a Swiss Trauma Center. *Emergency Medicine International, 2012,* 1–7. doi:10.1155/2012/167698

Pliskin, N. H., Ammar, A. N., Fink, J. W., Hill, S. K., Malina, A. C., Ramati, A., . . . Lee, R. C. (2006). Neuropsychological changes following electrical injury. *Journal of the International Neuropsychological Society, 12*(1), 17–23.

Pliskin, N. H., Meyer, G. J., Dolske, M. C., Heilbronner, R. L., Kelley, K. M., & Lee, R. C. (1994). Neuropsychiatric aspects of electrical injury: A review of neuropsychological research [Review, 13 References]. *Annals of the New York Academy of Sciences,* 219–223.

Price, T. C., & Cooper, M. A. (2013). Electrical and lightning injuries. In J. Marx, R. Walls, & R. Hockberger (Eds.), *Rosen's emergency medicine: Concepts and clinical practice* (pp. 1906–1914). Philadelphia, PA: Elsevier Saunders.

Primeau, M. (2005). Neurorehabilitation of behavioral disorders following lightning and electrical trauma. *NeuroRehabilitation, 20*(1), 25–33.

Ramati, A., Rubin, L. H., Wicklund, A., Pliskin, N. H., Ammar, A. N., Fink, J. W., & Kelley, K. M. (2009). Psychiatric morbidity following electrical injury and its effects on cognitive functioning. *General Hospital Psychiatry, 31*(4), 360–366. doi:10.1016/j.genhosppsych.2009.03.010

Ritenour, A. E., Morton, M. J., McManus, J. G., Barillo, D. J., & Cancio, L. C. (2008). Lightning injury: A review. *Burns, 34,* 585–594. doi:10.1016/j.burns.2007.11.006

Silversides, J. (1964). The neurological sequelae of electrical injury. *Canadian Medical Association Journal, 91*(5), 195.

Spies, C., & Trohman, R. G. (2006). Narrative review: Electrocution and life-threatening electrical injuries. *Annals of Internal Medicine, 145*(7), 531–537.

Theman, K., Singerman, J., Gomez, M., & Fish, J. S. (2008). Return to work after low voltage electrical injury. *Journal of Burn Care & Research, 29*(6), 959–964. doi:10.1097/bcr.0b013e31818b9eb6

Terrio, H., Brenner, L. A., Ivins, B. J., Cho, J. M., Helmick, K., Schwab, K., . . . Warden, D. (2009). Traumatic brain injury screening: Preliminary findings in a U.S. Army Brigade Combat Team. *Journal of Head Trauma Rehabilitation, 24*(1), 14–23.

Wesner, M. L., & Hickie, J. (2013). Long-term sequelae of electrical injury. *Canadian Family Physician, 59,* 935–939.

Yarnell, P. R., & Lammertse, D. P. (1995). Neurorehabilitation of lightning and electrical injuries. *Seminars in Neurology, 15*(4), 391–396.

CHAPTER 9

Acquired Brain Injury Secondary to Substance Use Disorder

BENJAMIN A. PYYKKONEN

OVERVIEW

The *Diagnostic and Statistical Manual of Mental Disorders* (5th ed.; *DSM-5*; American Psychiatric Association [APA], 2013) identifies 10 separate classes of substances related to significant substance abuse concerns (p. 481). Each of these separate classes of substances has unique cognitive and behavioral profiles and sequelae. Of the 10 separate substance classes, four have more clearly documented patterns of pathophysiological sequelae and demonstrated impact on cognitive functioning. These substance categories include alcohol, inhalants, sedatives/hypnotics/anxiolytics, and stimulants. The following chapter discusses the specific impact of each of these separate classes of drugs and related acquired brain injury on cognitive and emotional functioning. The remaining six substance clusters include caffeine, cannabis, opioids, hallucinogens, tobacco, and other or unknown substances. Although these classes present with clear short-term cognitive, behavioral, and emotional impact, their cognitive impact is relatively transient in nature in comparison to the permanence of the impact associated with the other substance classes just noted. As such, the current review specifically examines only the impact of these four substance classes with clearly demonstrated cognitive profiles associated with acquired brain injury.

In addition, substance use and related inebriation puts one at remarkably increased risk for acquired brain injury secondary to head injury. Although in many cases this type of injury may be closely related to substance abuse, this manner of acquired head injury is not discussed here, but will be discussed in other chapters of this text (see Chapters 1 and 2).

HISTORY

The profound cost of substance use disorders is immense and has been documented to be in excess of several hundreds of billions of dollars annually (Kalechstein & van Gorp, 2007). Kalechstein and van Gorp (2007) also report a remarkably large number of admissions for substance misuse, with more than 1.7 million substance treatment-related admissions in 2003. These admissions likely reflect more acute intervention and not the chronic impact of substance misuse, and therefore underrepresent the actual impact. Although significant variation exists in the proportions of substance misuse from specific substance clusters, substance misuse is considerable across all geographic, ethnic, racial, financial, and age categories.

As already noted, substance use disorders, as described by the *DSM-5*, pertain to 10 distinct clusters of substance, in which there is problematic use characterized by four criteria (*DSM-5*, p. 485). Whereas previous classification systems emphasized tolerance and withdrawal symptoms, the current system emphasizes problematic use whether there is related dependence or not. The *DSM-5* criteria include impaired control (use exceeding intended use, cravings, unsuccessful attempts to reduce use, time spent acquiring, using, and recovering from substance use), social impairment (failure to fulfill major role obligations), risky use (physical hazard associated with use, persistent use despite experiencing negative consequences), and pharmacological criteria (increased tolerance to the substance and signs/symptoms of withdrawal) (5th ed.; *DSM-5*; APA, 2013).

Despite these well-documented consequences associated with it, substance use appears to have been evident in the archaeological records for many millennia around the world. Despite the long history of substance use and misuse, actual prevalence has fluctuated over time, and more recent data suggest that both use and misuse may be in slight decline after increases in previous decades (samhsa.gov). It is, however, worth noting that these Substance Abuse and Mental Health Services Administration (SAMHSA) data were collected largely prior to recent changes in state laws in which recreational marijuana use was decriminalized. Despite the political and legal attention given to marijuana use, this chapter focuses on other classes of drugs with a more clearly identified relationship to acquired brain injury or impact.

PATHOPHYSIOLOGY

The pathophysiology of each aforementioned substance class (alcohol, inhalants, sedatives, and stimulants) will be discussed in turn by class in the sections that follow.

Alcohol

Alcohol is a central nervous system (CNS) depressant. The CNS depressant effects of alcohol may cause impaired coordination, gait ataxia, slurred speech, and impaired saccadic movements of the eyes. In addition to the physical presentation associated with the acute effects of alcohol, intoxicated individuals demonstrate reduced capacity for response inhibition, which has been identified in studies of event-related potentials (ERP; Oscar-Berman & Marinković, 2007). However, of greater significance to acquired brain injury are the effects of long-term alcohol abuse/misuse characterized by dependence and withdrawal. The most extreme presentation of alcohol-related cognitive deficits is reflected in Wernicke–Korsakoff's syndrome in which profound anterograde memory loss is evident. Wernicke–Korsakoff's syndrome is attributable to a deficiency of thiamine caused by a dietary pattern in which the vast majority of calories consumed are alcohol related rather than more nutrient-rich foods. This thiamine deficiency results in "bilateral necrosis of the mammillary bodies and of a variety of medial diencephalic and other periventricular nuclei" (Blumenfeld, 2002). This deficiency and related Wernicke–Korsakoff's syndrome characterized by gait ataxia, acute confusion, lasting and profound impairment in memory consolidation, and confabulation represent the most significant cognitive presentation of acquired brain injury secondary to alcohol misuse. However, less significant cognitive presentations are associated with cerebral atrophy, white and gray matter loss, and reduced volume in the prefrontal cortex (Allen, Frantom, Forrest, & Strauss, 2006). In addition to the direct impact of prolonged exposure of the brain to alcohol, the indirect impact of alcohol on the brain caused by impaired liver functioning is also a significant potential source of acquired brain injury associated with alcohol exposure. Allen et al. (2006) identify significant impairment of memory, eye tracking, and hand–eye coordination in individuals with cirrhosis related to alcohol use when compared with individuals with non–alcohol-induced cirrhosis.

In addition to the potential long-term impact on the individual consuming alcohol, significant dysfunction of the CNS, craniofacial anomalies, disrupted free and postnatal growth, and markedly increased risk of intellectual disability and behavioral problems are associated with prenatal alcohol exposure, and may be described as fetal alcohol syndrome (FAS) or alcohol-related neurodevelopmental disorder (ARND) (Guerri, Bazinet, & Riley, 2009). These significant impairments and developmental disruption may be attributable to impaired functioning of glial cells, resulting in hypoplasia of the corpus callosum and anterior commissure, and microglial apoptosis (Wilhelm & Guizzetti, 2016).

Inhalants

Inhalants are broad and varied with regard to chemical type. The National Institute on Drug Abuse (NIDA, 2012) defines inhalants as "the wide variety of substances—including solvents, aerosols, gases, and nitrites—that are rarely, if ever, taken via any other route of administration" (www.drugabuse.gov/publications/drugfacts/inhalants). The pathophysiology of the particular inhalants is varied and related specifically to the particular inhalant. However, the most commonly inhaled substances for recreational use is toluene, which has a direct effect on the CNS as it readily passes through the blood–brain barrier, where it inhibits glutamate-activated ion channels (Cruz, Rivera-García, & Woodward, 2014). "In rat studies, acute and repeated toluene exposure markedly reduces metabolic function in the brain, especially the hippocampus, pons and thalamus. Toluene also increases dopamine release and the activity of dopaminergic neurons. Repeated exposure to toluene can lead to white matter damage (solvent vapor/toluene leukoencephalopathy), which may involve axonal damage rather than demyelination" (McKeown & Tarabar, 2015). Poor oxygenation related to inhalant use is also a strong risk factor for significant cognitive impairment and death due to anoxia (Cruz et al., 2014). Inhalant abuse can cause cardiac arrhythmias, hypoxia, hypothermia, and "sudden sniffing death" (Cruz et al., 2014). Organic solvent exposure (toluene being the most common), because of its lipophilic nature, preferentially impacts white matter (Yucel, Takagi, Walterfang, & Lubman, 2008). Periventricular white matter appears to be at particular risk in chronic toluene exposure (Yucel et al., 2008).

Sedatives/Hypnotics/Anxiolytics

Sedatives are a group of central nerve depressants that work primarily by facilitating the inhibitory gamma-aminobutyric acid (GABA) (Weaver, 2015). Sedative intoxication is manifest by unsteady gait, slowed reflexes, and nystagmus (Weaver, 2015). Severe overdose may result in impaired autonomic control of respiration and may cause anoxic injury, coma, or death (Weaver, 2015). Anoxic injury most significantly impacts areas of the brain that metabolize oxygen at higher rates and have reduced blood flow in comparison to other regions. The regions of the brain most sensitive to anoxia include the hippocampus, frontal regions, and thalamus (Mendoza & Foundas, 2008). Of these regions, those involved in memory (hippocampus) and executive functioning (neocortex, frontal regions, and thalamus) are most likely impacted by sedative overdose.

Stimulants

The stimulant class of substances includes drugs such as cocaine and methamphetamine. Each of the stimulant medications has its own particular risk profile. Among the greatest risks to cognitive and functional capacity from this class of substances is the increased risk for cerebral infarct and stroke related to the use of these substances. Cocaine, in particular, is a significant risk factor for stroke because of its capacity as a vasoconstrictor (Allen et al., 2006). Furthermore, cocaine use has been correlated with long-term reductions in cerebral metabolism in multiple regions including the orbitofrontal cortex, the anterior cingulate, dorsolateral prefrontal cortex, amygdala, putamen, and cerebellum (Bolla & Cadet, 2007). In their review, Bolla and Cadet (2007) identified the impact on multiple neurotransmitters including dopamine, serotonin, and norepinephrine. This constriction reduces arterial volume, thereby increasing blood pressure and risk for hemorrhage and stroke. Cocaine and amphetamine users are also at increased risk for seizures, which in turn may cause cell death. Amphetamines such as MDMA (ecstasy) may cause permanent damage to serotonergic systems through excitotoxicity. Further cellular damage may occur because of disruption of temperature regulation, causing hyperthermia, which may result in diffuse brain damage, coma, or death.

ETIOLOGY

Inherent to the ideology of acquired brain injury secondary to substance use is substance misuse. In general, the risk is directly proportionate to the amount of the substance used. Despite this rather direct and positive correlation between quantity and risk of acquired brain injury, there is significant interindividual variability in the risk of developing a pattern of habitual misuse, the development of tolerance to the substance, and chronicity of misuse. Allen et al. (2006) identify many risk factors for substance abuse including increased age as it relates to risk for abuse and dependence on benzodiazepines and younger age for alcohol and non–prescription drug misuse. It is also worth noting that there is a certain circular nature to the risk for substance use, as the acute and short-term deficits associated with substance misuse, namely impaired judgment and decreased inhibition, increase the likelihood of subsequent misuse/abuse.

EPIDEMIOLOGY

- Costs associated with substance use exceed 300 billion US dollars annually (Allen et al., 2006).
- The harmful use of alcohol results in 3.3 million deaths each year (World Health Organization [WHO], 2012).
- According to the annual report of the WHO (2012), individuals 15 years old or older consume 6.2 L of pure alcohol per year. This average consumption is noted in the context of large percentages of the world's population drinking little, if any, alcohol, which suggests that 38.3% of the population consumes an average 17 L of pure alcohol annually (United Nations Office on Drugs and Crime [UNODC], 2012; WHO, 2012).
- Alcohol consumption (UNODC, 2012; WHO, 2012):

- Worldwide, 61.7% of the population aged 15 years or older did not drink alcohol in 12 months preceding the survey. In all WHO regions, females are more often lifetime abstainers than males. There is considerable variation in the prevalence of abstention across WHO regions.
- 16.0% of drinkers aged 15 years or older engage in regular heavy episodic drinking (UNODC, 2012; WHO, 2012).

- Documented health consequences of alcohol consumption (UNODC, 2012; WHO, 2012):
  - Approximately 3.3 million deaths, or 5.9% of deaths, globally, were attributable to alcohol consumption.
  - Significant gender-based differences in the proportion of deaths throughout the world are attributable to alcohol, with men being at roughly twice the risk for injury related to alcohol use/misuse.
- Non–alcohol substance use (UNODC, 2012; WHO, 2012):
  - Recent estimates from 2008 suggest that 155 to 250 million people, or 3.5% to 5.7% of the world's population aged 15 to 64, used other psychoactive substances, including cannabis, amphetamines, cocaine, opioids, and nonprescribed psychoactive prescription medication. Cannabis continues to be the most commonly used substance of abuse, followed by amphetamine-type stimulants, then cocaine and opioids. Within this there is marked variability regionally.
  - With estimated annual prevalence rates ranging from 0.6% to 0.8% of the population aged 15 to 64 years, the use of opioids has remained stable (UNODC, 2012).
- Benzodiazepines:
  - Epidemiological data reviewed by Crowe and Barker (2007) indicate somewhere between 1.6% and 5% of the adult population regularly use benzodiazepines.
- Amphetamine/Stimulants:
  - Data published from a survey conducted in 2008 by the National Institute on Drug Abuse (2010) estimate 1.4 million Americans met the criteria for cocaine abuse/dependence over a 12-month period.

174 ACQUIRED BRAIN INJURY

- Data published from the 2012 National Survey on Drug Use and Health (SAMHSA, 2013) estimate that more than 12 million individuals aged 12 years or older have used methamphetamine in their lifetimes and 1.2 million used methamphetamine in the last year.

CLINICAL PRESENTATION

The clinical presentation associated with acquired brain injury related to substance use/misuse is variable. Important considerations related to this presentation include the amount used, the time over which this is used, and the time since use of the substance. Each of these classes of drugs mentioned earlier has distinct neurological, cognitive, and behavioral profiles related to the amount of time since the particular substance was used. Each of the substances will be discussed using the descriptors utilized by Allen et al. (2006): acute deficits, short-term deficits, and long-term deficits with respect to the time since exposure to the substance.

Alcohol

Acute Deficits
The acute neurocognitive deficits associated with short-term alcohol withdrawal (approximately 1 week following initial cessation) are characterized by significant improvement after initial demonstration of significant and broad deficits including memory, visuospatial ability, and general intellectual functioning (Allen et al., 2006).

Short-Term Deficits
The short-term neurocognitive deficits (2–5 weeks following initial cessation) associated with alcohol consumption include deficits across multiple aspects of executive functioning (abstract reasoning, problem solving), verbal memory, nonverbal memory, visuospatial ability, and impairment in gait and balance (Allen et al., 2006).

Long-Term Deficits
In individuals maintaining sobriety longer than 5 weeks, significant improvement across multiple cognitive domains, verbal abilities in particular, can be expected. However, ongoing impairment in aspects of executive functioning, motor, and memory are evident,

especially in individuals who have a longer history of alcohol abuse (Allen et al., 2006). In addition to these specific domain-based deficits, individuals with habitual alcohol use are at increased risk for global cognitive decline later in life.

Inhalants

The acute intoxication of toluene (a representative inhalant) is not dissimilar to that of inebriation caused by excessive alcohol substance. Individuals using toluene demonstrate impaired orientation to time, motor coordination, a euphoric state, emotional lability, slurred speech, blurred vision, and even illusions and hallucinations (Cruz et al., 2014). In addition to the acute effects associated with the "high" of toluene misuse, a well-documented pattern of chronic impairment has been demonstrated including impairment in memory, cognitive processing speed, attention/concentration, and executive functioning (Cruz et al., 2014). This impairment in cognition is in addition to increased risk for neurological symptoms including cerebellar ataxia, nystagmus, and hearing loss (Cruz et al., 2014). In addition to significant impairment evident in intentional misuse of toluene, there is evidence of long-term cognitive deficits resulting from occupational exposure in printers. Nordling, Karlson, Nise, Malmberg, and Orbaek (2010) examined CNS effects in printers 20 years after exposure, identifying declines in verbal memory, attention, and reasoning beyond that of a comparison group. In addition, the exposed group of printers reported slightly higher symptoms of depression than comparison controls.

Sedatives/Hypnotics/Anxiolytics

Benzodiazepines, a drug class with sedative, hypnotic, and anxiolytic qualities, will be reviewed with regard to its impact on cognitive performance.

Acute and Short-Term Cognitive Effects

In acute benzodiazepine intoxication, significant anterograde amnesia characterized by deficits in explicit memory, immediate and delayed recall may be seen, as well as impairment in verbal fluency tasks, psychomotor speed, effortful processing, and attention/working memory (Crowe & Barker, 2007). Not surprisingly, the degree of impairment appears to be dose dependent (Crow & Barker, 2007).

Long-Term Effects

In addition to the impact of short-term intoxication, the effects of long-term benzodiazepine use with no evidence of intoxication are significant. In a review of a series of meta-analytic studies, Crowe and Barker (2007) identified a pattern of significant cognitive impairment associated with chronic benzodiazepine use. In individuals with ongoing benzodiazepine use, significant impairment relative to controls was evident across multiple cognitive domains including "sensory processing, psychomotor speed, nonverbal memory, visuospatial awareness, speed of processing, problem solving, attention/concentration, verbal memory, general intelligence, motor control/performance, working memory, and verbal reasoning" (Crowe & Barker, 2007).

Long-Term Effects Post Withdrawal

Benzodiazepine use is associated with long-term cognitive deficits while actively being used. Although relatively few studies per cognitive domain were analyzed in the study, an additional meta-analytic review of studies examining cognitive performance in individuals with a history of long-term benzodiazepine use who are no longer using benzodiazepines revealed impaired verbal memory, psychomotor speed, speed of processing, motor control/performance, working memory, visuospatial, general intelligence, attention/concentration, and nonverbal memory (Barker, Greenwood, Jackson, & Crowe, 2004).

Stimulants

Cocaine

Acute effects

Immediately after administration of cocaine, significant improvement in performance on measures of attention and speed of information processing have been reported (Bolla & Cadet, 2007). This improvement is evident only in the acute stage. A pattern of impairment is, however, noted in studies examining longer term effects.

Short-term effects

In well-controlled studies examining cognitive functioning in cocaine abusers who have been abstinent for weeks, impaired performance has been found on measures of executive functioning, attention, impulsivity, visuoperception, psychomotor speed, manual dexterity, and verbal learning and memory (Bolla & Cadet, 2007)

In a systematic quantitative review of 46 studies, Potvin, Stavro, Rizkallah, and Pelletier (2014) identified a pattern of impairment across multiple cognitive domains including executive functions, impulsivity, verbal learning/memory, visuospatial ability, and working memory. This same meta-analytic review identified significant, but less robust, deficits in attention and speed of processing deficits in individuals with short-term abstinences, which were identified as short term by virtue of the participants' positive drug tests.

Long-term effects
In their review of cognitive functioning in cocaine abuse, Bolla and Cadet (2007) report a pattern of long-term deficits in performance across multiple cognitive domains in chronic cocaine abusers, including deficits in executive functioning, visuospatial processing, memory, concentration, and motor functioning after 6 months of abstinence. This is consistent with imaging results suggesting long-term impact of cocaine use upon brain atrophy with a fairly clear correlation with length of cocaine use history (Allen et al., 2006). In their meta-analytic review of cognitive performance in chronic cocaine abusers, Potvin et al. (2014) identified ongoing deficits at 12 and 20 weeks of abstinence. Deficits in cognitive performance at 12 weeks were identified across multiple cognitive domains including attention, executive functioning, impulsivity, language, speed of processing, verbal learning, verbal memory, visual learning, visual memory, visuospatial abilities, and working memory. In this same meta-analysis, although insufficient data were available for analysis at 20 weeks to look at specific domains, global impairment was documented (Potvin et al., 2014).

Methamphetamine

Acute effects
Low to moderate doses of methamphetamine may cause euphoria, arousal, and behavioral disinhibition; and in smaller therapeutic doses, short-term improvement in cognitive performance and anxiety may be seen; higher doses may precipitate psychotic episodes (Courtney et al., 2012), and paranoia, delirium, and anxiety are also noted in increased frequency with higher doses (Scott et al., 2007).

Short-term effects
Methamphetamine withdrawal is associated with significant depressive symptoms, irritability, anxiety, and hypersomnia, but is most often resolved in 14 days (Courtney et al., 2012).

Long-term effects

In a quantitative meta-analysis, Scott et al. (2007) identified moderate impairment associated with chronic methamphetamine use in episodic memory, executive functions, and information-processing speed, and lesser but still significant impact on motor skills, language, and visuoconstructional abilities. The pattern of impairment is described as "consistent with a frontostriatal neuropathogenesis, neurotoxicity along with perhaps more modest contributions from neurotoxicity in the posterior parietal and medial temporal cortices" (Scott et al., 2007). In another review, Allen et al. (2006) report verbal memory, executive function, attention/concentration, verbal fluency, and visual scanning persisting 1 year post abstinence.

DIAGNOSTIC CONSIDERATIONS

The fifth edition of the *Diagnostic and Statistical Manual of Mental Disorders* (*DSM-5*) provides diagnostic criteria for substance use disorder. In the previous edition (*DSM-IV*; APA, 2000), substance abuse and dependence were identified as separate categories, whereas in the current manual, these categories are collapsed into one category—substance use disorder (APA, 2013). This new single category classifies substance use disorder on a continuum from mild to severe. The new diagnostic category is divided into three degrees of severity: mild, moderate, and severe. The severity classification is based on the number of diagnostic criteria present; accordingly, cases with two to three present are classified as mild; four to five as moderate; and six to seven as severe substance use disorder. Whereas the *DSM-IV* emphasized the importance of abuse versus dependence/tolerance, the *DSM-5* appropriately identifies significant functional impact as evidence of abuse without tolerance/dependence. Whether associated with the number of diagnostic criteria or dependence/withdrawal, the overall exposure as it relates to cognitive dysfunction is largely consistent with a dose-dependent response independent of the drug category—more use results in increased risk for associated deficits in cognitive performance. Although by definition all substance use disorders cause significant functional and emotional distress/dysfunction, four specific substances classes have more clear cognitive profiles and have been discussed thus far. These classes specifically include alcohol, inhalants, sedatives/hypnotics/anxiolytics, and stimulants (e.g., cocaine/amphetamine). Finally, as it relates to understanding and diagnosing cognitive impairment related to substance use disorder, it is worth noting that cognitive inefficiencies/deficits are a risk factor for substance use disorder, which in turn is a risk factor for further cognitive impairment.

TREATMENT

Treatment of substance use disorder and related acquired brain injury is going to be highly specific to the injuries sustained, as well as the substance class that is misused. Despite this significant variability, similarities emerge when reviewing the existing literature. First, abstinence appears to arrest further progression of cognitive difficulties—alcohol-induced dementia is a notable exception to this. In this case, the alcohol consumption appears to accelerate the onset of other dementing conditions. Second, abstinence should be pursued under the treatment of a physician skilled and experienced in treating withdrawal symptoms. The withdrawal itself can be dangerous and should be monitored for safety. Treatment should include careful neuropsychological evaluation to identify the nature, presence, or severity of cognitive deficits by domain, which may be associated with chronic substance use or potentially related medical conditions such as stroke, epilepsy, and anoxia. In addition, consideration might be given to employing remediating and compensatory strategies related to any acquired cognitive impairment resulting from substance misuse. As noted earlier, the most commonly impacted domains are verbal memory and executive function/attention, and as such, these domains should be explicitly addressed in these rehabilitative approaches. This intervention is helpful not only because of its increased functionality, but may be especially helpful in the case of executive functioning and response inhibition as it relates to sobriety maintenance.

PROGNOSIS

The prognosis concerning recovery from acquired brain injury secondary to substance misuse is somewhat guarded. The reason for this guarded prognosis is related to difficulties in maintaining sobriety for individuals who have misused substances to such a degree as to cause significant cognitive impairment. This is particularly true, as already noted, because the domains and regions impacted by substance misuse from the classes reviewed (alcohol, inhalants, sedatives/hypnotics/anxiolytics, and stimulants) are the very domains/regions required to inhibit drug use and promote the development of coping strategies and alternatives. However, according to the literature, if abstinence can be achieved, some recovery of cognitive function can be expected in the months following cessation of substance misuse. Nevertheless, significant declines in performance across cognitive domains relative to controls and normative data can be expected in the long term.

CLINICAL SYNOPSIS

- Substance misuse/abuse is a significant risk factor for acquired brain injury. However, this relationship is not necessarily definitive, and individuals who abuse/misuse substances may not demonstrate cognitive impairment.
- Although unclear for other abused substances, the very long-term effects and risk for dementing conditions are well established for alcohol abuse/misuse.
- Shorter term deficits are evident in substance abuse and are largely consistent with a dose-dependent response related to degree of drug exposure and duration of exposure.
- Performance decrements on measures of cognitive ability are greatest in the acute and short-term abstinence from substance use. Notable reductions in cognitive impairment are present throughout the first year of abstinence.
- Although significant improvement following maintenance of abstinence can be expected, ongoing cognitive deficits, especially related to verbal memory, attention, concentration, executive functioning, and cognitive processing speed are often evident in individuals with a history of chronic substance misuse/abuse.
- Alcohol abuse is associated with increased risk for early "brain aging" characterized by brain atrophy and cognitive decline as well as increased risk for developing a dementing condition. This is true even after maintaining sobriety for many years.
- Further research is needed to clarify the very long-term (2 or more years of sobriety) expectations following abuse/misuse of substances other than alcohol.

CASE STUDY

The patient was a 38-year-old male with a long history of panic disorder without agoraphobia and more recent benzodiazepine abuse/misuse. He has repeatedly "taken extra" pills and has required additional prescriptions from his treating psychiatrist on numerous occasions. He has changed psychiatrists on many occasions owing to his consistent pattern of significantly overusing his anxiolytic (clonazepam). In response to concerns about his benzodiazepine use (specifically clonazepam), his current treating psychiatrist suggested admission to an inpatient unit to "detox" from clonazepam. In the recent past, the patient presented for physical therapy because of balance difficulties and vertigo. The vertigo and balance difficulties were first evident following an attempt to reduce clonazepam use. He described being very fearful of future reduction, and stated that he "needs" the clonazepam to function and has needed increased amounts over the past 4 years. He reported attempting to find a psychiatrist who was willing to "work with him" to get additional clonazepam. He has also requested multiple prescriptions from his primary care physician. He also reports often feeling foggy or overly tired at work, which he attributes to taking more than his recommended dosage of clonazepam. This tiredness and grogginess has been noted by his immediate supervisor. He has had to leave work early on many occasions alternately because of his anxiety and building sense of panic and his grogginess. He presented rather disheartened in response to his panic symptoms and reliance on increasing levels of clonazepam to help him cope with his panic.

With regard to *DSM-5* criteria for substance use disorder (APA, 2013), this patient met the diagnostic criteria for moderate substance use disorder (4–5 criteria).

- He reported an increased need for clonazepam to manage his anxiety and panic symptoms and that he would often take more of the medication than prescribed, despite not intending to do so.
- He has unsuccessfully attempted to reduce his use of clonazepam, but, instead, has only increased it further.
- He reported that his pattern of clonazepam use has negatively impacted his occupational activities.
- A clear pattern of tolerance was evident, as he had taken more and more of the medication to manage his anxiety.

Treatment

Most importantly, the patient will need to gradually reduce his benzodiazepine use so as not to facilitate "rebound anxiety." Rebound anxiety, a sharp increase in anxiety-related symptomatology, is not uncommon when reducing benzodiazepine usage, and is characterized by a sharp increase in anxiety-related symptoms after benzodiazepine usage has been decreased. This phenomenon is related to withdrawal symptoms and can be rather distressing for the individual. More gradual declines in benzodiazepine use reduce the risk of rebound anxiety. Consideration should be given to anxiolytic medications that are not benzodiazepines, as well as to cognitive behavioral therapy, potentially including interceptive exposure. With regard to the cognitive effects of benzodiazepine misuse, the patient has, fortunately, not had any seizures related to withdrawal when he has attempted to reduce medication usage on his own. However, there was some evidence of reduced efficiency in problem solving and attention. If these cognitive factors present as a growing impediment to treatment, consideration should be given to ordering a neuropsychological evaluation in order to better understand the nature, presence, or severity of domain-based deficits as they might be related to treatment and occupational/social functioning. This domain-based analysis might also inform therapeutic clinical work so that it might be better tailored to the patient's strengths. Should any particular personal or normative deficits be evident, long-term neuropsychological follow-up would be recommended.

REFERENCES

Allen, D. N., Frantom, L. V., Forrest, T. J., & Strauss, G. P. (2006). Neuropsychology of substance use disorders. In P. J. Snyder, P. D. Nussbaum, & D. L. Robbins (Eds.), *Clinical neuropsychology: A pocket handbook for assessment*. Washington, DC: American Psychological Association.

American Psychiatric Association. (2000). *Diagnostic and statistical manual of mental disorders* (4th ed., text revision). Washington, DC: Author.

American Psychiatric Association. (2013). *Diagnostic and statistical manual of mental disorders* (5th ed.). Arlington, VA: American Psychiatric Publishing.

Barker, M. J., Greenwood, K. M., Jackson, M., & Crowe, S. F. (2004). Persistence of cognitive effects after withdrawal from long-term benzodiazepine use: A meta-analysis. *Archives of Clinical Neuropsychology, 19*(3), 437–454. doi:10.1016/S0887-6177(03)00096-9

Blumenfeld, H. (2002). *Neural anatomy through clinical cases*. Sunderland, MA: Sinauer Associates.

Bolla, K. I., & Cadet, J. L. (2007). Cocaine. In A. Kalechstein & W. G. van Gorp (Eds.), *Neuropsychology and substance use: State-of-the-art and future directions*. New York, NY: Taylor & Francis.

Courney, K., Arelano, R., Barkley-Levenson, E., Galvan, A., Poldrack, R., Mackillop, J., . . . Ray, L. (2012). The relationship between measures of impulsivity and alcohol misuse: An integrative structural equation approach. *Alcohol Clinical Experimental Research, 36*(6), 923–931.

Crowe, S. F., & Barker, M. J. (2007). Benzodiazepines. In A. Kalechstein & W. G. van Gorp (Eds.). *Neuropsychology and substance use: State-of-the-art and future directions*. New York, NY: Taylor & Francis.

Cruz, S. L., Rivera-García, M. T., & Woodward, J. J. (2014). Review of toluene action: Clinical evidence, animal studies and molecular targets. *Journal of Drug and Alcohol Research, 3*, 1–15.

Guerri, C., Bazinet, A., & Riley, E. P. (2009). Foetal alcohol spectrum disorders and alterations in brain and behaviour. *Alcohol and Alcoholism, 44*(2), 108–114. doi:10.1093/alcalc/agn105

Kalechstein, A., & van Gorp, W. (2007). *Neuropsychology and substance use: State-of-the-art and future directions*. New York, NY: Taylor & Francis.

McKeown, N., & Tarabar, A. (2015). *Toluene toxicity*. Retrieved from http://emedicine.medscape.com/article/818939-overview

Mendoza, J., & Foundas A. (2008). *Clinical neuroanatomy: A neurobehavioral approach*. New York, NY: Springer.

National Institute on Drug Abuse. (2010). *Research report series: Cocaine abuse and addiction*. Bethesda, MD: National Institutes of Health, U.S. Department of Health and Human Services.

National Institute on Drug Abuse. (2012). *DrugFacts: Inhalants*. Retrieved from www.drugabuse.gov/publications/drugfacts/inhalants

Nordling, N., Karlson, B., Nise, G., Malmberg, B., & Orbaek, P. (2010). Delayed manifestations of CNS effects in formerly exposed printers—A 20-year follow-up. *Neurotoxicology and Teratology, 32*(6), 620–626.

Oscar-Berman, M.,& Marinkovic, K. (2007). Alcohol: Effects on neurobehavioral functions and the brain. *Neuropsychology Review, 17*(3), 239–257.

Potvin, S., Stavro, K., Rizkallah, E., & Pelletier, J. (2014). Cocaine and cognition: A systematic quantitative review. *Journal of Addiction Medicine, 8*(5), 368–376. doi:10.1097/ADM.0000000000000066

Scott, J. C., Woods, S. P., Matt, G. E., Meyer, R. A., Heaton, R. K., Atkinson, J. H., & Grant, I. (2007). Neurocognitive effects of methamphetamine: A critical review and meta-analysis. *Neuropsychology Review, 17*(3), 275–297. doi:10.1007/s11065-007-9031-0

Substance Abuse and Mental Health Services Administration. (2013). *Results from the 2012 National Survey on Drug Use and Health: Summary of national findings* (NDSUH Series H-46, HHS). Rockville, MD: Author.

United Nations Office on Drugs and Crime. (2012). *World Drug Report 2012*. Retrieved from https://www.unodc.org/documents/data-and-analysis/WDR2012/WDR_2012_web_small.pdf

Weaver, M. F. (2015). Prescription sedative misuse and abuse. *The Yale Journal of Biology and Medicine, 88*(3), 247–256.

Wilhelm, C. J., & Guizzetti, M. (2016). Fetal alcohol spectrum disorders: An overview from the glia perspective. *Frontiers in Integrative Neuroscience, 9*, 65. doi:10.3389/fnint.2015.00065

World Health Organization. (2012). *Facts and figures*. Geneva, Switzerland: Author. Retrieved from www.who.int/substance_abuse/facts/en

Yucel, M., Takagi, M., Walterfang, M., & Lubman, D. (2008). Toluene misuse and long-term harms: A systematic review of the neuropsychological and neuroimaging literature. *Neuroscience and Neurobehavioral Reviews, 32*, 910–926.

CHAPTER 10

Post–Acquired Brain Injury Headaches

MAURICIO F. VILLAMAR
JONATHAN H. SMITH

OVERVIEW

Headache (HA) attributed to acquired brain injury (ABI), and particularly HA attributed to traumatic brain injury (TBI), is among the most common secondary HA disorders (Headache Classification Committee of the International Headache Society, 2013). Although posttraumatic headache (PTH) can occur in isolation, it is often a component of postconcussion syndrome (PCS), an entity that includes multiple somatic, cognitive, and psychological symptoms. These may include HA, fatigue, memory and concentration deficits, sleep disturbances, mood changes, anxiety, dizziness, blurred vision, among others (Dikmen, Machamer, Fann, & Temkin, 2010) (see Chapter 1).

Interestingly, HA and other pain disorders are more frequent in milder as compared with more severe TBI (Nampiaparampil, 2008; Yamaguchi, 1992). This is thought to be secondary to damage to central nervous system (CNS) structures involved in affective pain processing seen in severe TBI (Riechers, Walker, & Ruff, 2015), or also thought to be caused by a higher likelihood of developing a sensitization effect after mild injury (Miller, 2000). However, it is also possible that pain is underrecognized in people with deficits in communication or cognition as a consequence of severe brain injury.

The presence of post-ABI HA does not necessarily imply coexistence of severe underlying anatomical abnormalities. However,

HA can be a manifestation of disorders such as intracranial or extra-axial hematomas or other mass lesions, carotid–cavernous fistulas, communicating hydrocephalus, dural leaks, and/or ventriculoperitoneal shunt malfunction. In the appropriate setting, the foregoing should be considered part of the evaluation of HA.

HISTORY

- HA disorders have been written about throughout the centuries, with references to sick-headaches in Sumerian poems, Egyptian papyrus, and in the writings of Hippocrates (c.460–c.370 BCE).
- Hippocrates described complications of head injury, with later authors referring to the effects of *commotio cerebri* after trauma (McCrory & Berkovic, 2001).

PATHOPHYSIOLOGY

The pathophysiology of post-ABI HA is yet to be fully understood. The genesis of chronic pain after CNS injury appears to be related in part to the increased expression of certain sodium channel subtypes, leading to neuronal hyperexcitability, particularly in the thalamus and in other regions involved in pain processing (Waxman & Hains, 2006). Activation of microglia and production of prostaglandin E_2 perpetuates sodium channel overexpression (Zhao, Waxman, & Hains, 2007).

Episodic tension–type HA appears to be secondary to nociceptive stimuli originating from pericranial myofascial tissues. If such noxious stimuli persist over a prolonged period of time, sensitization of pain pathways in the CNS such as the spinal dorsal horn and the trigeminal nucleus may ensue, leading to HA chronification. Decreased antinociceptive activity from supraspinal structures, impairing the descending inhibition of pain, may also be a contributing factor (Bendtsen & Jensen, 2009).

Pathogenesis of post-ABI migraine-like HA is complex, and many mechanisms have been involved. These include increased cortical excitability secondary to proinflammatory and excitatory molecules leading to spreading depression; structural damage to the meninges and blood vessels; and dysfunctional activation of the trigeminal nucleus caudalis (Riechers et al., 2015).

Cervicogenic HA may develop as a consequence of injury to the cervical vertebrae and cervical paraspinal muscles. This is particularly common in acceleration–deceleration or rotational injuries affecting the head and neck (Riechers et al., 2015).

ETIOLOGY

HA may occur in the setting of multiple causes of ABI. These may all be identified through an appropriate clinical history and neurologic examination.

Traumatic Brain Injury

- TBI is defined as a structural or functional lesion secondary to the effect of external forces on the head, such as blunt trauma, acceleration/deceleration movements (e.g., whiplash), penetrating injuries, blasts or explosions (see Chapters 1 and 2).
- HA is among the commonest sequelae of TBI, and most of the information discussed in this chapter is centered on this topic.

Cerebrovascular Disease

- HA that occurs in the setting of an acute onset, focal neurologic deficit should prompt concern for a medical emergency, such as ischemic stroke or intracranial hemorrhage.
- HA that is abrupt in onset and progression ("thunderclap onset") requires immediate emergency evaluation to screen for aneurysmal subarachnoid hemorrhage.

Meningoencephalitis/Encephalitis

- HA is the commonest and often the first symptom of meningitis and encephalitis (see Chapter 5).
- The diagnosis should be suspected when HA is accompanied by neck stiffness, fever, altered mental status, and/or seizures.
- Early, aggressive treatment with antimicrobial agents is critical to reducing morbidity and mortality resulting from CNS infections.

- Release of bacterial toxins and inflammatory mediators directly stimulate sensory terminals in the meninges. Increased intracranial pressure can occur in encephalitis and also have a role in the genesis of HA (Headache Classification Committee of the International Headache Society, 2013).

EPIDEMIOLOGY

Prevalence of HA immediately following TBI can be as high as 90% (Obermann, Keidel, & Diener, 2010). It can persist beyond 6 months in up to 44% of patients (Martelli, Grayson, & Zasler, 1999), and beyond 1 year in 18% to 33% (Lew et al., 2006).

Mild TBI has been linked to a higher risk of developing PTH as compared with moderate or severe TBI. Another significant risk factor is the preexistence of HA before injury (Lew et al., 2006). Older age appears to be protective and, although some evidence suggests a higher likelihood of developing PTH in females, there are no clear differences between genders (Lucas, Hoffman, Bell, & Dikmen, 2014).

The prevalence of PTH differs between civilian and military populations. Among civilians, HA has been reported to persist for more than 3 months in 15% of mild TBI patients (Faux & Sheedy, 2008). This contrasts with a prevalence of 52% to 55% among Operation Iraqi Freedom and Operation Enduring Freedom veterans 1 year after suffering mild combat TBI (Lew et al., 2009; Ruff, Riechers, Wang, Piero, & Ruff, 2012). This may be related, at least in part, to differences in brain injury mechanisms. For instance, exposure to blasts is much more frequent in the latter population, and has been associated with neuronal dysfunction even in the absence of obvious structural lesions (Kato et al., 2007). Likewise, the concurrent presence of mental health conditions (e.g., depression and posttraumatic stress disorder), which is higher in military populations, may play a role.

CLINICAL PRESENTATION

Clinical presentations of PTH are variable. Multiple HA subtypes have been described, including those with characteristics of tension-type HA, migraine, cervicogenic HA and, more rarely, cluster HA, hemicrania continua, and chronic paroxysmal hemicrania (Finkel, Yerry, Scher, & Choi, 2012).

In civilians, tension-type HA appears to be the most frequent semiology (37%–85% of all PTH) (Evans, 2004; Lew et al., 2006), although some studies suggest that migraine may be the predominant type (Lucas, Hoffman, Bell, Walker, & Dikmen, 2012). Cervicogenic HA is less common, and approximately 10% of PTH cannot be classified as a diagnosable syndrome (Lucas et al., 2014). Among military populations, as well as in children, most PTH (55%–78%) are described as migraine-type (Kuczynski, Crawford, Bodell, Dewey, & Barlow, 2013; Theeler & Erickson, 2009; Theeler, Flynn, & Erickson, 2010).

The most common semiologies of post-ABI HA are characterized by the following features:

- *Migraine phenotype:* Location preferentially unilateral, but can change sides. Pain described as throbbing or pulsating. Frequently associated with nausea, vomiting, or dizziness. Tends to worsen with exertion and exposure to loud sounds or bright lights. Can be preceded by transient neurologic symptoms (i.e., aura). Moderate to severe intensity.
- *Tension-type phenotype:* Location bilateral, predominantly occipital, although commonly holocephalic, helmet- or band-like. Pain typically dull, pressure-like, pulling, or dragging but not pulsating. Absence of associated nausea or vomiting, and less frequent environmental sensitivities as compared to migraine. Not worsened by physical activity. Mild to moderate intensity.

DIAGNOSTIC CONSIDERATIONS

A careful clinical assessment is essential in the evaluation of HA. HA diaries are also critical in establishing HA characteristics, triggers, premonitory signs, severity, frequency, and duration.

Brain imaging studies are not ordered routinely in all patients with post-ABI HA. However, certain signs and symptoms can suggest the presence of intracranial lesions or elevated intracranial pressure that warrant neuroimaging. These may include HA that awakens the patient from sleep, HA that worsens with Valsalva maneuver or when lying down, or the concomitant presence of double vision, seizures, gait difficulty, or papilledema (optic disk swelling). Any abnormality on the neurologic examination should prompt further investigation.

If symptoms develop acutely after the injury, a CT scan of the head is the initial test of choice, particularly to evaluate for hemorrhagic complications. When evaluating the patient days, weeks, or longer after the injury, MRI is of much higher yield.

Traumatic Brain Injury

- According to the third edition of *The International Classification of Headache Disorders* (ICHD-3), HA is arbitrarily attributed to traumatic injury if it develops within 7 days of either (a) head injury, (b) regaining consciousness following head injury, or (c) discontinuation of drugs that impair ability to sense or report HA following injury (Headache Classification Committee of the International Headache Society, 2013).
- Temporal relation is easy to establish when HA occurs shortly after trauma. However, in a study of civilians with mild to moderately severe TBI, approximately 28% of new HA had its onset 3 or more months after the injury (Hoffman et al., 2011). Among war veterans, only 27% of HA had its onset within the first 7 days of injury (Theeler & Erickson, 2009), all of which complicates the diagnosis of post-ABI HA.
- Temporal classification of HA attributed to TBI:
  - *Acute:* if HA duration is less than 3 months.
  - *Persistent:* if HA continues for more than 3 months after injury and cannot be better explained by another ICHD-3 diagnosis.
- When HA following trauma becomes persistent, the possibility of medication-overuse HA should be considered.

Cerebrovascular Disease

- HA with acute onset neurologic deficits requires emergency room evaluation with CT scan of the head to screen for intracranial hemorrhage.
- The clinical history of a thunderclap HA (rapidly peaking, typically within 1 minute) requires a standard emergency room approach with a CT, sometimes followed by a lumbar puncture to screen for a ruptured aneurysm.

Meningoencephalitis/Encephalitis

- The classic triad of HA, fever, and neck stiffness seen in meningitis is relatively uncommon, although the presence of two of these features is relatively sensitive for the diagnosis (Attia, Hatala, Cook, & Wong, 1999).
- The diagnosis requires empiric treatment with intravenous antimicrobials, along with blood cultures and spinal fluid evaluation. Patients who are older (>60), immunocompromised, and/or have an abnormal neurologic examination should undergo CT imaging of the head before lumbar puncture out of concern for precipitating brain herniation.

TREATMENT

The treatment of post-ABI HA should be determined by the predominant HA phenotype (i.e., migraine, tension-type) (Seifert & Evans, 2010). To date, there have been no class I studies supporting treatment of post-ABI HA. Most therapeutic approaches are empiric or anecdotal (Watanabe, Bell, Walker, & Schomer, 2012).

Neither the severity of the initial injury nor the duration of HA has been found to serve as a marker that assists in the choice of optimal HA treatment. Interdisciplinary care, comprising pharmacologic, nonpharmacologic, behavioral, and educational approaches, appears to be most effective. Choice of medications should be based on HA characteristics, medication side effects, and presence of comorbidities in a patient (see Tables 10.1 and 10.2).

Pharmacologic Interventions

- In general, acute pharmacologic treatment is more successful when taken at the onset of the HA attack rather than waiting until symptoms have begun to worsen.
- Opiates (oxycodone, codeine, morphine, among others) and combination medications containing barbiturates (Fioricet, Fiorinal) are only rarely used in the treatment of post-ABI HA in view of the risk of medication-overuse HA. Medication-overuse HA, a pattern of worsening HA with overuse of acute pain medications, can be seen from use of barbiturates for as little as 5 days per month, and 8 days per month for opioids (Bigal & Lipton, 2009). In addition, prolonged use

TABLE 10.1 COMMON ABORTIVE MEDICATIONS USED FOR THE ACUTE TREATMENT OF POST–ACQUIRED BRAIN INJURY HEADACHE

Headache Type	Medication Class	Comments
Tension-type	Acetaminophen (paracetamol)	• Avoid total doses of acetaminophen of more than 4 g/d owing to risk of liver toxicity.
	NSAIDs (i.e., ibuprofen, diclofenac, naproxen)	• Naproxen, which has a long half-life, is less associated with medication-overuse HA and has a better cardiovascular profile with long-term use. • Prolonged use should be avoided in patients with renal or peptic ulcer disease.
Migraine	NSAIDs	• NSAIDs can be given parenterally (ketorolac) or as suppositories (indomethacin).
	Triptans (i.e., sumatriptan, eletriptan, rizatriptan, frovatriptan, naratriptan)	• Triptans are available in different formulations that are preferred in certain patients. These can include orally disintegrating tablets for those with difficulty swallowing or significant nausea and vomiting, as well as intranasal and subcutaneous formulations for faster onset of action. • Naratriptan and frovatriptan have the longest half-life and lowest side-effect profile. • Triptans can cause vasoconstriction and are contraindicated in patients with uncontrolled hypertension, stroke, or coronary artery disease. • Are associated with medication-overuse HA if taken more than 9 d/mo.

(continued)

TABLE 10.1 COMMON ABORTIVE MEDICATIONS USED FOR THE ACUTE TREATMENT OF POST–ACQUIRED BRAIN INJURY HEADACHE (*continued*)

Migraine (*continued*)	Dopamine receptor 2 antagonists (metoclopramide, prochlorperazine, promethazine)	• Are particularly helpful in patients who experience significant nausea and/or vomiting. • Are not associated with rebound HA. • Prolonged use has been associated with extrapyramidal side effects, which include a variety of drug-induced movement disorders.
	Combination analgesics (i.e., Excedrin migraine)	• Are associated with increased risk of medication-overuse HA if used more than 10 d/mo.

HA, headache; NSAIDs, nonsteroidal anti-inflammatory drugs.

    is associated with tolerance and dependence, sedation, and sometimes withdrawal seizures.

- An overview of abortive medications commonly used for the acute treatment of post-ABI HA is presented in Table 10.1.
- Prophylactic, or preventive medications, should be considered in patients who experience frequent episodes of post-ABI HA (approximately two to three or more per week). Table 10.2 describes some of the medications used for this indication.
- Among "natural" treatments, magnesium, butterbur (Petasites), vitamin B_{12}, and coenzyme Q10 have been used as prophylactic interventions, particularly for migraine. Magnesium and Petasites have the strongest evidence (Holland et al., 2012), but the latter has been associated with the risk of liver toxicity, which could limit its long-term use.

Nonpharmacologic Interventions

- Use of nonpharmacologic interventions of post-ABI HA can be considered either alone or in combination with medication. In general, nonpharmacologic treatments tend to be

TABLE 10.2 COMMON PROPHYLACTIC MEDICATIONS FOR POST–ACQUIRED BRAIN INJURY HEADACHE

Headache Type	Medication Class	Comments
Tension-type	TCAs (amitriptyline, nortriptyline)	• Amitriptyline is drug of choice for tension-type HA prophylaxis. • TCAs should preferably be taken at night due to sedation. Can help treat insomnia. • Should use low dose and titrate up slowly. • Can decrease seizure threshold; avoid in epilepsy patients. • Can be cardiotoxic in high dosages. Use cautiously in patients with history of suicide attempts.
	Other antidepressants (i.e., mirtazapine, venlafaxine)	• Mirtazapine and venlafaxine are drugs of second choice. • Selective serotonin reuptake inhibitors, such as citalopram and sertraline, have not been found to be more effective than placebo for tension-type HA prophylaxis.
Migraine	Beta-blockers (i.e., propranolol, metoprolol)	• Beta-blockers are contraindicated in patients with asthma or chronic obstructive pulmonary disease because they can cause bronchoconstriction. • It is necessary to monitor heart rate because they cause bradycardia. • There is conflicting evidence on whether beta-blockers can increase risk of depression.

(continued)

TABLE 10.2 COMMON PROPHYLACTIC MEDICATIONS FOR POST–ACQUIRED BRAIN INJURY HEADACHE (continued)

Migraine (continued)	Antiepileptic drugs (topiramate, valproic acid, gabapentin)	• Valproic acid and topiramate are category D in pregnancy owing to risk of fetal malformations. If at all possible, avoid in reproductive-age women. • Valproic acid can be an adjunct in treatment of mood disorders. • There is strong evidence for topiramate in prevention of HA. Can lead to weight loss, kidney stones, and cognitive changes. • Gabapentin can be helpful in the treatment of neuropathic pain.
	Botulinum toxin	• FDA approved for the treatment of chronic migraine. • Local injections tend to be well tolerated. Very rare side effects include allergic reactions, and distal spread of toxin causing muscle weakness, double vision, difficulty in swallowing.

HA, headache; TCAs, tricyclic antidepressants.

preferred when patients have poor medication tolerance or contraindications to their use, are pregnant or nursing, have suboptimal relief from medication use, are experiencing symptoms of medication-overuse HA, or simply prefer to try nonpharmacologic alternatives.

- In general, most nonpharmacologic treatments are aimed at preventing or decreasing HA frequency and severity rather than being used for acute HA treatment.
- Behavioral treatments have the most robust evidence to support their use in post-ABI HA prophylaxis. Some of the most common evidence-based approaches include cognitive behavioral therapy, relaxation, and biofeedback (Nicholson, Buse, Andrasik, & Lipton, 2011).

- Among complementary and alternative medicine interventions, use of acupuncture in migraine and tension-type HA is supported by systematic reviews (Linde et al., 2009a, 2009b).
- Although physical therapy is often not a first line of treatment, its use can be very effective for certain types of HA, particularly cervicogenic. Interventions most often consist of exercises targeting cervical alignment and musculature, and can help identify "trigger points" that can precipitate HA (Riechers et al., 2015).
- There is no evidence to establish spinal manipulative therapies or massage as a first-line therapy (Nicholson et al., 2011). Homeopathy is ineffective in HA treatment (Ernst, 1999).
- Surgery and different neuromodulation techniques can be considered when more conservative management fails (Villamar, Santos Portilla, Fregni, & Zafonte, 2012).

Lifestyle Modifications

- Identification of HA triggers and their subsequent avoidance can be helpful in decreasing HA severity and frequency. A HA diary can be an excellent way to identify them.
- Common triggers may include sleep deprivation, stress, bright lights, loud noises, and certain foods such as monosodium glutamate, nitrates, aspartame, excess caffeine, and alcohol (particularly red wine). Other triggers, which are more difficult to avoid, can include hormonal and weather changes.

Addressing Comorbidity

- Among patients with post-ABI chronic HA, addressing patient-specific factors such as medication-overuse HA, caffeine overuse, etiologies of disrupted sleep, comorbid psychiatric conditions (especially posttraumatic stress disorder), obesity, and tobacco dependence are important measures to decrease HA frequency and severity and to improve the overall quality of life.

PROGNOSIS

The prevalence of HA immediately following TBI can be as high as 90% (Obermann et al., 2010). It can persist beyond 6 months in up to 44% of patients (Martelli et al., 1999), and beyond 1 year in 18% to 33% (Lew et al., 2006). HA will meet the criteria for persistent post-ABI HA if it continues for more than 3 months after injury and cannot be better explained by another ICHD-3 diagnosis. There is usually improvement in HA severity and frequency after the first 6 months. However, many patients with persistent HA at this time could continue to suffer HA indefinitely (Riechers et al., 2015).

Among patients with moderate to severe TBI, the presence or absence of anatomical abnormalities during the acute postinjury phase does not appear to correlate with the risk of developing post-ABI HA at 1 year (Lucas, Devine, Hoffman, & Dikmen, 2013). HA appears to be more severe and have a greater functional impact in patients who suffer penetrating as opposed to closed-head injuries (Walker et al., 2013).

When evaluating patients for persistent HA, the possibility of medication-overuse HA needs to be considered because more than 70% of patients with PTH use over-the-counter medication (DiTommaso et al., 2014).

Litigation has been linked to persistence of PTH. Neuropsychological testing has shown a direct relationship between greater amount of potential compensation and increasing rate of failure on malingering indicators in individuals who suffered mild TBI (Seifert & Evans, 2010). Similarly, "when tort compensation in Saskatchewan, Canada was changed to a no-fault system without payments for pain and suffering, the number of claims decreased by about 25%" (Cassidy et al., 2000). Occasionally, patients' HA fails to recover even after claim settlement. The extent to which this can be secondary to reinforcement of behavior or due to persistence of somatic symptoms is unclear (Seifert & Evans, 2010).

CLINICAL SYNOPSIS

- Post-ABI HA is one of the most common secondary HA disorders.
- Post-ABI HA does not have specific clinical features. Diagnosis is based primarily on temporal relation to the injury, and the etiopathogenesis of the injury (i.e., meningitis, physical trauma).
- Neuroimaging is not part of the routine workup for patients with chronic post-ABI HA. However, it needs to be considered if there are signs or symptoms suggestive of intracranial lesions or elevated intracranial pressure.

- Tension-type and migraine HA are the most frequent semiologies encountered in civilians, military populations, and children.
- Choice of medications should be based on HA characteristics, medication side effects, and patient comorbidities.
- Pharmacologic interventions in post-ABI HA are of two types: those used for the acute treatment of HA, and those that aim at preventing HA recurrence.
- Multiple nonpharmacologic interventions can be helpful adjuncts in the treatment of post-ABI HA. Among these, behavioral treatments such as cognitive-behavioral therapy, relaxation, and biofeedback have the strongest evidence.
- Comorbidities, such as posttraumatic stress disorder, should be screened for and treated concurrently with HA to optimize quality of life.
- There is usually improvement in HA severity and frequency after the first 6 months following the injury. However, many patients who have persistent HA at this time could continue to suffer HA indefinitely. Litigation may play a role in some cases.

CASE STUDY

A 42-year-old woman presented to the clinic with persistent HA 2 years following a motor vehicle collision, where she briefly lost consciousness. She reported a history of infrequent episodic migraine HA since childhood, but now has daily, severe, holocephalic HA associated with nausea, light-and-sound sensitivity. She reported treating her HA with daily over-the-counter combination analgesics containing acetaminophen, caffeine, and aspirin. In addition, she reported flashbacks and nightmares related to the injury.

After being reassured by a normal neurologic examination, one can diagnose her with chronic posttraumatic HA, which is presenting with a migrainous phenotype. One can suspect medication overuse and probable posttraumatic stress disorder as comorbidities that are likely aggravating her condition. Prescription consideration includes topiramate to an initial target dose of 50 mg twice daily, recommendation of withdrawal from the combination analgesic, and then referring her to a counselor for the mood disorder. Additional considerations for prescriptions include naproxen sodium, sumatriptan, and prochlorperazine for abortive treatment.

At 3 months' follow-up, she reported HA-free days for the first time since her injury, and an overall 50% improvement in HA frequency and intensity.

REFERENCES

Attia, J., Hatala, R., Cook, D. J., & Wong, J. G. (1999). The rational clinical examination: Does this adult patient have acute meningitis? *JAMA, 282*(2), 175–181.

Bendtsen, L., & Jensen, R. (2009). Tension-type headache. *Neurologic Clinics, 27*(2), 525–535. doi:10.1016/j.ncl.2008.11.010

Bigal, M. E., & Lipton, R. B. (2009). Overuse of acute migraine medications and migraine chronification. *Current Pain and Headache Reports, 13*(4), 301–307.

Cassidy, J. D., Carroll, L. J., Cote, P., Lemstra, M., Berglund, A., & Nygren, A. (2000). Effect of eliminating compensation for pain and suffering on the outcome of insurance claims for whiplash injury. *The New England Journal of Medicine, 342*(16), 1179–1186. doi:10.1056/NEJM200004203421606

Dikmen, S., Machamer, J., Fann, J. R., & Temkin, N. R. (2010). Rates of symptom reporting following traumatic brain injury. *Journal of the International Neuropsychological Society, 16*(3), 401–411. doi:10.1017/S1355617710000196

DiTommaso, C., Hoffman, J. M., Lucas, S., Dikmen, S., Temkin, N., & Bell, K. R. (2014). Medication usage patterns for headache treatment after mild traumatic brain injury. *Headache, 54*(3), 511–519.

Ernst, E. (1999). Homeopathic prophylaxis of headaches and migraine? A systematic review. *Journal of Pain and Symptom Management, 18*(5), 353–357.

Evans, R. W. (2004). Post-traumatic headaches. *Neurologic Clinics, 22*(1), 237–249, viii. doi:10.1016/S0733-8619(03)00097-5

Faux, S., & Sheedy, J. (2008). A prospective controlled study in the prevalence of posttraumatic headache following mild traumatic brain injury. *Pain Medicine, 9*(8), 1001–1011. doi:10.1111/j.1526-4637.2007.00404.x

Finkel, A. G., Yerry, J., Scher, A., & Choi, Y. S. (2012). Headaches in soldiers with mild traumatic brain injury: Findings and phenomenologic descriptions. *Headache, 52*(6), 957–965. doi:10.1111/j.1526-4610.2012.02167.x

Headache Classification Committee of the International Headache Society. (2013). The International Classification of Headache Disorders, 3rd edition (beta version). *Cephalalgia, 33*(9), 629–808. doi:10.1177/0333102413485658

Hoffman, J. M., Lucas, S., Dikmen, S., Braden, C. A., Brown, A. W., Brunner, R., ... Bell, K. R. (2011). Natural history of headache after traumatic brain injury. *Journal of Neurotrauma, 28*(9), 1719–1725. doi:10.1089/neu.2011.1914

Holland, S., Silberstein, S. D., Freitag, F., Dodick, D. W., Argoff, C., Ashman, E., ...The American Headache Society. (2012). Evidence-based guideline update: NSAIDs and other complementary treatments for episodic migraine prevention in adults: Report of the Quality Standards Subcommittee of the American Academy of Neurology and the American Headache Society. *Neurology, 78*(17), 1346–1353. doi:10.1212/WNL.0b013e3182535d0c

Kato, K., Fujimura, M., Nakagawa, A., Saito, A., Ohki, T., Takayama, K., & Tominaga, T. (2007). Pressure-dependent effect of shock waves on rat brain: Induction of neuronal apoptosis mediated by a caspase-dependent pathway. *Journal of Neurosurgery, 106*(4), 667–676. doi:10.3171/jns.2007.106.4.667

Kuczynski, A., Crawford, S., Bodell, L., Dewey, D., & Barlow, K. M. (2013). Characteristics of post-traumatic headaches in children following mild traumatic brain injury and their response to treatment: A prospective cohort. *Developmental Medicine and Child Neurology, 55*(7), 636–641. doi:10.1111/dmcn.12152

Lew, H. L., Lin, P. H., Fuh, J. L., Wang, S. J., Clark, D. J., & Walker, W. C. (2006). Characteristics and treatment of headache after traumatic brain injury: A focused review. *American Journal of Physical Medicine & Rehabilitation, 85*(7), 619–627. doi:10.1097/01.phm.0000223235.09931.c0

Lew, H. L., Otis, J. D., Tun, C., Kerns, R. D., Clark, M. E., & Cifu, D. X. (2009). Prevalence of chronic pain, posttraumatic stress disorder, and persistent postconcussive symptoms in OIF/OEF veterans: Polytrauma clinical triad. *Journal of Rehabilitation Research and Development, 46*(6), 697–702.

Linde, K., Allais, G., Brinkhaus, B., Manheimer, E., Vickers, A., & White, A. R. (2009a). Acupuncture for migraine prophylaxis. *Cochrane Database of Systematic Reviews,* (1), CD001218. doi:10.1002/14651858.CD001218.pub2

Linde, K., Allais, G., Brinkhaus, B., Manheimer, E., Vickers, A., & White, A. R. (2009b). Acupuncture for tension-type headache. *Cochrane Database of Systematic Reviews,* (1), CD007587. doi:10.1002/14651858.CD007587

Lucas, S., Devine, K. B., Hoffman, J., & Dikmen, S. (2013). *Acute neuroimaging abnormalities associated with post-traumatic headache following traumatic brain injury.* Paper presented at the American Academy of Neurology Annual Meeting, San Diego, CA.

Lucas, S., Hoffman, J. M., Bell, K. R., & Dikmen, S. (2014). A prospective study of prevalence and characterization of headache following mild traumatic brain injury. *Cephalalgia, 34*(2), 93–102. doi:10.1177/0333102413499645

Lucas, S., Hoffman, J. M., Bell, K. R., Walker, W., & Dikmen, S. (2012). Characterization of headache after traumatic brain injury. *Cephalalgia, 32*(8), 600–606. doi:10.1177/0333102412445224

Martelli, M. F., Grayson, R. L., & Zasler, N. D. (1999). Posttraumatic headache: Neuropsychological and psychological effects and treatment implications. *The Journal of Head Trauma Rehabilitation, 14*(1), 49–69.

McCrory, P. R., & Berkovic, S. F. (2001). Concussion: The history of clinical and pathophysiological concepts and misconceptions. *Neurology, 57*(12), 2283–2289.

Miller, L. (2000). Neurosensitization: A model for persistent disability in chronic pain, depression, and posttraumatic stress disorder following injury. *NeuroRehabilitation, 14*(1), 25–32.

Nampiaparampil, D. E. (2008). Prevalence of chronic pain after traumatic brain injury: A systematic review. *JAMA, 300*(6), 711–719. doi:10.1001/jama.300.6.711

Nicholson, R. A., Buse, D. C., Andrasik, F., & Lipton, R. B. (2011). Nonpharmacologic treatments for migraine and tension-type headache: How to choose and when to use. *Current Treatment Options in Oncology, 13*(1), 28–40. doi:10.1007/s11940-010-0102-9

Obermann, M., Keidel, M., & Diener, H. C. (2010). Post-traumatic headache: Is it for real? Crossfire debates on headache: Pro. *Headache, 50*(4), 710–715. doi:10.1111/j.1526-4610.2010.01644.x

Riechers, R. G., II, Walker, M. F., & Ruff, R. L. (2015). Post-traumatic headaches. *Handbook of Clinical Neurology, 128*, 567–578. doi:10.1016/B978-0-444-63521-1.00036-4

Ruff, R. L., Riechers, R. G., II, Wang, X. F., Piero, T., & Ruff, S. S. (2012). For veterans with mild traumatic brain injury, improved posttraumatic stress disorder severity and sleep correlated with symptomatic improvement. *Journal of Rehabilitation Research and Development, 49*(9), 1305–1320.

Seifert, T. D., & Evans, R. W. (2010). Posttraumatic headache: A review. *Current Pain and Headache Reports, 14*(4), 292–298. doi:10.1007/s11916-010-0117-7

Theeler, B. J., & Erickson, J. C. (2009). Mild head trauma and chronic headaches in returning US soldiers. *Headache, 49*(4), 529–534. doi:10.1111/j.1526-4610.2009.01345.x

Theeler, B. J., Flynn, F. G., & Erickson, J. C. (2010). Headaches after concussion in US soldiers returning from Iraq or Afghanistan. *Headache, 50*(8), 1262–1272. doi:10.1111/j.1526-4610.2010.01700.x

Villamar, M. F., Santos Portilla, A., Fregni, F., & Zafonte, R. (2012). Noninvasive brain stimulation to modulate neuroplasticity in traumatic brain injury. *Neuromodulation, 15*(4), 326–338. doi:10.1111/j.1525-1403.2012.00474.x

Walker, W. C., Marwitz, J. H., Wilk, A. R., Ketchum, J. M., Hoffman, J. M., Brown, A. W., & Lucas, S. (2013). Prediction of headache severity (density and functional impact) after traumatic brain injury: A longitudinal multicenter study. *Cephalalgia, 33*(12), 998–1008. doi:10.1177/0333102413482197

Watanabe, T. K., Bell, K. R., Walker, W. C., & Schomer, K. (2012). Systematic review of interventions for post-traumatic headache. *PM&R: The Journal of Injury, Function, and Rehabilitation, 4*(2), 129–140. doi:10.1016/j.pmrj.2011.06.003

Waxman, S. G., & Hains, B. C. (2006). Fire and phantoms after spinal cord injury: Na+ channels and central pain. *Trends in Neurosciences, 29*(4), 207–215. doi:10.1016/j.tins.2006.02.003

Yamaguchi, M. (1992). Incidence of headache and severity of head injury. *Headache, 32*(9), 427–431.

Zhao, P., Waxman, S. G., & Hains, B. C. (2007). Extracellular signal-regulated kinase-regulated microglia-neuron signaling by prostaglandin E_2 contributes to pain after spinal cord injury. *Journal of Neuroscience, 27*(9), 2357–2368. doi:10.1523/JNEUROSCI.0138-07.2007

CHAPTER 11

Post–Acquired Brain Injury Epilepsy

ERIN PLUMLEY
ROBERT J. KOTLOSKI
BRUCE HERMANN

OVERVIEW

Epilepsy resulting from an acquired brain injury (ABI), that is acquired epilepsy, is a significant clinical problem that is likely to increase in the future owing to medical advances that will allow for improved survival following ABI and to shifts in demographics resulting in the growth of elderly populations at high risk for ABI and epilepsy. Although the capacity of ABI to cause epilepsy has been known for millennia, our understanding of the pathophysiology of acquired epilepsy and our abilities to diagnose and to treat remain severely limited. However, with increased awareness of ABI and its sequelae, including epilepsy, it can be reasonably hoped that improvements will be forthcoming.

In this chapter, we will overview acquired epilepsy with a focus on posttraumatic epilepsy (PTE), including epidemiology, pathophysiology, and clinical care. In addition, we will briefly discuss other common etiologies of post-ABI epilepsy, including poststroke epilepsy and tumor-associated epilepsy (TAE). A case study will be provided at the end of the chapter to provide further consideration of disability and life-altering consequences of ABI and epilepsy.

204 ACQUIRED BRAIN INJURY

INTRODUCTION

To address the issue of epilepsy resulting from an ABI, it is important to first review the definitions of relevant terms. As noted so far in this book, ABI refers to a wide spectrum of brain injuries resulting from nongenetic and noncongenital causes, typically divided into traumatic or nontraumatic etiologies. ABIs include traumatic brain injury (TBI) or cerebral concussion, stroke, anoxia, tumor, intracranial and intracerebral hemorrhage, encephalitis, or other acquired insults (Teasell et al., 2007b). Common sequelae of ABIs include well-known cognitive, emotional, and behavioral changes, though there may also be a variety of less visible consequences, including epileptogenesis. Epileptogenesis refers to the process whereby a nonepileptic brain transitions to a brain with an enduring predisposition to generate unprovoked seizures (i.e., an epileptic brain) (Jensen, 2009). Seizures are an abnormal, excessive, or synchronous neuronal activity in the brain resulting in signs or symptoms (Fisher et al., 2005). As defined by the International League Against Epilepsy (ILAE), epilepsy is defined by any of

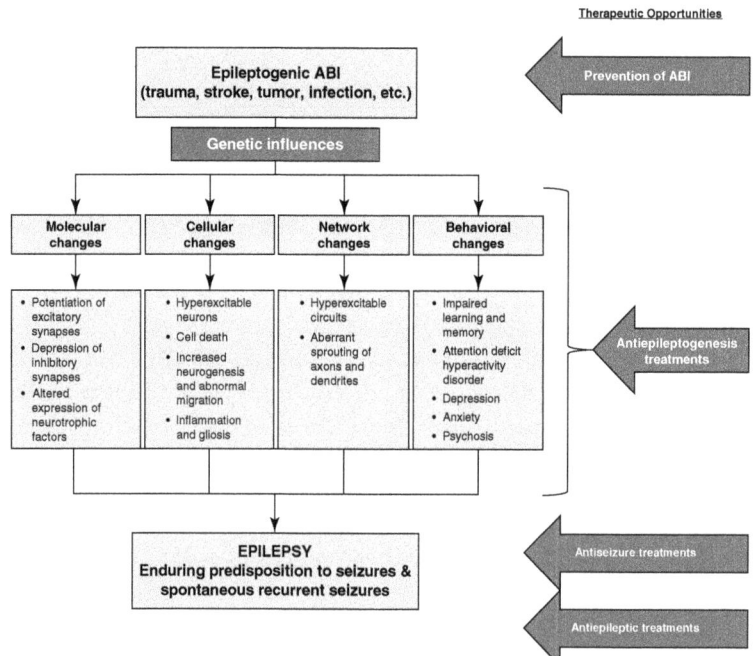

Figure 11.1. Progression of epileptogenic acquired brain injury (ABI) and therapeutic opportunities.

the following conditions: (a) at least two unprovoked (or reflex) seizures occurring greater than 24 hours apart; (b) one unprovoked (or reflex) seizure and a probability of further seizures similar to the general recurrence risk after two unprovoked seizures, occurring over 10 years; and (c) a diagnosis of an epilepsy syndrome (Fisher et al., 2014). Figure 11.1 demonstrates the progression of epileptogenic acquired brain injury and therapeutic opportunities.

Epilepsy is estimated to affect approximately 70 million individuals worldwide, with a lifetime incidence of up to 5 per 1,000 in developed countries and two- to threefold greater in developing countries (Ngugi, Bottomley, Kleinschmidt, Sander, & Newton, 2010). The impact of unpredictable seizures in epilepsy has a significant effect on the quality of life, which can result in serious injuries, limitations on activities including driving restrictions, and stigma, which can further limit employment and social interactions (Jacoby & Austin, 2007). Furthermore, cognitive deficits and mental health disorders are frequently seen as comorbidities with epilepsy (LaFrance, Kanner, & Hermann, 2008), even outside the setting of ABI. Current pharmacological therapies fail to control seizures in 25% to 30% of individuals (Kwan & Brodie, 2000; Mattson, Cramer, & Collins, 1996), and despite the introduction of several new antiseizure medications, including those with novel mechanisms of action, the proportion of medically intractable cases remains stable (Boon, Chauvel, Pohlmann-Eden, Otoul, & Wroe, 2002; Cross & Riney, 2009; Leppik, 2002; Matsuo & Riaz, 2009). Additionally, antiseizure medications are known to have a variety of significant adverse effects (Swann, 2001), including impairing cognitive functioning (Park & Kwon, 2008), which may be particularly problematic in the setting of ABI.

ETIOLOGY AND EPIDEMIOLOGY

Posttraumatic Epilepsy

PTE is a common as well as particularly debilitating long-term consequence of TBI that accounts for nearly 20% of all acquired epilepsies in the general population (Agrawal, Timothy, Pandit, & Manju, 2006; Teasell, Bayona, Lippert, Villamere, & Hellings, 2007a). ABI and TBI are recently gaining recognition as major health concerns (Annegers, Grabow, Kurland, & Laws, 1980). For example, in military populations, TBI accounts for a third of all combat-related injuries, and TBI is seen in 60% of veterans with a blast-related injury (Okie, 2005). In all, 500,000 individuals suffer from PTE in the United States and the European Union (Pitkänen, Bolkvadze, & Immonen, 2011). Epilepsy following TBI is particularly challenging as other sequelae of TBI are exacerbated by unpredictable seizures and the potential adverse effects of antiseizure medications. PTE, with acute and chronic changes resulting from TBI and epileptogenesis, and with focal and global structural pathology, is a prototype for epileptogenesis in other forms of ABI-related epilepsy in which the more extensive nature of the disease is often more difficult to appreciate.

Over the past several decades, clinical research into the various aspects of acquired epilepsy have included diagnostic methodology, risk factors, recurrence, treatment, and experimental models. A TBI is defined by the Department of Defense and the Department of Veterans Affairs (Traumatic Brain Injury Task Force, 2007) as any traumatically induced structural injury and/or physiological disruption of brain function as a result of an external force that is indicated by new onset or worsening of at least one of the following clinical signs, immediately following the event: (a) any period of loss of or a decreased level of consciousness; (b) any loss of memory for events immediately before or after the injury; (c) any alteration in mental state at the time of injury; (d) neurological deficits that may or may not be transient; (e) intracranial lesion. Recent data from nonmilitary populations (Faul, Xu, Wald, & Coronado, 2010) estimate that 1.7 million people sustain a TBI each year in the United States. Of those individuals, 52,000 die as a result of their injury, which contributes to nearly one-third of all injury-related deaths (Institute of Medicine Committee on Gulf War and Health, 2008). Another 275,000 are hospitalized, and the remaining 1.365 million are treated and released from the emergency department. Furthermore, TBI-related emergency department visits have increased 14.4% and hospitalizations have increased 19.5% from 2002 to 2006. The number of TBIs that do not receive medical care is also not known, but is estimated to be significant for mild injuries. The costs of TBI in the United States are estimated to be $60 billion annually, which includes the significant costs due to TBI-related disability. As the vast majority of those suffering from TBI survive (greater than 95%), these individuals are at risk for long-term consequences, such as PTE. And as the incidence of TBI-related emergency department visits and hospitalizations has been increasing, the mortality from TBI has been declining, likely due to preventative measures such as helmets and seat belts as well as improved treatment (Coronado et al., 2011). Therefore, more individuals survive TBI and potentially suffer long-term consequences, such as PTE.

Following a TBI, seizures can occur immediately (<24 hours), early (1–7 days), or late (>7 days). While immediate and early seizures are thought to relate to the acute severity of the TBI, late seizures suggest that epileptogenesis secondary to TBI has occurred and produced a permanent propensity for seizures. The length of time between injury and the emergence of clinical seizures is variable and may be prolonged, with 12.6% of veterans presenting with a first seizure more than 14 years after the TBI (Raymont et al., 2010). As the definition of epilepsy is a brain with an enduring predisposition to generate seizures and at least one unprovoked seizure (Fisher et al., 2014), those with at least one unprovoked, late seizure following TBI could qualify for a diagnosis of PTE. Furthermore, in those with TBI who suffer a single late seizure, 86% will have a second seizure within 2 years (Haltiner, Temkin, & Dikmen, 1997). Data from the Vietnam conflict demonstrate that over 50% of individuals with penetrating head trauma develop PTE (Raymont et al., 2010; Salazar et al., 1985). Other studies (Annegers, Hauser, Coan, & Rocca, 1998) have demonstrated the 30-year cumulative incidence of epilepsy following TBI is 2.1% for mild injuries, 4.2% for moderate injuries, and 16.7% for severe injuries. Therefore, even the least affected group of TBI demonstrates a two- or threefold increase in the risk for epilepsy. The risk of developing new onset epilepsy following a mild TBI is increased even 10 years following the injury (Christensen et al., 2009).

With these continuing risks and the debilitating features of PTE, and likely increase in prevalence in the future due to a variety of factors, there is major unmet clinical need for improved understanding about the vulnerabilities to late effects of TBI and identification of therapeutic targets to prevent PTE. Currently there are no good predictors of PTE, other than risk based on the severity of the initial injury, and no treatments exist to modify the development of PTE despite significant efforts (Beghi, 2003; Temkin, 2009; Temkin et al., 1990; Temkin et al., 1999). Furthermore, PTE is often pharmaco-resistant to available antiseizure drugs (Herman, 2002), which magnifies the impact of PTE once seizures begin.

PATHOPHYSIOLOGY

As previously stated, epileptogenesis is the process of structural and functional changes, including the collective molecular-, cellular-, and systems-level mechanisms, that transform the normal brain to one that generates spontaneous recurrent seizures occurring following a brain insult, such as TBI, stroke, infection, and status epilepticus (Dudek & Sutula, 2007; Pitkänen & Lukasiuk, 2009; Vezzani et al., 2016). The "latentcy period" is a concept suggesting that after ABI occurs, there is a variable critical period of time from or during the time of the brain insult before the occurrence of the first spontaneous seizure (Pitkänen & Lukasiuk, 2009; Vezzani et al., 2016), which suggests a progressive series of cellular changes may be involved as well as different pathophysiological processes (Agrawal et al., 2006; Hunt, Boychuk, & Smith, 2013). The latent period may last months or years, and during this time the structure and physiology of the brain experiences epileptogenic changes that result in the development of epilepsy (Vezzani et al., 2016). Furthermore, many molecular and cellular studies have been oriented to the analysis of changes that may occur during the latent period (Dudek & Staley, 2011).

The presence of spontaneous burst discharges that develop after a mechanical brain insult seems to be a necessary minimal criterion for the human "PTE" model (Hunt et al., 2013). It is likely that other models of epilepsy and epileptogenesis, in which a slowly evolving process leads to circuit plasticity with permanent structural and functional changes and eventually to spontaneous seizures such as the kindling model (McNamara, 1986; Morimoto, Fahnestock, & Racine, 2004), share many mechanisms with PTE. Additionally, the molecular mechanisms activated in response to ABI overlap with mechanisms identified as important for epileptogenesis. For example, the neurotrophin brain-derived neurotrophic factor (BDNF) and its receptor TrkB have been demonstrated to play an important role in epileptogenesis in the kindling model (Binder, Routbort, Ryan, Yancopoulos, & McNamara, 1999; He et al., 2004; Kotloski & McNamara, 2010) and following TBI (Hu et al., 2004; Rostami et al., 2014). BDNF has been demonstrated to activate the JAK-STAT pathway, which regulates transcription of GABA-A receptor subunits (Lund et al., 2008), and the JAK-STAT pathway is also activated following TBI (Raible, Frey, & Brooks-Kayal, 2014; Raible, Frey, Cruz Del Angel, Russek, & Brooks-Kayal,

2012). Tau, an axonal protein with a microtubule-binding domain in its phosphorylated forms, has been demonstrated to aggregate into intracellular tangles following brain trauma (Corsellis, Bruton, & Freeman-Browne, 1973; McKee et al., 2009), as well as in other chronic neurologic diseases including Alzheimer's disease (Grundke-Iqbal et al., 1986). Tau has also been linked to hyperexcitability (Holth et al., 2013), and genetic removal of tau decreases seizures in a mouse model of Alzheimer's disease (Roberson et al., 2011), perhaps due to loss of GABAergic interneurons (Andrews-Zwilling et al., 2010; Li et al., 2009). Plaques of Aβ protein have also been shown in numerous studies of TBI (Ikonomovic et al., 2004; Roberts, Allsop, & Bruton, 1990; Roberts et al., 1994). The burden of Aβ in the brain has also been shown to increase seizure susceptibility in mouse models of Alzheimer's disease, and the apoE4 mice develop spontaneous tonic-clonic seizures (Hunter et al., 2012). Microglial activation, as measured by glial fibrillary acidic protein (GFAP) immunoreactivity, increases following TBI (Carbonell & Grady, 1999; Regner et al., 2001; Shitaka et al., 2011), and GFAP in serum has been proposed as a biomarker of TBI in humans (Schiff, Hadker, Weiser, & Rausch, 2012). Microglial activation is also seen following seizures (Shapiro, Wang, & Ribak, 2008), and microglial activation is hypothesized to participate in cerebral inflammation that leads to hyperexcitability and seizures (Vezzani, Friedman, & Dingledine, 2013). Animal models used to study the epileptogenesis mechanisms due to infection can be complicated because most of the infectious agents that cause encephalitis in rodents are associated with high mortality (Vezzani et al., 2016). Mice infected with the Theiler's murine encephalomyelitis virus (TMEV) respond differently. For example, SJL/J mice exhibiting mononuclear cell infiltration into the CNS with demyelination in response to the infection are used as a model of multiple sclerosis, whereas C57BL/6J mice infected with TMEV develop acute and late seizures as well as hippocampal damage (Vezzani et al., 2016). The mechanisms of early seizures during the acute symptomatic period after an infection is often multifactorial and varies depending on the type of infection (Vezzani et al., 2016). A common underlying factor in most CNS infections (i.e., meningitis and encephalitis) is the triggering of the inflammatory cascade with release of inflammatory cytokines (Vezzani et al., 2016). Furthermore, the mechanisms of epilepsy following CNS infections are not well established, but data from advances in experimental models may enhance our knowledge of the mechanisms (Vezzani et al., 2016). Individuals with brain infections may demonstrate structural damage, such as infarction, cortical necrosis, and gliosis, which may represent epileptogenic foci (Vezzani et al., 2016).

POSTSTROKE EPILEPSY

Stroke is a common ABI that may result in epileptogenesis and epilepsy. In the elderly, stroke is the most commonly identified etiology for new onset seizures (Annegers, Hauser, Lee, & Rocca, 1995; Loiseau et al., 1990; Stephen & Brodie, 2000). Even in apparently idiopathic cases, cerebrovascular disease is likely a contributor, as these individuals have elevated risk factors for stroke including hypertension, hyperlipidemia, coronary artery disease, and peripheral vascular disease (Li et al., 1997). Factors that increase the likelihood of poststroke epilepsy include stroke severity, large infarct size, and hemorrhagic transformation (Keller, Hobohm, Zeynalova, Classen, & Baum, 2015) as well as cortical involvement (Conrad et al., 2013). Retrospectively, 30% to 40% of elderly with seizures have had a stroke (W. Allen Hauser, Hesdorffer, & Epilepsy Foundation of America., 1990). Prospectively, 8.6% of those with ischemic stroke suffered a seizure within 9 months after the stroke, while 10.6% of those with a hemorrhagic stroke had a seizure within the same period (Bladin et al., 2000). In those with a poststroke seizure, the risk of a second seizure, and thereby a suggestion of an enduring predisposition to epilepsy, may be as high as 20% (Silverman, Restrepo, & Mathews, 2002). Likely secondary to the strong link between stroke and epilepsy, prescriptions for statins are associated with a decreased risk of new-onset epilepsy (Pugh et al., 2009).

Tumor-Associated Epilepsy

Brain tumors are another common cause of new-onset epilepsy. Estimates suggest that tumors represent the etiology for 10% to 12% of epilepsy in the elderly, the population most likely to suffer from cancer (Mousali et al., 2009; Roberts, Godfrey, & Caird, 1982). Seizures can often be the presenting symptom in patients with brain tumors, whether primary or metastatic and whether intra-axial or extra-axial (Hamasaki et al., 2013). The probability that seizures will be associated with a CNS tumor depends on the tumor type, grade, and its location within the brain or, if extra-axial, its location within the cranial vault (van Breemen et al., 2007). While all types of primary and secondary tumors may present with seizures (Lee et al., 2013; Lu-Emerson & Eichler, 2012; Rajneesh & Binder, 2009), tumors of glial origin are very likely to be associated with seizures, with astrocytomas having seizure rates in the 50% to 80% range, and oligodendroglioma with rates of 46% to 78% (Chang et al., 2008; Hamasaki et al., 2013; Kahlenberg et al., 2012). These gliomas grow slowly, invading the surrounding tissue and causing gliosis and chronic inflammatory response. With their growth rate, high-grade tumors such as glioblastoma multiforme (GBM) likely effect epileptogenic changes in the peritumoral region due to mass effect and as a result of local neuronal network disruption. An incidence rate of 22% to 62% (Chaichana et al., 2011; Hamasaki et al., 2013; Kerkhof et al., 2013) is seen in individuals with GBM. Meningiomas, although common (Ostrom et al., 2013), are among the least epileptogenic intracranial tumors with a reported seizure rate between 13% and 26% (Chaichana et al., 2013; Lieu & Howng, 2000). Nearly half of those with TAE from metastatic disease did not have a diagnosis of cancer previously (Lynam et al., 2007). Overall, lower-grade tumors are more likely to present with seizures than higher-grade or metastatic tumors (Johnston & Smith, 2010), and when the inherent epileptogenicity of the tumors is combined with prevalence, gliomas, meningiomas, and metastatic tumors are the most common causes of TAE (Roberts et al., 1982; Sundaram, 1989). The mechanisms behind TAE are likely multifactorial, involving metabolic and pH changes, alterations in levels of neurotransmitters and their receptors, and disruption of localized neural networks in the region of brain tissue surrounding the tumor (Cowie & Cunningham, 2014).

Postinfectious Epilepsy

In patients following central nervous system (CNS) infection, seizures are characterized into early seizures (1–2 weeks following injury), which are believed to represent acute symptomatic seizures; and late seizures (months or years following injury), which occur spontaneously and represent the clinical onset of acquired epilepsy (Vezzani et al., 2016). The mechanisms of early and late seizures are thought to be different. As previously stated, posttraumatic seizures are characterized into immediate or impact-associated (<24 hours after injury), early (1–7 days after injury), or late (> 7 days after injury) (Agrawal et al., 2006; Annegers et al., 1998; Frey, 2003; Pitkänen et al., 2014), and this classification scheme is also believed to represent different underlying pathophysiological processes (Agrawal et al., 2006). Furthermore, when studying patients after brain injury from the acute phase to 1 year, Angeleri et al. (1999) found that in all patients, early seizures, which in their protocol referred to the 4 weeks' interval following injury, occurred within the first 10 days with a subsequent free period of >1 month. This suggested that the interval period was due to two types of seizures having different epileptogenic processes (Angeleri et al., 1999; Phillips, 1954).

CLINICAL PRESENTATION

The clinical presentation of seizures is variable and may include difficulty with speech, confusion, tonic-clonic convulsions, automatisms, head turning, hemiclonic movements, staring, fluttering of the eyes, and a multitude of other symptoms/signs. The most recent revised classification of seizures and epilepsy syndromes by the ILAE divides seizures into focal and generalized categories. Focal seizures, previously termed "partial seizures," are conceptualized as originating within networks localized or more widely distributed to one hemisphere and may originate in subcortical structures (Berg et al., 2010). Some patients have more than one seizure type involving more than one network, though with each seizure type having a consistent site of onset (Berg et al., 2010). For each focal seizure, the ictal onset is consistent from one seizure to another, with preferential propagation patterns that can involve the contralateral hemisphere (Berg et al., 2010). Focal onset seizures are characterized by one or more subjective symptoms (i.e., epigastric sensation, olfactory or gustatory sensations, autonomic) and altered (dyscognitive) or retained awareness (Jette et al., 2015). Generalized seizures are conceptualized as originating at a point within, and rapidly employing, bilaterally distributed networks including cortical and subcortical structures, but may not include the entire cortex (Berg et al., 2010). While individual generalized seizures can be asymmetric, the localization/lateralization are not consistent from one seizure to the next (Berg et al., 2010). Generalized seizures are characterized by tonic-clonic, absence, clonic, tonic, atonic, or myoclonic activity (Jette et al., 2015).

DIAGNOSTIC CONSIDERATIONS

To gain a better understanding of subtypes of PTE, Gupta et al. (2014) retrospectively reviewed patients from a 10-year period with moderate to severe TBI and subsequent drug-resistant epilepsy who had been evaluated by video-electroencephalography (video EEG) in an epilepsy-monitoring unit (EMU). One hundred twenty-three patients were identified with PTE, which represented 4.3% of all patients evaluated in the EMU. Most were identified as having localization-related epilepsy, which included 3% with parietal and occipital lobe epilepsy, 35% with frontal lobe epilepsy, and 57% with temporal lobe epilepsy (TLE). Of those patients with TLE, 26% had temporal neocortical lesions, 30% were nonlesional, and 44% had mesial temporal sclerosis (Gupta et al., 2014).

Neuropsychological assessment is a consult service utilized in epilepsy centers to evaluate cognitive and psychological functioning of patients with epilepsy. Neuropsychological assessment may be used as a diagnostic tool to identify cognitive impairment that may assist physicians in identifying lateralization or localization of the epilepsy syndrome. In addition, neuropsychological evaluation can help differentiate between neurological, psychological, behavioral, and social processes and are reflective in the clinical picture (Wilson et al., 2015). In addition, the ILAE Diagnostic Methods Commission charged with the Neuropsychology Task Force developed a set of recommendations that endorsed routine screening of cognition, mood, and behavior in new-onset epilepsy as well as identifying a core set of cognitive and psychological domains that should be used to provide an objective account of the patient's cognitive, psychological, and emotional functioning (Wilson et al., 2015).

TREATMENT

PTE can contribute to additional brain damage as seizures have been shown to result in hypoxia, increased intracranial pressure, cerebral edema, intracerebral hemorrhage, increased metabolic demand within brain, and glutamate excitotoxicity (Agrawal et al., 2006). Therefore, prophylaxis is important in the management of acute seizures and PTE. Current clinical guidelines encourage clinicians to prescribe prophylactic antiepileptic medications early in the hospital course, typically for the first 7 days, for individuals with severe brain injury (Rao & Parko, 2015). Prophylaxis medications used for treatment target different pathways; therefore, injury severity, patient status, and side effects should be considered before administering medications (Salazar et al., 1985). A recommendation published in *The New England Journal of Medicine* in 1990 recommended phenytoin for 7 days following a TBI (Temkin et al., 1990). In severe TBI, phenytoin was found to reduce the incidence of early seizures from 14.2% to 3.6% (Temkin et al., 1990). Phenytoin demonstrated a significant benefit in reducing the seizure rate by 73% within the first week following a brain injury (Haltiner, Temkin, Winn, & Dikmen, 1996), but was not found to benefit patients treated with phenytoin when compared with the placebo group in the development of late seizures (Young et al., 1983). Furthermore, a randomized control trial demonstrated a trend toward higher mortality when used at later time points (Agrawal et al., 2006).

Additional medications used for prophylaxis include carbamazepine, valproate, and phenobarbital. A preliminary study revealed that carbamazepine reduced posttraumatic seizures by 61% (Torbic, Forni, Anger, Degrado, & Greenwood, 2013). Valproate has demonstrated similar efficacy compared to phenytoin (Torbic et al., 2013); however, it has increased mortality in patients with posttraumatic seizures (Temkin et al., 1999). Phenobarbital has not shown a statistically significant reduction in long-term prevention of seizures following severe TBI (Torbic et al., 2013).

Despite these findings, a meta-analysis, including 10 randomized controlled trials (RCT) with 2,326 participants, reviewed pharmacological treatments for preventing epilepsy following moderate to severe TBI and found that an antiseizure medication, when compared with a placebo or standard care, demonstrated low-quality evidence of reducing the risk of early posttraumatic seizures (Thompson, Pohlmann-Eden, Campbell, & Abel, 2015). Although the benefit was not statistically significant, the authors found the risk of late-seizure occurrence was reduced by antiseizure medication treatment compared with placebo or usual care (Thompson et al., 2015). The authors identified limitations that included variable quality of evidence as the randomization process was not clearly identified in some studies as well as the risk of selective reporting bias. Overall, the authors determined the findings should be interpreted cautiously.

Given that antiepileptic medications may have suboptimal results, patients with drug-resistant epilepsy (DRE) have used alternative therapies for seizure management. Resection surgery is considered to treat PTE when the genesis of the seizure is local and focal (Chen, Ruff, Eavey, & Wasterlain, 2009). However, if the genesis of the seizures has multiple cortical epileptic foci or is generalized, then resection surgery is not an option. When a patient suffers from DRE, additional treatments may be considered, such as deep brain stimulation or vagus nerve stimulation (Chen et al., 2009). In addition, deep brain stimulation has been considered following failure of resective surgery and/or vagus nerve stimulation (Ge, Hu, Liu, Zhang, & Meng, 2013). The ketogenic diet is a more common alternative approach that has demonstrated anticonvulsant effects by decreasing the number of seizures in patients with epilepsy (Masino, Kawamura, Wasser, Pomeroy, & Ruskin, 2009). A suggested alternative approach to preventing seizures following TBI that has been evaluated in preclinical trials is hypothermia. Hypothermia has been recognized as a potential neuroprotective strategy as well as being associated with protective biochemical and behavioral effects in preclinical and clinical studies of neural injury (Lucke-Wold et al., 2015).

PROGNOSIS

Seizures may immediately follow a mild head trauma, such as a concussion, with the prognosis believed to be good as there is agreement that treatment with antiseizure medications is not indicated (McCrory & Berkovic, 2000; Perron, Brady, & Huff, 2001). For example, in a retrospective study of concussive convulsions in a cohort of 22 Australian rugby players, the convulsions did not result in PTE over a mean follow-up of 3.5 years (McCrory, Bladin, & Berkovic, 1997). On the contrary, as stated previously, seizure prophylaxis with antiseizure medications are standard during the acute phase of a moderate to severe brain injury. Unfortunately, early treatments with antiseizure medications do not decrease the risk of PTE (Temkin, 2009).

PTE is heterogeneous and the prognosis is variable. Furthermore, patients may suffer from drug-resistant epilepsy, which occurs when the individual has failed to remain seizure-free with the two antiseizure medications (Kwan & Brodie, 2000). In patients with drug-resistant epilepsy, surgical resection of the damaged tissue may be effective (Wiebe et al., 2001) and evidence supports early consideration of surgical treatment (Engel et al., 2012). In a retrospective review of 57 patients receiving surgical treatment for PTE with 30 of those patients undergoing medial temporal lobe resection, it was found that patients with PTE in the medial temporal lobe responded favorably to surgical treatment (Hartzfeld, Elisevich, Pace, Smith, & Gutierrez, 2008). In addition, epilepsy is often complicated by psychiatric, cognitive, and social comorbidities that impact quality of life and may have an adverse effect on the course of the disorder (Lin, Mula, & Hermann, 2012). In patients with PTE, cognitive impairment may be secondary to the initial brain injury or complicated by the epilepsy. Cognitive screening has been advocated for as a component of clinical care (Lin et al., 2012).

CLINICAL SYNOPSIS

- Epilepsy that develops after an ABI is currently a clinically important condition that is expected to grow in significance.
- The etiologies for acquired epilepsy are diverse and include TBI/cerebral concussion, stroke, anoxia, hemorrhage, tumors, encephalitis, as well as a myriad of other "acquired" insults.
- Epilepsy is a disease of the brain defined by any of the following conditions: at least two unprovoked (or reflex) seizures occurring greater than 24 hours apart; one unprovoked (or reflex) seizure and a probability of further seizures similar to the general recurrence risk after two unprovoked seizures, occurring over 10 years; or, a diagnosis of an epilepsy syndrome. Epileptogenesis is the processes (molecular, cellular, network, etc.) by which a normal brain becomes an epileptic brain.
- PTE is a prototypical acquired epilepsy, with both provoked seizures in the immediate/impact-associated (<24 hours after injury) and early (1–7 days after injury) periods resulting from the acute effects of the injury, and late (>7 days after injury) seizures resulting from epileptogenesis.
- Stroke, brain tumors, and CNS infections are also frequent etiologies for post-ABI epilepsy.
- While seizures can be treated/prevented in both the acute and late time periods with current antiseizure medications,

no diagnostic tests or therapeutic interventions are available for epileptogenesis following ABI.

CASE STUDY

The patient is a 28-year-old, right-handed man with an otherwise unremarkable antecedent medical history who suffered a severe TBI secondary to an unhelmeted motorcycle accident that resulted in bilateral subdural hematomas, right frontal intraparenchymal hemorrhage, and occipital and clival fractures. He underwent emergent craniectomy, and during his hospital course a ventriculperitoneal shunt was placed to treat hydrocephalus. He demonstrated sympathetic storming during his hospitalization and rehabilitation. The patient was observed to have myoclonic jerks following the injury. The patient received seizure prophylaxis that included levetiracetam as well as continuous EEG monitoring, which demonstrated an asymmetric suppression-burst pattern with the amplitudes of cerebral activities over the right greater than over the left hemisphere, though no electrographic seizures were recorded.

One month following the injury, the patient was alert, moved all extremities, squeezed hands on command, and presented thumbs up, but was slow to respond. EEG 2 months following the injury was moderately to severely abnormal and demonstrated unreactive persistent hemispheric asymmetry, with delta slowing over the right hemisphere with dampened voltages, and some higher amplitude slowing seen over the left hemisphere, not exceeding the mid-theta band. There were no epileptiform discharges or electrographic seizures, and the EEG remained unchanged from previous studies.

Approximately 3 months following the accident, the patient was observed to have episodes of staring with unresponsiveness and stiffening bilaterally in his legs followed by a postictal period lasting a few minutes. Nine months following the accident, the patient's levetiracetam was discontinued and subsequently he had two episodes of unresponsiveness associated with generalized tonic-clonic activity. He was represcribed levetiracetam and the dosage was increased. One and a half years following the accident, EEG was abnormal due to the presence of focal slowing of the right frontotemporal region indicative of underlying area of structural abnormality as well as high-amplitude faster frequencies seen over the right temporal leads, which clinically represented an area of skull defect consistent with breach rhythm. In addition, CT scan revealed hydrocephalus with VP shunt in place, encephalomalacia in the bilateral orbital frontal lobes, and left subdural hygroma. Neuropsychological testing 3 years following the brain injury revealed average intelligence, average or higher language and perceptual skills, average or higher verbal and visual learning and memory with no evidence of accelerated forgetting, and multiple abnormalities in executive functioning (inattention with impulsivity, decreased speeded mental flexibility, abnormal novel problem solving, and psychomotor slowing). The abnormalities cluster in the area of executive functioning with clear sparing of memory function, suggesting integrity of the mesial temporal/hippocampal systems bilaterally. Impairments in executive function were consistent with the localization of his brain lesions (encephalomalacia in bilateral orbital frontal lobes and left subdural hygroma). The diagnostic impression included mild neurocognitive disorder due to TBI and PTE.

REFERENCES

Agrawal, A., Timothy, J., Pandit, L., & Manju, M. (2006). Post-traumatic epilepsy: An overview. *Clinical Neurology and Neurosurgery, 108*(5), 433–439. doi:10.1016/j.clineuro.2005.09.001

Andrews-Zwilling, Y., Bien-Ly, N., Xu, Q., Li, G., Bernardo, A., Yoon, S. Y., . . . Huang, Y. (2010). Apolipoprotein E4 causes age- and Tau-dependent impairment of GABAergic interneurons, leading to learning and memory deficits in mice. *The Journal of Neuroscience, 30*(41), 13707–13717. doi:10.1523/jneurosci.4040-10.2010

Angeleri, F., Majkowski, J., Cacchiò, G., Sobieszek, A., D'Acunto, S., Gesuita, R., . . . Salvolini, U. (1999). Posttraumatic epilepsy risk factors: One-year prospective study after head injury. *Epilepsia, 40*(9), 1222–1230. Retrieved from www.ncbi.nlm.nih.gov/pubmed/10487184

Annegers, J. F., Grabow, J. D., Kurland, L. T., & Laws, E. R. (1980). The incidence, causes, and secular trends of head trauma in Olmsted County, Minnesota, 1935-1974. *Neurology, 30*(9), 912–919.

Annegers, J. F., Hauser, W. A., Coan, S. P., & Rocca, W. A. (1998). A population-based study of seizures after traumatic brain injuries. *The New England Journal of Medicine, 338*(1), 20–24. doi:10.1056/NEJM199801013380104

Annegers, J. F., Hauser, W. A., Lee, J. R., & Rocca, W. A. (1995). Incidence of acute symptomatic seizures in Rochester, Minnesota, 1935-1984. *Epilepsia, 36*(4), 327–333.

Beghi, E. (2003). Overview of studies to prevent posttraumatic epilepsy. *Epilepsia, 44*(Suppl. 10), 21–26.

Berg, A. T., Berkovic, S. F., Brodie, M. J., Buchhalter, J., Cross, J. H., van Emde Boas, W., . . . Scheffer, I. E. (2010). Revised terminology and concepts for organization of seizures and epilepsies: Report of the ILAE Commission on Classification and Terminology, 2005–2009. *Epilepsia, 51*(4), 676–685. doi:10.1111/j.1528-1167.2010.02522.x

Binder, D. K., Routbort, M. J., Ryan, T. E., Yancopoulos, G. D., & McNamara, J. O. (1999). Selective inhibition of kindling development by intraventricular administration of TrkB receptor body. *The Journal of Neuroscience, 19*(4), 1424–1436.

Bladin, C. F., Alexandrov, A. V., Bellavance, A., Bornstein, N., Chambers, B., Coté, R., . . . Norris, J. W. (2000). Seizures after stroke: A prospective multicenter study. *Archives of Neurology, 57*(11), 1617–1622.

Boon, P., Chauvel, P., Pohlmann-Eden, B., Otoul, C., & Wroe, S. (2002). Dose-response effect of levetiracetam 1000 and 2000 mg/day in partial epilepsy. *Epilepsy Research, 48*(1/2), 77–89.

Carbonell, W. S., & Grady, M. S. (1999). Regional and temporal characterization of neuronal, glial, and axonal response after traumatic brain injury in the mouse. *Acta Neuropathologica, 98*(4), 396–406.

Chen, J. W., Ruff, R. L., Eavey, R., & Wasterlain, C. G. (2009). Posttraumatic epilepsy and treatment. *Journal of Rehabilitation Research and Development, 46*(6), 685–696. Retrieved from www.ncbi.nlm.nih.gov/pubmed/20104398

Christensen, J., Pedersen, M. G., Pedersen, C. B., Sidenius, P., Olsen, J., & Vestergaard, M. (2009). Long-term risk of epilepsy after traumatic brain injury in children and young adults: A population-based cohort study. *Lancet, 373*(9669), 1105–1110. doi:10.1016/S0140-6736(09)60214-2

Conrad, J., Pawlowski, M., Dogan, M., Kovac, S., Ritter, M. A., & Evers, S. (2013). Seizures after cerebrovascular events: Risk factors and clinical features. *Seizure, 22*(4), 275–282. doi:10.1016/j.seizure.2013.01.014

Coronado, V. G., Xu, L., Basavaraju, S. V., McGuire, L. C., Wald, M. M., Faul, M. D., . . . Centers for Disease Control and Prevention. (2011). Surveillance for traumatic brain injury-related deaths—United States, 1997-2007. *MMWR Surveillance Summaries, 60*(5), 1–32.

Corsellis, J. A., Bruton, C. J., & Freeman-Browne, D. (1973). The aftermath of boxing. *Psychological Medicine, 3*(3), 270–303.

Cross, J. H., & Riney, C. J. (2009). Topiramate. In S. Shorvon, E. Perucca, & J. Engel (Eds.), *The treatment of epilepsy* (pp. 673–683). West Sussex, UK: Wiley-Blackwell.

Dudek, F. E., & Staley, K. J. (2011). The time course of acquired epilepsy: Implications for therapeutic intervention to suppress epileptogenesis. *Neuroscience Letters, 497*(3), 240–246. doi:10.1016/j.neulet.2011.03.071

Dudek, F. E., & Sutula, T. P. (2007). Epileptogenesis in the dentate gyrus: A critical perspective. *Progress in Brain Research, 163,* 755–773. doi:10.1016/S0079-6123(07)63041-6

Engel, J., Jr., McDermott, M. P., Wiebe, S., Langfitt, J. T., Stern, J. M., Dewar, S., . . . Early Randomized Surgical Epilepsy Trial Study Group. (2012). Early surgical therapy for drug-resistant temporal lobe epilepsy: A randomized trial. *JAMA, 307*(9), 922–930. doi:10.1001/jama.2012.220

Faul, M., Xu, L., Wald, M., & Coronado, V. (2010). *Traumatic brain injury in the United States: Emergency department visits, hospitalizations, and deaths.* Atlanta, GA: Centers for Disease Control and Prevention, National Center for Injury Prevention and Control.

Fisher, R. S., Acevedo, C., Arzimanoglou, A., Bogacz, A., Cross, J. H., Elger, C. E., . . . Wiebe, S. (2014). ILAE official report: A practical clinical definition of epilepsy. *Epilepsia, 55*(4), 475–482. doi:10.1111/epi.12550

Fisher, R. S., van Emde Boas, W., Blume, W., Elger, C., Genton, P., Lee, P., & Engel, J. (2005). Epileptic seizures and epilepsy: Definitions proposed by the International League Against Epilepsy (ILAE) and the International Bureau for Epilepsy (IBE). *Epilepsia, 46*(4), 470–472. doi:10.1111/j.0013-9580.2005.66104.x

Frey, L. C. (2003). Epidemiology of posttraumatic epilepsy: A critical review. *Epilepsia, 44*(Suppl. 10), 11–17. Retrieved from www.ncbi.nlm.nih.gov/pubmed/14511389

Ge, Y., Hu, W., Liu, C., Zhang, J. G., & Meng, F. G. (2013). Brain stimulation for treatment of refractory epilepsy. *Chinese Medical Journal, 126*(17), 3364–3370. Retrieved from www.ncbi.nlm.nih.gov/pubmed/24033966

Grundke-Iqbal, I., Iqbal, K., Tung, Y. C., Quinlan, M., Wisniewski, H. M., & Binder, L. I. (1986). Abnormal phosphorylation of the microtubule-associated protein tau (tau) in Alzheimer cytoskeletal pathology. *Proceedings of the National Academy of Sciences of the United States of America, 83*(13), 4913-4917.

Gupta, P. K., Sayed, N., Ding, K., Agostini, M. A., Van Ness, P. C., Yablon, S., . . . Diaz-Arrastia, R. (2014). Subtypes of post-traumatic epilepsy: Clinical, electrophysiological, and imaging features. *Journal of Neurotrauma, 31*(16), 1439–1443. doi:10.1089/neu.2013.3221

Haltiner, A. M., Temkin, N. R., & Dikmen, S. S. (1997). Risk of seizure recurrence after the first late posttraumatic seizure. *Archives of Physical Medicine and Rehabilitation, 78*(8), 835–840.

Haltiner, A. M., Temkin, N. R., Winn, H. R., & Dikmen, S. S. (1996). The impact of posttraumatic seizures on 1-year neuropsychological and psychosocial outcome of head injury. *Journal of the International Neuropsychological Society, 2*(6), 494–504. Retrieved from www.ncbi.nlm.nih.gov/pubmed/9375153

Hartzfeld, P., Elisevich, K., Pace, M., Smith, B., & Gutierrez, J. A. (2008). Characteristics and surgical outcomes for medial temporal posttraumatic epilepsy. *British Journal of Neurosurgery, 22*(2), 224–230. doi:10.1080/02688690701818901

Hauser, W. A., Hesdorffer, D. C., & Epilepsy Foundation of America. (1990). *Epilepsy: Frequency, causes and consequences.* New York, NY: Demos Medical.

He, X. P., Kotloski, R., Nef, S., Luikart, B. W., Parada, L. F., & McNamara, J. O. (2004). Conditional deletion of TrkB but not BDNF prevents epileptogenesis in the kindling model. *Neuron, 43*(1), 31–42. doi:10.1016/j.neuron.2004.06.019

Herman, S. T. (2002). Epilepsy after brain insult: Targeting epileptogenesis. *Neurology, 59*(9, Suppl. 5), S21–26.

Holth, J. K., Bomben, V. C., Reed, J. G., Inoue, T., Younkin, L., Younkin, S. G., . . . Noebels, J. L. (2013). Tau loss attenuates neuronal network hyperexcitability in mouse and Drosophila genetic models of epilepsy. *The Journal of Neuroscience, 33*(4), 1651–1659. doi:10.1523/JNEUROSCI.3191-12.2013

Hu, B., Liu, C., Bramlett, H., Sick, T. J., Alonso, O. F., Chen, S., & Dietrich, W. D. (2004). Changes in trkB-ERK1/2-CREB/Elk-1 pathways in hippocampal mossy fiber organization after traumatic brain injury. *Journal of Cerebral Blood Flow & Metabolism, 24*(8), 934–943. doi:10.1097/01.WCB.0000125888.56462.A1

Hunt, R. F., Boychuk, J. A., & Smith, B. N. (2013). Neural circuit mechanisms of post-traumatic epilepsy. *Frontiers in Cellular Neuroscience, 7,* 89. doi:10.3389/fncel.2013.00089

Hunter, J. M., Cirrito, J. R., Restivo, J. L., Kinley, R. D., Sullivan, P. M., Holtzman, D. M., . . . Paul, S. M. (2012). Emergence of a seizure phenotype in aged apolipoprotein epsilon 4 targeted replacement mice. *Brain Research, 1467,* 120–132. doi:10.1016/j.brainres.2012.05.048

Ikonomovic, M. D., Uryu, K., Abrahamson, E. E., Ciallella, J. R., Trojanowski, J. Q., Lee, V. M., . . . DeKosky, S. T. (2004). Alzheimer's pathology in human temporal cortex surgically excised after severe brain injury. *Experimental Neurology, 190*(1), 192–203. doi:10.1016/j.expneurol.2004.06.011

Institute of Medicine Committee on Gulf War and Health. (2008). *Brain injury in veterans and long-term health outcomes.* Washington, DC: National Academies Press.

Jacoby, A., & Austin, J. K. (2007). Social stigma for adults and children with epilepsy. *Epilepsia, 48*(Suppl. 9), 6–9. doi:10.1111/j.1528-1167.2007.01391.x

Jensen, F. E. (2009). Introduction: Posttraumatic epilepsy: Treatable epileptogenesis. *Epilepsia, 50*(Suppl. 2), 1–3. doi:10.1111/j.1528-1167.2008.02003.x

Jette, N., Beghi, E., Hesdorffer, D., Moshe, S. L., Zuberi, S. M., Medina, M. T., & Bergen, D. (2015). ICD coding for epilepsy: Past, present, and future—A report by the International League Against Epilepsy Task Force on ICD codes in epilepsy. *Epilepsia, 56*(3), 348–355. doi:10.1111/epi.12895

Keller, L., Hobohm, C., Zeynalova, S., Classen, J., & Baum, P. (2015). Does treatment with t-PA increase the risk of developing epilepsy after stroke? *Journal of Neurology, 262*(10), 2364–2372. doi:10.1007/s00415-015-7850-0

Kotloski, R., & McNamara, J. O. (2010). Reduction of TrkB expression de novo in the adult mouse impairs epileptogenesis in the kindling model. *Hippocampus, 20*(6), 713–723. doi:10.1002/hipo.20673

Kwan, P., & Brodie, M. J. (2000). Early identification of refractory epilepsy. *The New England Journal of Medicine, 342*(5), 314–319. doi:10.1056/NEJM200002033420503

LaFrance, W. C., Kanner, A. M., & Hermann, B. (2008). Psychiatric comorbidities in epilepsy. *International Review of Neurobiology, 83*, 347–383. doi:10.1016/S0074-7742(08)00020-2

Leppik, I. E. (2002). Three new drugs for epilepsy: Levetiracetam, oxcarbazepine, and zonisamide. *Journal of Child Neurology, 17*(Suppl. 1), S53-57.

Li, G., Bien-Ly, N., Andrews-Zwilling, Y., Xu, Q., Bernardo, A., Ring, K., . . . Huang, Y. (2009). GABAergic interneuron dysfunction impairs hippocampal neurogenesis in adult apolipoprotein E4 knockin mice. *Cell Stem Cell, 5*(6), 634–645. doi:10.1016/j.stem.2009.10.015

Li, X., Breteler, M. M., de Bruyne, M. C., Meinardi, H., Hauser, W. A., & Hofman, A. (1997). Vascular determinants of epilepsy: The Rotterdam Study. *Epilepsia, 38*(11), 1216–1220.

Lin, J. J., Mula, M., & Hermann, B. P. (2012). Uncovering the neurobehavioural comorbidities of epilepsy over the lifespan. *Lancet, 380*(9848), 1180–1192. doi:10.1016/S0140-6736(12)61455-X

Lucke-Wold, B. P., Nguyen, L., Turner, R. C., Logsdon, A. F., Chen, Y. W., Smith, K. E., . . . Richter, E. (2015). Traumatic brain injury and epilepsy: Underlying mechanisms leading to seizure. *Seizure, 33*, 13–23. doi:10.1016/j.seizure.2015.10.002

Lund, I. V., Hu, Y., Raol, Y. H., Benham, R. S., Faris, R., Russek, S. J., & Brooks-Kayal, A. R. (2008). BDNF selectively regulates GABAA receptor transcription by activation of the JAK/STAT pathway. *Science Signaling, 1*(41), ra9. doi:10.1126/scisignal.1162396

Masino, S. A., Kawamura, M., Wasser, C. D., Pomeroy, L. T., & Ruskin, D. N. (2009). Adenosine, ketogenic diet and epilepsy: The emerging therapeutic relationship between metabolism and brain activity. *Current Neuropharmacology, 7*(3), 257–268. doi:10.2174/157015909789152164

McCrory, P. R., & Berkovic, S. F. (2000). Video analysis of acute motor and convulsive manifestations in sport-related concussion. *Neurology, 54*(7), 1488–1491. Retrieved from www.ncbi.nlm.nih.gov/pubmed/10751264

McCrory, P. R., Bladin, P. F., & Berkovic, S. F. (1997). Retrospective study of concussive convulsions in elite Australian rules and rugby league footballers: Phenomenology, aetiology, and outcome. *BMJ, 314*(7075), 171–174. Retrieved from www.ncbi.nlm.nih.gov/pubmed/9022428

McKee, A. C., Cantu, R. C., Nowinski, C. J., Hedley-Whyte, E. T., Gavett, B. E., Budson, A. E., . . . Stern, R. A. (2009). Chronic traumatic encephalopathy in athletes: Progressive tauopathy after repetitive head injury. *Journal of Neuropathology & Experimental Neurology, 68*(7), 709–735. doi:10.1097/NEN.0b013e3181a9d503

McNamara, J. O. (1986). Kindling model of epilepsy. In A. V. Delgado-Escueta (Ed.), *Basic mechanisms of the epilepsies: Molecular and cellular approaches (Advances in Neurology)* (Vol. 44, pp. 303–318). New York, NY: Raven Press.

Morimoto, K., Fahnestock, M., & Racine, R. J. (2004). Kindling and status epilepticus models of epilepsy: Rewiring the brain. *Progress in Neurobiology, 73*(1), 1-60. doi:10.1016/j.pneurobio.2004.03.009

Ngugi, A. K., Bottomley, C., Kleinschmidt, I., Sander, J. W., & Newton, C. R. (2010). Estimation of the burden of active and life-time epilepsy: A meta-analytic approach. *Epilepsia, 51*(5), 883–890. doi:10.1111/j.1528-1167.2009.02481.x

Okie, S. (2005). Traumatic brain injury in the war zone. *The New England Journal of Medicine, 352*(20), 2043–2047. doi:10.1056/NEJMp058102

Park, S. P., & Kwon, S. H. (2008). Cognitive effects of antiepileptic drugs. *Journal of Clinical Neurology, 4*(3), 99–106. doi:10.3988/jcn.2008.4.3.99

Perron, A. D., Brady, W. J., & Huff, J. S. (2001). Concussive convulsions: Emergency department assessment and management of a frequently misunderstood entity. *Academic Emergency Medicine, 8*(3), 296–298. Retrieved from www.ncbi.nlm.nih.gov/pubmed/11229957

Phillips, G. (1954). Traumatic epilepsy after closed head injury. *Journal of Neurology, Neurosurgery, and Psychiatry, 17*(1), 1–10. Retrieved from www.ncbi.nlm.nih.gov/pubmed/13131074

Pitkänen, A., Bolkvadze, T., & Immonen, R. (2011). Anti-epileptogenesis in rodent post-traumatic epilepsy models. *Neuroscience Letters, 497*(3), 163–171. doi:10.1016/j.neulet.2011.02.033

Pitkänen, A., Kemppainen, S., Ndode-Ekane, X. E., Huusko, N., Huttunen, J. K., Gröhn, O., . . . Bolkvadze, T. (2014). Posttraumatic epilepsy—Disease or comorbidity? *Epilepsy & Behavior, 38*, 19c24. doi:10.1016/j.yebeh.2014.01.013

Pitkänen, A., & Lukasiuk, K. (2009). Molecular and cellular basis of epileptogenesis in symptomatic epilepsy. *Epilepsy & Behavior, 14*(Suppl. 1), 16–25. doi:10.1016/j.yebeh.2008.09.023

Pugh, M. J. V., Knoefel, J. E., Mortensen, E. M., Amuan, M. E., Berlowitz, D. R., & Van Cott, A. C. (2009). New-onset epilepsy risk factors in older veterans. *Journal of the American Geriatrics Society, 57*(2), 237–242. doi:10.1111/j.1532-5415.2008.02124.x

Raible, D. J., Frey, L. C., & Brooks-Kayal, A. R. (2014). Effects of JAK2-STAT3 signaling after cerebral insults. *JAK-STAT, 3*, e29510. doi:10.4161/jkst.29510

Raible, D. J., Frey, L. C., Cruz Del Angel, Y., Russek, S. J., & Brooks-Kayal, A. R. (2012). GABA(A) receptor regulation after experimental traumatic brain injury. *Journal of Neurotrauma, 29*(16), 2548–2554. doi:10.1089/neu.2012.2483

Rao, V. R., & Parko, K. L. (2015). Clinical approach to posttraumatic epilepsy. *Seminars in Neurology, 35*(1), 57–63. doi:10.1055/s-0035-1544239

Raymont, V., Salazar, A. M., Lipsky, R., Goldman, D., Tasick, G., & Grafman, J. (2010). Correlates of posttraumatic epilepsy 35 years following combat brain injury. *Neurology, 75*(3), 224–229. doi:10.1212/WNL.0b013e3181e8e6d0

Regner, A., Alves, L. B., Chemale, I., Costa, M. S., Friedman, G., Achaval, M., . . . Emanuelli, T. (2001). Neurochemical characterization of traumatic brain injury in humans. *Journal of Neurotrauma, 18*(8), 783–792. doi:10.1089/08977150131691948

Roberson, E. D., Halabisky, B., Yoo, J. W., Yao, J., Chin, J., Yan, F., . . . Mucke, L. (2011). Amyloid-β/Fyn-induced synaptic, network, and cognitive impairments depend on tau levels in multiple mouse models of Alzheimer's disease. *The Journal of Neuroscience, 31*(2), 700–711. doi:10.1523/JNEUROSCI.4152-10.2011

Roberts, G. W., Allsop, D., & Bruton, C. (1990). The occult aftermath of boxing. *Journal of Neurology, Neurosurgery, & Psychiatry, 53*(5), 373–378.

Roberts, G. W., Gentleman, S. M., Lynch, A., Murray, L., Landon, M., & Graham, D. I. (1994). Beta amyloid protein deposition in the brain after severe head injury: Implications for the pathogenesis of Alzheimer's disease. *Journal of Neurology, Neurosurgery, & Psychiatry, 57*(4), 419–425.

Roberts, M. A., Godfrey, J. W., & Caird, F. I. (1982). Epileptic seizures in the elderly: I. Aetiology and type of seizure. *Age and Ageing, 11,* 24–28.

Rostami, E., Krueger, F., Plantman, S., Davidsson, J., Agoston, D., Grafman, J., & Risling, M. (2014). Alteration in BDNF and its receptors, full-length and truncated TrkB and p75(NTR) following penetrating traumatic brain injury. *Brain Research, 1542,* 195–205. doi:10.1016/j.brainres.2013.10.047

Salazar, A. M., Jabbari, B., Vance, S. C., Grafman, J., Amin, D., & Dillon, J. D. (1985). Epilepsy after penetrating head injury: I: Clinical correlates: A report of the Vietnam Head Injury Study. *Neurology, 35*(10), 1406–1414. Retrieved from www.ncbi.nlm.nih.gov/pubmed/3929158

Schiff, L., Hadker, N., Weiser, S., & Rausch, C. (2012). A literature review of the feasibility of glial fibrillary acidic protein as a biomarker for stroke and traumatic brain injury. *Molecular Diagnosis & Therapy, 16*(2), 79–92. doi:10.2165/11631580-000000000-00000

Shapiro, L. A., Wang, L., & Ribak, C. E. (2008). Rapid astrocyte and microglial activation following pilocarpine-induced seizures in rats. *Epilepsia, 49*(Suppl. 2), 33–41. doi:10.1111/j.1528-1167.2008.01491.x

Shitaka, Y., Tran, H. T., Bennett, R. E., Sanchez, L., Levy, M. A., Dikranian, K., & Brody, D. L. (2011). Repetitive closed-skull traumatic brain injury in mice causes persistent multifocal axonal injury and microglial reactivity. *Journal of Neuropathology & Experimental Neurology, 70*(7), 551–567. doi:10.1097/NEN.0b013e31821f891f

Silverman, I. E., Restrepo, L., & Mathews, G. C. (2002). Poststroke seizures. *Archives of Neurology, 59*(2), 195–201.

Stephen, L. J., & Brodie, M. J. (2000). Epilepsy in elderly people. *Lancet, 355*(9213), 1441–1446. doi:10.1016/S0140-6736(00)02149-8

Swann, A. C. (2001). Major system toxicities and side effects of anticonvulsants. *Journal of Clinical Psychiatry, 62*(Suppl. 14), 16–21.

Teasell, R., Bayona, N., Lippert, C., Villamere, J., & Hellings, C. (2007a). Post-traumatic seizure disorder following acquired brain injury. *Brain Injury, 21*(2), 201–214. doi:10.1080/02699050701201854

Teasell, R., Bayona, N., Marshall, S., Cullen, N., Bayley, M., Chundamala, J., . . . Tu, L. (2007b). A systematic review of the rehabilitation of moderate to severe acquired brain injuries. *Brain Injury, 21*(2), 107–112. doi:10.1080/02699050701201524

Temkin, N. R. (2009). Preventing and treating posttraumatic seizures: The human experience. *Epilepsia, 50*(Suppl. 2), 10–13. doi:10.1111/j.1528-1167.2008.02005.x

Temkin, N. R., Dikmen, S. S., Anderson, G. D., Wilensky, A. J., Holmes, M. D., Cohen, W., . . . Winn, H. R. (1999). Valproate therapy for prevention of posttraumatic seizures: A randomized trial. *Journal of Neurosurgery, 91*(4), 593–600. doi:10.3171/jns.1999.91.4.0593

Temkin, N. R., Dikmen, S. S., Wilensky, A. J., Keihm, J., Chabal, S., & Winn, H. R. (1990). A randomized, double-blind study of phenytoin for the prevention of post-traumatic seizures. *The New England Journal of Medicine, 323*(8), 497–502. doi:10.1056/NEJM199008233230801

Thompson, K., Pohlmann-Eden, B., Campbell, L. A., & Abel, H. (2015). Pharmacological treatments for preventing epilepsy following traumatic head injury. *Cochrane Database of Systematic Reviews,* (8), CD 009900. doi: 10.1002/14651858.CD009900

Torbic, H., Forni, A. A., Anger, K. E., Degrado, J. R., & Greenwood, B. C. (2013). Use of antiepileptics for seizure prophylaxis after traumatic brain injury. *American Journal of Health-System Pharmacy, 70*(9), 759–766. doi:10.2146/ajhp120203

Traumatic Brain Injury Task Force. (2007). *Report to the (Army) Surgeon General: Traumatic Brain Injury Task Force.* Retrieved from http://www.dcoe.mil/content/Navigation/Documents/TBITaskForceReportJanuary2008.pdf

Vezzani, A., Friedman, A., & Dingledine, R. J. (2013). The role of inflammation in epileptogenesis. *Neuropharmacology, 69,* 16–24. doi:10.1016/j.neuropharm.2012.04.004

Vezzani, A., Fujinami, R. S., White, H. S., Preux, P. M., Blümcke, I., Sander, J. W., & Löscher, W. (2016). Infections, inflammation and epilepsy. *Acta Neuropathologica, 131*(2), 211–234. doi:10.1007/s00401-015-1481-5

Wiebe, S., Blume, W. T., Girvin, J. P., Eliasziw, M., & Effectiveness and Efficiency of Surgery for Temporal Lobe Epilepsy Study Group. (2001).

A randomized, controlled trial of surgery for temporal-lobe epilepsy. *The New England Journal of Medicine, 345*(5), 311–318. doi:10.1056/NEJM200108023450501

Wilson, S. J., Baxendale, S., Barr, W., Hamed, S., Langfitt, J., Samson, S., . . . Smith, M. L. (2015). Indications and expectations for neuropsychological assessment in routine epilepsy care: Report of the ILAE Neuropsychology Task Force, Diagnostic Methods Commission, 2013–2017. *Epilepsia, 56*(5), 674–681. doi:10.1111/epi.12962

Young, B., Rapp, R. P., Norton, J. A., Haack, D., Tibbs, P. A., & Bean, J. R. (1983). Failure of prophylactically administered phenytoin to prevent late posttraumatic seizures. *Journal of Neurosurgery, 58*(2), 236–241. doi:10.3171/jns.1983.58.2.0236

CHAPTER 12

Post–Acquired Brain Injury Movement Disorders

HANNAH L. COMBS
KATHRYN J. DUNHAM
BRITTANY D. WALLS
AMELIA J. ANDERSON-MOONEY

OVERVIEW

It is widely accepted that movement disorders (MD) can develop as a consequence of an acquired brain injury (ABI) (Krauss & Jankovic, 2002), although challenges abound in the determination of etiology, appropriate assessment techniques, and effective treatments. Post-ABI MDs can vary significantly in symptom presentation and underlying pathogenesis on the basis of the influence of injury-related and patient-related factors, rendering understanding of those factors critical to treatment. A brief discussion of such pertinent factors is provided in what follows.

HISTORY

Review of historical writings reveals a variety of case reports on posttraumatic MDs. The possible link between trauma and development of a MD can be traced back as far as James Parkinson's (1817) *Essay on the Shaking Palsy*. In this work, he observed that patients with what would eventually be termed Parkinson's disease (PD) denied experiencing any traumatic injuries that could damage the brain stem, which would have been expected to cause disordered movement. Martland (1928) described the development of "punch drunk" syndrome with both behavioral and movement features after repeated boxing-related head injuries. Elaborating on this finding, Kremer, Russell, and Smyth (1947) reviewed a case series of seven patients that developed parkinsonian features after midbrain injuries of varying etiology, suggesting that the cause of the trauma is not as substantial as the affected area secondary to severe trauma. Continued case reports and reviews regarding posttraumatic MDs have been published (Koller, Wong, & Lang, 1989; O'Suilleabhain & Dewey, 2004) since the second half of the 20th century, highlighting increasing specificity regarding the neuroanatomical structures and pathways involved in post-ABI MDs.

PATHOPHYSIOLOGY

When focal lesions are present, MD symptoms following ABI typically result secondary to strategic lesions in the basal ganglia or cerebellum, although lesions throughout the motor system have been implicated in the development of MD post ABI.

- *Tremor*, which appears to be the most common symptom occurring after severe injuries (Krauss, Trankle, & Kopp, 1996), has been linked to lesions in the substantia nigra, thalamus, and cerebellum (Krauss et al., 1995).
- *Dystonia* is typically the result of a lesion in the caudate, putamen, subthalamic nucleus, and thalamus (Krauss et al., 1992; Krauss, Mohadjer, Nobbe, & Mundinger, 1994).
- *Dyskinesia* can result from lesions of the subthalamus, striatum, or thalamus (Koller, Weiner, Nausieda, & Klawans, 1979).

Post-ABI MD may also develop in the absence of focal lesions. For instance, there is some evidence that prior ABI with loss of consciousness increases the risk of later developing PD with its associated synuclein-related pathology (Bower et al., 2003). In addition, although some data suggest no increased risk for MDs in individuals exposed to repeated head injuries (Savica, Parisi, Wold, Josephs, & Ahlskog, 2012), other work has classified a disorder named "chronic traumatic encephalopathy" (CTE; formerly known as "dementia pugilistica") in individuals who indeed develop MDs after chronic, repeated head injuries.

Although the literature remains controversial, as a clinical syndrome, CTE is characterized as a progressive tauopathy, involving cortical neurofibrillary tangles as well as damage to the cerebellum, septum pellucidum, and substantia nigra (Corsellis, Bruton, & Freeman-Browne, 1973; DeKosky, Blennow, Ikonomovic, & Gandy, 2013; Jordan, 2013). Two separate classification systems have been developed to differentiate stages of CTE pathology after repeated ABI in which movement symptoms or damage to brain structures related to movement are involved (McKee et al., 2013; Omalu et al., 2011).

ETIOLOGY

However, the belief that any MD develops secondarily to preceding trauma is, by nature, always speculative. Generally, the milder the injury and the longer the interval between injury and onset of MD, the more speculative the causality becomes (O'Suilleabhain & Dewey, 2004).

Specifically, there is a strong research base to support the relationship between MDs and severe ABI, but the relationship with mild ABI is less strongly established (Curran & Lang, 1995; Jankovic, 1994; Krauss & Jankovic, 2002). Determining etiology by timeline is also flawed, because post-ABI MDs may have a delayed onset and variable progression over time (Katz, 1990). Despite this, some injury-specific connections are present in the literature.

- *CTE:* When pathologically confirmed CTE is present, it is usually associated with repeated blows to the head, often due to sporting injuries in high-contact (e.g., football, boxing, and hockey) and/or high-velocity (e.g., motor racing) sports.
- *Moderate to severe ABIs:* Links may be more definitively made between moderate to severe ABIs and MDs (Bazarian, Cernak, Noble-Haeusslein, Potolicchio, & Temkin, 2009; Johnson & Hall, 1992). MDs may develop particularly often secondary to penetrating injuries or hemorrhages occurring after diffuse impact (Krauss et al., 1995; Krauss & Jankovic, 1997).

EPIDEMIOLOGY

- *Severe ABI:* Krauss, Trankle, and Heinz-Kopp (1996) reviewed the prevalence of MD in a sample of 221 adults with severe ABI, with follow-up occurring 3.9 years post injury on average. In this group, 22.6% of patients developed MDs, the most common symptom of which was tremor (19%) and dystonia (4.1%). Prevalence may be higher in children after severe ABI, with literature reflecting rates from 13% to 66% (Krauss & Jankovic, 2002). One survey including 289 children after severe ABI demonstrated a 45% rate of tremor specifically (Johnson & Hall, 1992).

- *Moderate and Mild ABI:* MDs are thought to occur less commonly in this group. Although transient tremors that do not require intervention may be more common, rates of persistent tremor are estimated to be approximately half of those after severe ABI, with one study estimating the maximum prevalence of persistent, mild tremors after mild to moderate ABI at 10% (Krauss, Trankle, & Kopp, 1997). This sample included both children and adults.

CLINICAL PRESENTATION

- *Neurodegenerative disorders:* Beyond the known increased risk of Alzheimer's disease associated with both moderate and severe ABI (Plassman et al., 2000), patients with a positive ABI history can also develop progressive neurodegenerative disorders involving movement. The most commonly recognized neurodegenerative disorders developing after ABI are CTE and PD, with characteristic disease courses and symptom presentations.
    - *CTE*: Onset of clinical symptoms of CTE can be quite delayed. In athletes, symptoms may not emerge until 10 to 20 years after the end of an athlete's career (Bazarian et al., 2009). By definition, CTE includes the presence of motor symptoms, which typically present as slurring of speech, uncoordinated gait, tremor, or spasticity in addition to headache, mood changes, and cognitive changes (Jordan, 2013). The movement pattern may appear to be parkinsonian in some patients (Krauss & Jankovic, 2002).
    - *PD*: Pathogenic connections between PD and ABI are inconsistent in the literature, although some available evidence is compelling. The risk of PD is elevated with more complicating symptoms, including loss of consciousness or more severe injury overall (Bower et al., 2003).

In an examination of 93 twin pairs (both monozygotic and dizygotic), a history of ABI with amnesia or loss of consciousness was associated with a greater risk for PD, which was compounded when those injuries required hospitalization or were followed by additional ABI (Goldman et al., 2006). PD itself is characterized by a distinctive pattern of levodopa-responsive movement symptoms, including asymmetrical resting tremor, bradykinesia, rigidity, and postural instability (Lang & Lozano, 1998).

- *Nondegenerative movement disorders:* The presentation of MD that are not related to PD or CTE can be highly varied, including tremors and other symptoms and clinical courses that can confound even skilled diagnosticians.
  - *Onset timelines*: Onset of MD symptoms may be significantly delayed after the ABI occurs, with latencies of weeks to years after injury (Krauss & Jankovic, 2002). In some samples, tremors were noted to develop between 2 weeks and 6 months post ABI, and dystonia developed between 2 months and 2 years afterward (Krauss et al., 1997).
  - *Symptoms*: Post-ABI movement symptoms often occur with spasticity, generalized weakness, and apraxia (O'Suilleabhain & Dewey, 2004). Beyond this, tremors and dystonia are among the most consistently noted symptoms, particularly after severe ABI (Curran & Lang, 1995; Jankovic, 1994).
  - *Spasticity:* Commonly experienced after moderate to severe ABI, spasticity is characterized by increased muscle tone that interferes with usual muscle contractures. This can be severe enough to interfere with independence in activities of daily living, including basic mobility and self-care (Elovic, Simone, & Zafonte, 2004).
  - *Myoclonus:* Myoclonic movements involve sudden jerking movements that may be unpredictable. These movements are often less rhythmic and smaller in amplitude when compared with tremors (O'Suilleabhain & Dewey, 2004).
  - *Tremor:* Post-ABI tremors include both postural and kinetic tremors, the latter often being more disabling. Often affecting the arms, such tremors can be present at rest and

during action, increasing in amplitude toward the action's end point. Tremors often range in frequency from 2.5 to 4 Hz, but can be very coarse, with amplitudes larger than 10 cm (Krauss & Jankovic, 2002).

- *Dystonia:* Involuntary muscle contractures resulting in twisted or contorted postures can occur, typically involving one side of the body (*hemidystonia*). This may co-occur with tremor or myoclonus and be present at rest (Krauss & Jankovic, 2002).
- *Other posttraumatic hyperkinesias:* Although occurring less frequently, additional hyperkinetic symptoms may develop post ABI, including ballism, chorea, and tics/ tourettism (Krauss & Jankovic, 2002).

DIAGNOSTIC CONSIDERATIONS

Beyond the diagnoses just discussed, clinicians must also be keenly aware of the potential for psychogenic MDs post ABI. Prevalence data estimate that 2% to 20% of MDs are actually psychogenic in nature (Edwards & Bhatia, 2012; Thenganatt & Jankovic, 2014).

- *Symptom presentation:* Of patients with psychogenic MDs, 50% have psychogenic tremor and an additional 20% demonstrate psychogenic myoclonus (Edwards & Bhatia, 2012; Thenganatt & Jankovic, 2014). Symptoms may indeed have an acute onset associated with some sort of adverse event, including infections and minor peripheral injuries, which can complicate identification of the symptoms as psychogenic. However, psychogenic movement symptoms often differ in critical ways that can aid diagnostic accuracy (Morgante, Edwards, & Espay, 2013). In an examination of 127 patients with psychogenic tremor, the symptoms were noted to ameliorate or cease with distracting maneuvers (72.4% of patients), and were more inconsistent and variable in their presentation. For instance, symptoms beginning in one limb may resolve and then recur in a different limb (Thenganatt & Jankovic, 2014).
- *Risk factors:* Data suggest that psychogenic MDs are more common in women and in individuals with a history of childhood trauma or neglect (Thenganatt & Jankovic, 2014). Patients may display other physical difficulties that are difficult to

identify and treat, such as fibromyalgia, atypical chest pain, and irritable bowel syndrome. They may also occur in the context of frankly psychiatric symptoms, such as panic attacks (Thenganatt & Jankovic, 2014).

TREATMENT

Although treatments for post-ABI MDs indeed focus on effective management of motor symptoms, treatment techniques for idiopathic MDs may not be appropriate for post-ABI MDs (O'Suilleabhain & Dewey, 2004). Posttraumatic symptoms may not respond ideally to usual medical treatment: posttraumatic tremor can be especially difficult to treat, with weaker responses to medical intervention (Krauss & Jankovic, 2002). Further, other symptoms associated with ABI (e.g., impaired cognition, poor balance) can be worsened by standard MD treatment. However, both pharmacological and surgical treatments are available for various types of post-ABI movement symptoms.

Tremor

- *Medical treatments:* Drugs reported to improve post-ABI tremor include barbiturates (e.g., primidone), beta-blockers (e.g., propranolol), dopaminergic agents (e.g., L-dopa/carbidopa), antiepileptics (e.g., carbamazepine), anticholinergics, benzodiazepines (e.g., clonazepam), glutethimide, isoniazid, and L-tryptophan (Ellison, 1978; Harmon, Long, & Shirtz, 1991; Jacob & Pratap Chand, 1998; Katz, 1990; Remy et al., 1995). Botulinum toxin injections may be helpful to relieve tremor temporarily, but the high doses that must be administered to both proximal and distal muscles limit the utility of this treatment (Jankovic & Brin, 1991).

- *Surgical procedures:* Ablative functional stereotactic surgery within the ventrolateral (VL) thalamus and the subthalamic region (STN) can effectively lessen tremor (Krauss et al., 1994; Krauss & Jankovic, 2002). Thalamic deep brain stimulation (DBS) has been useful for some patients with post-ABI tremor (Andy, 1983; Benabid et al., 1996; Broggi, Brock, Franzini, & Geminiani, 1993; Nguyen & Degos, 1993; Vesper et al., 2000). However, DBS is typically considered much less effective post ABI than when used to treat idiopathic tremor in PD or essential tremor (Standhart, Pinter, Volc, & Alesch, 1998).

Posttraumatic Dystonia

- *Medical treatments:* Pharmacological treatment has been relatively ineffective in the few reported cases of post-ABI dystonia (Koller et al., 1989; Pettigrew & Jankovic, 1985). Anticholinergic medications have occasionally improved dystonic symptoms post ABI. However, botulinum toxin injections are the treatment of choice for patients with focal dystonia (Jankovic & Brin, 1991).

- *Surgical procedures:* If dystonia is related to subdural hematoma, draining the hemorrhage is often effective (Dressler & Schönle, 1990; Eaton, 1988; Nobbe & Krauss, 1997). Functional stereotactic surgery is an option for patients with disabling hemidystonia. Typical target sites include VL thalamus, STN, pulvinar nucleus, and the globus pallidus internus (GPi). Patients with secondary dystonia experience less improvement as compared with patients with primary dystonia, regardless of the target. Although there are a few reported cases that demonstrated improvement for post-ABI dystonia with DBS, the research is limited, and it is hard to determine the overall efficacy of the procedure in patients with post-ABI dystonia (Loher, Hasdemir, Burgunder, & Krauss, 2000; Sellal, Hirsch, Barth, Blond, & Marescaux, 1993).

Posttraumatic Parkinsonism

- *Medical treatments:* Dopaminergic medications, including levodopa and dopamine agonists, are the most effective drugs to treat posttraumatic parkinsonism (Marsden & Fahn, 1987). However, similar to the experience with treating other post-ABI MD, these agents are not as effective as when used to treat idiopathic PD.

- *Surgical procedures:* The usefulness of DBS in the treatment of post-ABI parkinsonism is not established. Subthalamic DBS may help motor symptoms to the extent that these symptoms respond to levodopa (O'Suilleabhain & Dewey, 2004).

Posttraumatic Hyperkinesias

- *Medical treatments:* Hyperkinetic movement symptoms may spontaneously resolve in the weeks following ABI, in which case, no treatment is necessary. For persistent chorea, neuroleptics or benzodiazepines have been recommended (Kant & Zeiler, 1996).
- *Surgical procedures:* Stereotactic ablative surgery to the thalamus has been demonstrated to be beneficial, especially in cases of hemiballism (Bullard & Nashold, 1984).

Posttraumatic Tics

- *Medical treatments:* Fewer than 1% of patients with ABI experience tics, and there is little evidence that demonstrates that tics seen post ABI are related to injury and would not have presented in the absence of the trauma (Krauss et al., 1996). If tics are significantly impairing, then neuroleptics, clonidine, and low-dose dopamine agonists may be helpful (O'Suilleabhain & Dewey, 2004). Owing to the rarity of this symptom post ABI, there is little evidence for surgical intervention.

PROGNOSIS

In general, acute ABI symptoms are more likely to resolve than delayed onset symptoms (Krauss et al., 1996). In addition, those patients who receive more intensive therapy within the first 5 months post ABI have been shown to experience better outcomes. Prognosis also varies significantly by predominant symptom type.

- *Posttraumatic tremor:* Post-ABI tremor may lessen or resolve spontaneously within 1 year after onset; nonetheless, the majority of post-ABI tremor will persist (Tan & Truong, 2009). Unfortunately, post-ABI tremor does not respond well to medical therapy, and the medications that have been described may provide only mild relief for the patient.
- *Posttraumatic dystonia:* The long-term prognosis of post-ABI dystonia has not been well researched. However, preliminary

evidence suggests that post-ABI dystonia is characterized by slow progression until stabilized (Tan & Truong, 2009). Fixed dystonic contractures are possible if physical therapy and other relaxation interventions are delayed. Medications and botulinum toxin injections to treat post-ABI dystonia are typically not as effective as when treating idiopathic dystonia (O'Suilleabhain & Dewey, 2004).

Posttraumatic parkinsonism: Although some patients with post-ABI parkinsonism respond well to treatment, most can be resistant to therapy (Marsden & Fahn, 1987). Similar to the experience with treating other post-ABI MD, medications to treat post-ABI parkinsonism are not typically as effective as when treating idiopathic PD. Parkinsonism as a result of repeated closed ABI (as in CTE) is progressive and is even less likely to respond to intervention (McKee et al., 2009).

Posttraumatic hyperkinesias: Preliminary evidence suggests treatment is effective with most posttraumatic hyperkinesias. However, given the rarity of post-ABI hyperkinesias, research is limited (Krauss & Jankovic, 2002). If choreiform movements or other hyperkinetic symptoms are related to subdural hematoma, prognosis is favorable if the hematoma is drained (Adler & Winston, 1984).

CLINICAL SYNOPSIS

- Post-ABI MD is a well-recognized clinical phenomenon that has been documented in clinical reports and empirical investigations for at least 200 years.
- Post-ABI MDs can occur because of lesions anywhere in the motor system or as a result of more widespread neurodegenerative pathologies.
- Tremor is the most frequent post-ABI movement symptom, although ABI can result in a multitude of varied disordered movements, ranging from limb weakness and spasticity to dystonia and ballismus.
- Neurodegenerative MD may also occur post ABI, most frequently CTE and PD.

- Prognosis depends on multiple factors, including the age of the patient, severity of initial injury, the therapy received after injury, predominant symptom type, and underlying pathophysiology.
- Patients with post-ABI movement symptoms may respond more poorly to the medical treatments routinely used to address those symptoms in idiopathic patient groups. Effective medical treatments differ by symptom.
- Some surgical procedures, including ablative and functional stimulation, have demonstrated patient benefit, although available evidence varies by symptom.

CASE STUDY

Broggi, Brock, Franzini, and Geminiani (1993) described the case of a 19-year-old male who had a motorcycle accident at age 17. Injuries included cerebral edema, "modest" subarachnoid hemorrhage, and diffuse contusions and foci of intraparenchymal hemorrhage. He regained consciousness after a 40-day coma with right-sided tremor, worse in the arm, and slight paresis in his right hemisphere of the body. The patient's movement status improved little over the following 2 years, and follow-up imaging conducted when the patient presented for evaluation at age 19 indicated chronic lesions in multiple regions, including the left cerebral peduncle and substantia nigra.

On examination, right upper extremity tremor was slow and of medium amplitude (4–5 Hz), with predominant postural and action features. Tremor was also occasionally present at rest. A coarser action tremor was observed in the right leg, with mild to moderate bradykinesia observed in both the arm and the leg. Symptoms did not respond to usual medical therapy, including anticholinergic therapy with methoxine (an anticholinergic antispasmodic agent sometimes used for parkinsonism). Although symptoms were not eliminated completely, unilateral DBS of the ventral intermediate nucleus of the left thalamus resulted in notable symptom improvement, with amelioration of the right arm tremors and near eradication of the right leg tremors. Symptom improvement was noted to be consistent 10 months after surgery.

REFERENCES

Adler, J. R., & Winston, K. R. (1984). Chorea as a manifestation of epidural hematoma: Case report. *Journal of Neurosurgery, 60*(4), 856–857.

Andy, O. (1983). Thalamic stimulation for control of movement disorders. *Stereotactic and Functional Neurosurgery, 46*(1/4), 107–111.

Bazarian, J. J., Cernak, I., Noble-Haeusslein, L., Potolicchio, S., & Temkin, N. (2009). Long-term neurologic outcomes after traumatic brain injury. *Journal of Head Trauma Rehabilitation, 24*(6), 439–451. doi:10.1097/HTR.0b013e3181c15600

Benabid, A. L., Pollak, P., Gao, D., Hoffmann, D., Limousin, P., Gay, E., . . . Benazzouz, A. (1996). Chronic electrical stimulation of the ventralis intermedius nucleus of the thalamus as a treatment of movement disorders. *Journal of Neurosurgery, 84*(2), 203–214.

Bower, J., Maraganore, D., Peterson, B., McDonnell, S., Ahlskog, J., & Rocca, W. (2003). Head trauma preceding PD: A case-control study. *Neurology, 60*(10), 1610–1615.

Broggi, G., Brock, S., Franzini, A., & Geminiani, G. (1993). A case of post-traumatic tremor treated by chronic stimulation of the thalamus. *Movement Disorders, 8*(2), 206–208.

Bullard, D. E., & Nashold, B. S., Jr. (1984). Stereotaxic thalamotomy for treatment of posttraumatic movement disorders. *Journal of Neurosurgery, 61*(2), 316–321.

Corsellis, J., Bruton, C., & Freeman-Browne, D. (1973). The aftermath of boxing. *Psychological Medicine, 3*(03), 270–303.

Curran, T. G., & Lang, A. (1995). Trauma and tremor. In L. J. Findley & W. C. Koller (Eds.), *Handbook of tremor disorders* (pp. 411–428). New York, NY: Marcel Dekker.

DeKosky, S. T., Blennow, K., Ikonomovic, M. D., & Gandy, S. (2013). Acute and chronic traumatic encephalopathies: Pathogenesis and biomarkers. *Nature Reviews Neurology, 9*(4), 192–200.

Dressler, D., & Schönle, P. (1990). Bilateral limb dystonia due to chronic subdural hematoma. *European Neurology, 30*(4), 211–213.

Eaton, J. M. (1988). Hemidystonia due to subdural hematoma. *Neurology, 38*(3), 507–507.

Edwards, M. J., & Bhatia, K. P. (2012). Functional (psychogenic) movement disorders: Merging mind and brain. *Lancet Neurology, 11*(3), 250–260. doi:10.1016/S1474-4422(11)70310-6

Ellison, P. H. (1978). Propranolol for severe post-head injury action tremor. *Neurology, 28*(2), 197–197.

Elovic, E. P., Simone, L. K., & Zafonte, R. (2004). Outcome assessment for spasticity management in the patient with traumatic brain injury: The state of the art. *Journal of Head Trauma Rehabilitation, 19*(2), 155–177.

Goldman, S. M., Tanner, C. M., Oakes, D., Bhudhikanok, G. S., Gupta, A., & Langston, J. W. (2006). Head injury and Parkinson's disease risk in twins. *Annals of Neurology, 60*(1), 65–72.

Harmon, R. L., Long, D. F., & Shirtz, J. (1991). Treatment of post-traumatic midbrain resting-kinetic tremor with combined levodopa/carbidopa and carbamazepine. *Brain Injury, 5*(2), 213–218.

Jacob, P., & Pratap Chand, R. (1998). Posttraumatic rubral tremor responsive to clonazepam. *Movement Disorders, 13*(6), 977–978.

Jankovic, J. (1994). Post-traumatic movement disorders: Central and peripheral mechanisms. *Neurology, 44*(11), 2006–2006.

Jankovic, J., & Brin, M. (1991). Therapeutic uses of botulinum toxin. *The New England Journal of Medicine, 324*(17), 1186–1194.

Johnson, S., & Hall, D. (1992). Post-traumatic tremor in head injured children. *Archives of Disease in Childhood, 67*(2), 227–228.

Jordan, B. D. (2013). The clinical spectrum of sport-related traumatic brain injury. *Nature Reviews Neurology, 9*(4), 222–230.

Kant, R., & Zeiler, D. (1996). Hemiballismus following closed head injury. *Brain Injury, 10*(2), 155–158.

Katz, D. I. (1990). Movement disorders following traumatic head injury. *Journal of Head Trauma Rehabilitation, 5*(1), 86–90.

Koller, W. C., Weiner, W. J., Nausieda, P. A., & Klawans, H. L. (1979). Pharmacology of ballismus. *Clinical Neuropharmacology, 4*, 157–174.

Koller, W. C., Wong, G. F., & Lang, A. (1989). Posttraumatic movement disorders: A review. *Movement Disorders, 4*(1), 20–36.

Krauss, J. K., & Jankovic, J. (1997). Tics secondary to craniocerebral trauma. *Movement Disorders, 12*(5), 776–782.

Krauss, J. K., & Jankovic, J. (2002). Head injury and posttraumatic movement disorders. *Neurosurgery, 50*(5), 927–939; discussion 939–940.

Krauss, J. K., Mohadjer, M., Braus, D. F., Wakhloo, A. K., Nobbe, F., & Mundinger, F. (1992). Dystonia following head trauma: A report of nine patients and review of the literature. *Movement Disorders, 7*(3), 263–272.

Krauss, J. K., Mohadjer, M., Nobbe, F., & Mundinger, F. (1994). The treatment of posttraumatic tremor by stereotactic surgery: Symptomatic and functional outcome in a series of 35 patients. *Journal of Neurosurgery, 80*(5), 810–819.

Krauss, J. K., Trankle, R., & Kopp, K. H. (1996). Post-traumatic movement disorders in survivors of severe head injury. *Neurology, 47*(6), 1488–1492.

Krauss, J. K., Trankle, R., & Kopp, K. H. (1997). Posttraumatic movement disorders after moderate or mild head injury. *Movement Disorders, 12*(3), 428–431. doi:10.1002/mds.870120326

Krauss, J. K., Wakhloo, A. K., Nobbe, F., Tränkle, R., Mundinger, F., & Seeger, W. (1995). Lesion of dentatothalamic pathways in severe post-traumatic tremor. *Neurological Research, 17*(6), 409–416.

Kremer, M., Russell, W. R., & Smyth, G. (1947). A mid-brain syndrome following head injury. *Journal of Neurology, Neurosurgery, and Psychiatry, 10*(2), 49.

Lang, A. E., & Lozano, A. M. (1998). Parkinson's disease. *The New England Journal of Medicine, 339*(15), 1044–1053.

Loher, T. J., Hasdemir, M. G., Burgunder, J.-M., & Krauss, J. K. (2000). Long-term follow-up study of chronic globus pallidus internus stimulation for posttraumatic hemidystonia: Case report. *Journal of Neurosurgery, 92*(3), 457–460.

Marsden, C., & Fahn, S. (1987). *Movement disorders*. London, United Kingdom: Butterworth.

Martland, H. S. (1928). Punch drunk. *Journal of the American Medical Association, 91*(15), 1103–1107.

McKee, A. C., Cantu, R. C., Nowinski, C. J., Hedley-Whyte, E. T., Gavett, B. E., Budson, A. E., ... Stern, R. A. (2009). Chronic traumatic encephalopathy in athletes: Progressive tauopathy following repetitive head injury. *Journal of Neuropathology and Experimental Neurology, 68*(7), 709.

McKee, A. C., Stein, T. D., Nowinski, C. J., Stern, R. A., Daneshvar, D. H., Alvarez, V. E., ... Baugh, C. M. (2013). The spectrum of disease in chronic traumatic encephalopathy. *Brain, 136*(1), 43–64.

Morgante, F., Edwards, M. J., & Espay, A. J. (2013). Psychogenic movement disorders. *Continuum (Minneap Minn), 19*(5, Movement Disorders), 1383–1396. doi:10.1212/01.CON.0000436160.41071.79

Nguyen, J.-P., & Degos, J.-D. (1993). Thalamic stimulation and proximal tremor: A specific target in the nucleus ventrointermedius thalami. *Archives of Neurology, 50*(5), 498–500.

Nobbe, F. A., & Krauss, J. K. (1997). Subdural hematoma as a cause of contralateral dystonia. *Clinical Neurology and Neurosurgery, 99*(1), 37–39.

Omalu, B., Bailes, J., Hamilton, R. L., Kamboh, M. I., Hammers, J., Case, M., & Robert Fitzsimmons, J. (2011). Emerging histomorphologic phenotypes of chronic traumatic encephalopathy in American athletes. *Neurosurgery, 69*(1), 173–183.

O'Suilleabhain, P., & Dewey, R. B., Jr. (2004). Movement disorders after head injury: Diagnosis and management. *Journal of Head Trauma Rehabilitation, 19*(4), 305–313.

Parkinson, J. (1817). *An essay on the shaking palsy*. London, United Kingdom: Sherwood, Neely and Jones.

Pettigrew, L. C., & Jankovic, J. (1985). Hemidystonia: A report of 22 patients and a review of the literature. *Journal of Neurology, Neurosurgery and Psychiatry, 48*(7), 650–657.

Plassman, B. L., Havlik, R., Steffens, D., Helms, M., Newman, T., Drosdick, D., . . . Burke, J. (2000). Documented head injury in early adulthood and risk of Alzheimer's disease and other dementias. *Neurology, 55*(8), 1158–1166.

Remy, P., de Recondo, A., Defer, G., Loc'h, C., Amarenco, P., Plante-Bordeneuve, V., . . . Clanet, M. (1995). Peduncular 'rubral' tremor and dopaminergic denervation: A PET study. *Neurology, 45*(3), 472–477.

Savica, R., Parisi, J. E., Wold, L. E., Josephs, K. A., & Ahlskog, J. E. (2012). High school football and risk of neurodegeneration: A community-based study. *Mayo Clinic Proceedings, 87*(4), 335–340.

Sellal, F., Hirsch, E., Barth, P., Blond, S., & Marescaux, C. (1993). A case of symptomatic hemidystonia improved by ventroposterolateral thalamic electrostimulation. *Movement Disorders, 8*(4), 515–518.

Standhart, H., Pinter, M., Volc, D., & Alesch, F. (1998). Chronic electrical stimulation of the nucleus ventralis intermedius of the thalamus for the treatment of tremor. *Movement Disorders, 13*(Suppl. 3), 141.

Tan, L. C., & Truong, D. D. (2009). Post-traumatic movement disorders. In R. Lisak, D. Truong, W. Carroll, & R. Bhidayasiri (Eds.), *International neurology: A clinical approach* (pp. 659–660). Singapore: Wiley-Blackwell.

Thenganatt, M. A., & Jankovic, J. (2014). Psychogenic tremor: A video guide to its distinguishing features. *Tremor and Other Hyperkinetic Movements, 4*, 253. doi:10.7916/D8FJ2F0Q

Vesper, J., Funk, T., Kern, B., Wagner, F., Kestenbach, U., Jahnke, U., . . . Brock, M. (2000). Thalamic deep brain stimulation: Present state of the art. *Neurosurgery Quarterly, 10*(4), 252–260.

CHAPTER 13

Acquired Brain Injury in Children

ANA C. ALBUJA
ROBERT BAUMANN

OVERVIEW

Acquired brain injury (ABI) is defined as a postneonatal injury to the brain, most commonly as a result from a traumatic brain injury (TBI). Other etiologies include hypoxic–ischemic encephalopathy (HIE), cerebrovascular disease, and infection (van Tol, Gorter, DeMatteo, & Meester-Delver, 2011). *Brain injuries* that are present before the 28th day of postnatal life are classified as congenital, while those occurring past the 28th day are considered to be acquired. Since TBI, and concussion in particular, is the most common cause of ABI in children, this chapter will be focused on this topic.

HISTORY

The term "concussion" originates from the Latin verb *concutere*, "to shake violently" (McCrea, Hammeke, Olsen, Leo, & Guskiewicz, 2004). Acute management of TBI with trepanation, both for adults and for children, was already described in the writings of Hippocrates of Cos (c. 460–c. 370 BCE) (Missios, 2007) (see Chapter 1).

PATHOPHYSIOLOGY

TBI causes two injury types: primary and secondary. *Primary injury* is the mechanical damage that occurs at the time of trauma. It can lead to soft tissue lacerations, skull fractures, and a variety of central nervous system (CNS) lesions such as epidural or subdural hematomas, cerebral contusions, intracerebral hematomas, intraventricular hemorrhage, or diffuse axonal injury (see Chapters 1 and 2).

Immediately after the primary injury, TBI leads to a dysfunctional cascade involving multiple abnormalities in the CNS, which are collectively known as the *secondary injury*. These include molecular changes such as disruptions in adenosine triphosphate metabolism, release of glutamate, and accumulation of free radicals and intracellular calcium. At the cellular level, injury to the cytoskeleton, loss of cell membrane integrity, and dysfunctional axonal transport are also prominent phenomena. Finally, neuronal metabolism is affected by changes in cerebral blood flow (Rose, Weber, Collen, & Heyer, 2015). If severe enough, the ultimate outcome of the secondary injury may include cerebral infarction, edema, and brain herniation.

Once a primary injury occurs, most therapies aim at decreasing the extent and severity of the secondary injury. The view that children usually have more favorable outcomes after ABI due to greater potential for plasticity is now being challenged. When the developing brain of a child is injured, immature myelination and potential impairments in neuronal plasticity might ensue, increasing the likelihood of functional deficits later in life (Ajao et al., 2012).

ETIOLOGY

The mechanism of injury for pediatric TBI varies with age. In infants and young children, nonaccidental (abusive) TBI is an important etiology of brain injury and is commonly a repetitive insult (Duhaime, Christian, Rorke, & Zimmerman, 1998; Ewing-Cobbs et al., 2000). The incidence of nonaccidental TBI is underreported because only cases that are correctly diagnosed are conveyed in the general statistics (Mulpuri, Slobogean, & Tredwell, 2011). The main causes of accidental TBI in infants and children are falls and being struck by or against objects or other persons (Centers for Disease Control and Prevention [CDC], 2014; Quayle et al., 2014).

In the case of toddlers, falls are the main mechanism of injury. If the history and injury pattern are not consistent, nonaccidental trauma should be considered. When toddlers are involved in motor vehicle–related injuries, they are more frequently struck by a vehicle as pedestrians as opposed to being occupants in motor vehicle accidents.

School-aged children have fewer falls requiring hospitalization as they grow older. In this age group, there is a rise in injuries associated with bicycle crashes. The major causes of TBI in adolescents are assault, sports-related repetitive injury, and motor vehicle accidents (Langlois, Rutland-Brown, & Thomas, 2005; Quayle et al., 2014).

EPIDEMIOLOGY

ABI is a leading cause of death and permanent disability among children and young adults worldwide, with an estimated incidence of 240/100,000 per year (van Tol et al., 2011). TBI is by far the most common cause of ABI in children (Johnson, DeMatt, & Salorio, 2009) and is the most common cause of death in cases of childhood injury. Among all TBI cases, between 88% and 92% correspond to mild injury/concussion (Atabaki, 2013). The rate of emergency room visits is higher for younger children, but hospitalization and death are more frequent among older patients (Wing & James, 2013).

The sport most commonly associated with TBI is football (Atabaki, 2013). There are 1.1 million high school football players in the United States each year, of whom nearly 70,000 are diagnosed with concussion (Broglio et al., 2009). However, this prevalence is likely underreported (Atabaki, 2013; McCrea et al., 2004).

CLINICAL PRESENTATION

As a review from the earlier chapters, the 4th Concussion in Sport Group meeting defined concussion as "a complex pathophysiological process affecting the brain, induced by biomechanical forces" (McCrory et al., 2013). A concussion has to meet four basic requirements: (a) is caused by a direct blow to the head, face, neck, or other region of the body with a force spreading to the head; (b) results in rapid onset of neurological function impairment that lasts for a short period of time and resolves spontaneously; (c) is caused by a functional CNS disruption rather than a structural one; and (d) results in clinical symptoms that may or may not involve loss of consciousness (Echemendia, Giza, & Kutcher, 2015). TBI is a clinical diagnosis, and so history and physical examination are essential. If feasible, information should be obtained directly from the patient. Accurate information provided by witnesses is also very helpful (Atabaki, 2013).

History

- Relevant information to be obtained by health care providers includes circumstances of trauma (i.e., falls, motor vehicle accident), height of fall, type of object that caused impact to the head, speed of vehicle, degree of damage to vehicle and injuries to other occupants, whether protective equipment such as seatbelts were used, and so forth (Wing & James, 2013).
- Important clinical data to be collected include presence and duration of loss of consciousness, retrograde/anterograde amnesia, confusion, seizures (with as many descriptors as possible), headache, visual changes, nausea, and vomiting (Atabaki, 2013; Field, Collins, Lovell, & Maroon, 2003).
- Common signs and symptoms of concussion involve multiple domains:
    - Physical, such as headache, nausea, vomiting, balance problems, dizziness, problems with vision, sensitivity to lights or sounds, fatigue, numbness, tingling, and confusion
    - Cognitive, including problems with memory and concentration and feeling mentally foggy and slowed down
    - Psychological, namely, irritability, sadness, anxiety, and mood swings
    - Sleep related, such as increased or decreased sleepiness and insomnia (Atabaki, 2013)
- Although the aforementioned symptoms usually last 7 to 10 days after the insult, time to recovery may be longer in children and adolescents. Research shows that 80% to 90% of adolescents recover within 2 to 3 weeks after the injury (Covassin, Elbin, & Nakayama, 2010; Field et al., 2003; McCrea et al., 2004).
- Be aware that the initial symptoms of a concussion may appear several hours after the trauma, impairing the diagnosis at the time of injury (Echemendia et al., 2015).

Physical Examination

- Vital signs should be evaluated and managed accordingly. In particular, look for bradycardia, tachycardia, hypotension, and hypoxia.

TABLE 13.1 PEDIATRIC AND STANDARD GLASGOW COMA SCALE

Response	≤2 Yr Old	≥3 Yr Old	Score
Eye opening	Spontaneous	Spontaneous	4
	To speech	To speech	3
	To pain	To pain	2
	None	None	1
Best verbal response	Smiles, coos, babbles, age-appropriate speech	Oriented	5
	Irritable, cries	Confused	4
	Cries to pain	Inappropriate words	3
	Moans to pain	Incomprehensible sounds	2
	None	None	1
Best motor response	Normal spontaneous movement	Follows commands	6
	Withdraws to touch	Localizes pain	5
	Withdraws to pain	Withdraws to pain	4
	Abnormal flexion	Abnormal flexion	3
	Abnormal extension	Abnormal extension	2
	None	None	1

Modified from Lumba-Brown and Pineda (2014).

- Table 13.1 depicts the Pediatric and Standard Glasgow Coma Scale, which is used to quantify the severity of acute TBI.
- Examine the head, looking for scalp swelling, hematomas, abrasions, and lacerations.
- Palpate the scalp looking for obvious fracture or deformity, fontanel fullness in infants, bleeding or drainage from the ears or nose concerning for cerebrospinal fluid leakage.
- Also look for signs of fracture of the base of the skull, such as bruising over the mastoid (Battle's sign) or periorbital bruising (raccoon eyes).

- Examine pupils, looking for symmetry, size, and responsiveness.
- Perform a funduscopic examination to look for retinal hemorrhages and papilledema (swelling of the optic disc).
- Inspect and palpate the cervical spine, looking for potential step-offs or areas of focal tenderness.
- There should always be a complete neurological exam.
- Changes in the mental status examination should be monitored over time.
- The provider should ask the parents if the patient is acting at or close to his or her baseline, especially if the child is younger than 2 years of age (Wing & James, 2013).

DIAGNOSTIC CONSIDERATIONS

The initial evaluation by a health care provider should focus on determining the presence of a life-threatening injury. Emergent evaluation of severe TBI includes evaluation of airway, breathing, circulation, neurological deficits, and other concurrent injuries and is beyond the scope of this chapter (Atabaki, 2013) (see Chapter 2).

Several tools are available for health care providers for the evaluation of concussion. Some of these can be found in the CDC website: (CDC, 2016). The Post-Concussion Symptom Inventory (PCSI)–child/adolescent self-report and parent report forms are developmentally appropriate tools that can aid in the diagnosis and management of concussion (Gioia, Janusz, Isquith, & Vincent, 2008). In order to monitor response to treatment and resolution of symptoms, preinjury scores should be compared with postinjury symptoms. Psychometrically validated concussion-screening tools based on the history and physical examination, such as the Acute Concussion Evaluation (ACE) or the Sport Concussion Assessment Tool (SCAT3), can be used to perform an initial evaluation and diagnosis of patients with concussion (Gioia, Collins, & Isquith, 2008; McCrory et al., 2013).

A single tool or questionnaire is not sufficient for adequate evaluation of the injury. The skilled clinician should use the aforementioned information in the context of the child's developmental, medical, psychological, and family/school environment to help guide clinical decision making (Gioia, 2015).

Neuropsychological Testing

Baseline neuropsychological testing can be helpful when deciding when a patient should return to play, but it is not mandatory. Although these tests provide clinically significant information, they should not be the sole factor determining the return-to-play decision (Echemendia et al., 2015).

Imaging

The main use of computed tomography (CT) in the acute period after trauma is to rule out life-threatening injuries like skull/facial/spine fractures and the presence of blood products in the brain. CT scans have a significant cost and risks, including a three-fold increase in the risk of developing brain tumors later in life (Pearce et al., 2012).

In 2009, the Pediatric Emergency Care Applied Research Network (PECARN) issued validated prediction rules to identify children at very low risk of clinically important TBI, which is defined as TBI requiring neurosurgical intervention or leading to death (Kuppermann et al., 2009). These criteria allow for a more judicious use of imaging studies and can be found in Table 13.2. If the patient does not meet any of the criteria, the risk of clinically important TBI is very low and imaging is not recommended. Online calculators are also available.

For children younger than 2 years of age, this prediction rule had both a negative predictive value and sensitivity of 100%. For older children, negative predictive value was 99.95% and sensitivity 96.8%. When evaluating the patient days, weeks, or longer after the initial injury, magnetic resonance imaging (MRI) can help detect more subtle abnormalities but does not need to be done routinely (Atabaki, 2013). Functional MRI helps provide information regarding the pathophysiological mechanisms of the injury but is mostly used in research settings (Echemendia et al., 2015).

TREATMENT

Return to School

- One of the main challenges in the management of concussion in children and adolescents is preparing to return to school. Despite its importance, there is relatively little evidence regarding the return-to-school process (Gioia, 2015).

TABLE 13.2 PEDIATRIC EMERGENCY CARE APPLIED RESEARCH NETWORK (PECARN) CRITERIA FOR IDENTIFICATION OF PATIENTS WITH TBI WHO REQUIRE CT SCAN TO LOOK FOR LIFE-THREATENING INJURIES

Children Younger Than 2 Yr	Children Older Than 2 Yr
Glasgow Coma Scale < 15	
Altered mental status	
Severe mechanism of injury, including motor vehicle accident with patient ejection, death of another passenger, or rollover; person without helmet struck by motor vehicle, head struck by high-impact object, falls from >3 ft for <2 yr or from >5 ft for >2 yr	
History of loss of consciousness for >5 sec	History of loss of consciousness
Not acting normally per parent	History of vomiting
Palpable skull fracture	Signs of skull base fracture
Scalp hematoma in the occipital, parietal, or temporal region	Severe headache

CT, computed tomography; TBI, traumatic brain injury.
Modified from Kuppermann et al. (2009).

- Successful return to school requires a prepared system with trained medical providers and a team of school personnel who are trained in this field.
- The student should have an initial concussion evaluation by a health care provider, and the symptoms should be communicated to the trained school personnel.
- The family, health care provider, school, and athletics department should coordinate and communicate the student's status and progress. A school team that is qualified in this area should make necessary academic adjustments and accommodations to meet the student's needs.
- A program for management of concussion in school should focus on two areas:

- School accommodations or adaptations to the student's schedule in order to support areas of cognitive dysfunction after the concussion.
- Individualized evaluation and management of the student's cognitive exertional response. This response manifests by worsening in postconcussion symptoms such as headaches, fatigue, or decreased concentration triggered by the cognitive, emotional, and physical demands of the school setting. This varies from person to person (Gioia, 2015).
- In the past, the recommendation for the management of concussion was to allow the patient to rest completely until symptoms resolved. Currently, there is more evidence favoring an active rehabilitation model (Gagnon, Galli, Friedman, Grilli, & Iverson, 2009; Silverberg & Iverson, 2013). This type of therapy is especially helpful in patients who recover slowly such as children. If a child takes longer to recover and the activities are restricted for prolonged periods of time while using the first approach, there is a risk for developing secondary complications such as fatigue, deconditioning, and behavioral and emotional problems. Although there is limited clinical research focused on children with concussion, there is indirect evidence supporting an active rehabilitation approach (Gagnon et al., 2009; Leddy et al., 2010).
- The general treatment recommendation in the active rehabilitation model is to engage as much as possible in cognitive and physical activities while avoiding those that significantly worsen symptoms, especially in the initial phase of recovery (Gioia, 2015).
- Prolonged absence from school is not recommended. Absence for longer than 2 to 4 weeks can lead to difficulty interacting with classmates and readjusting to school routine (Barlow, 2014).

Return to Play

- Recommendations from different practice guidelines regarding the time when a patient should return to play comprise three settings: preparticipation counseling, management of suspected concussion, and management of diagnosed concussion.

- Preparticipation counseling: It is recommended that information about concussion risk be distributed to athletes, coaches, trainers, and families.
- Management of suspected concussion: Coaches and athletic trainers should ask the child to stop playing immediately. The basic rule is "sit it out, if in doubt." A concussed athlete should be observed closely during the first few hours after the injury to monitor for cognitive and/or physical worsening. An athlete who suffers a concussion should not return to compete on the same day (Echemendia et al., 2015). Reasons to proactively remove a child from play are to allow time for the healing process and to prevent neurocognitive consequences of reinjury and a rare complication, second-impact syndrome, that can present with cerebral edema, uncal herniation, and death (Atabaki, 2013; Bey & Ostick, 2009).
- Management of diagnosed concussion: Return to play should not be permitted until the athlete is asymptomatic in the absence of medications and until a skilled health care provider determines that the concussion has resolved.
- Current guidelines regarding when to return to play are individualized. However, the key factors are resolution of symptoms and return to baseline neurocognitive function.
- Return to play should be gradual. Patients should initially avoid physical activity, then start with some aerobic exercise, transition to a noncontact practice followed by full-contact practice, and finally return to play (Echemendia et al., 2015).

Medications

- Theoretically, pharmacological therapy can be useful for two purposes: to treat the symptoms of the concussion and/or to modulate the mechanisms underlying the secondary injury. However, at this time there is no evidence to support the use of any medications in particular for treatment of the secondary injury (Echemendia et al., 2015).
- Sequelae of concussion, such as headaches and seizures, should be treated with standard medications (see Chapters 10 and 11).

- Treatment of sleep disturbances is critical as it improves school performance and can decrease behavioral symptoms. Sleep hygiene should be encouraged. Use of caffeine or medications that affect sleep should be minimized. Management can include medications, such as melatonin or amitriptyline. However, cognitive behavioral therapy can be more effective than medications alone in the management of chronic insomnia (Barlow, 2014).

PROGNOSIS

- The range of outcomes in pediatric TBI is very broad, from full recovery to severe physical and/or intellectual disabilities.
- Regarding the prognosis after a concussion, the best evidence currently available suggests that postconcussion symptoms resolve over time in most patients (Hung et al., 2014). Between 13% and 29% of school-aged children remain symptomatic 3 months after the injury, and approximately 2% continue to show symptoms at 1 year (Barlow, 2014).
- Incapacitating sequelae can be seen following severe TBI. For example, children who sustain severe TBI have been found to have more behavioral problems and poorer intellectual, reading, and spelling ability 5 years after the injury (Catroppa, Anderson, Morse, Haritou, & Rosenfeld, 2008).
- A Glasgow Coma Scale of 5 or less shortly after the initial head trauma has been found to be the threshold at which a poor outcome is more probable (Chung et al., 2006).
- Children and adolescents who have suffered a TBI are at increased risk of social dysfunction. Studies show that these patients can have poor self-esteem, loneliness, maladjustment, reduced emotional control, and aggressive or antisocial behavior (Rosema, Crowe, & Anderson, 2012).
- It often takes months or years to fully appreciate the consequences of ABI in children, as developmental, educational, and social demands increase.
- The most significant predictors of long-term outcomes for children after an ABI include characteristics of the brain injury, such

as size and location; age at time of injury; premorbid function; and environmental factors such as family support and availability of rehabilitative resources (Gordon & di Maggio, 2012).

CLINICAL SYNOPSIS

- ABI is any injury to the brain that occurs after day 28 of postnatal life.
- The most common etiology is TBI. Other frequent causes include hypoxic ischemic encephalopathy, cerebrovascular disease, and infection.
- TBI causes significant morbidity and mortality in children and is an important public health concern.
- Early identification and management of TBI are essential in order to improve long-term outcomes.
- Shortly after injury, a careful clinical evaluation is critical. It can be used to define a risk stratification protocol to promote the judicious use of imaging studies while avoiding unnecessary expenses and radiation exposure for patients who do not have any red flags.
- Postconcussion syndrome includes a variety of somatic, cognitive, and psychological symptoms that can last for months if not treated adequately.
- Outcomes can be improved by strategies consisting of physical activity and cognitive approaches, as well as by a gradual return to sport and school. Treatment of associated sleep disturbances is of great importance.

CASE STUDY

A 12-year-old boy comes to your office for evaluation of headache and mood swings. One month earlier, he suffered a helmet-to-helmet collision with another player during a football game. He lost consciousness for a few seconds and then seemed to be confused. He was immediately removed from the game and evaluated in the emergency department. CT scan of the head showed no abnormalities. Patient was diagnosed with a concussion and discharged home. He rested for a few days after the trauma but then returned to school because his parents were afraid that he would get behind in his studies. Before the trauma, he was an honor roll student. Teachers are now concerned because his grades are dropping. You use different tools to evaluate the child and refer him for neuropsychological testing. His neurocognitive test results demonstrated impairments in learning and memory, attention/working memory, and processing speed. These results combined with his history were considered to be consistent with a mild traumatic brain injury. You schedule a meeting with parents and teachers, and a school plan is developed in which the boy has periodic rest periods from studying, has more time to take tests, and his homework is shorter.

You evaluate the boy 1 month later and his symptoms have improved significantly. His plan is modified again at that time. His rest periods are now less frequent. He is still allowed a longer time to take tests but has the same homework load as his classmates. Reevaluation with different tools and neuropsychological testing 3 months after the injury shows that patient is back to preconcussion state.

REFERENCES

Ajao, D. O., Pop, V., Kamper, J. E., Adami, A., Rudobeck, E., Huang, L., . . . Badaut, J. (2012). Traumatic brain injury in young rats leads to progressive behavioral deficits coincident with altered tissue properties in adulthood. *Journal of Neurotrauma, 29*(11), 2060–2074. doi:10.1089/neu.2011.1883

Atabaki, S. M. (2013). Updates in the general approach to pediatric head trauma and concussion. *Pediatric Clinics of North America, 60*(5), 1107–1122. doi:10.1016/j.pcl.2013.06.001

Barlow, K. M. (2014). Postconcussion syndrome: A review. *Journal of Child Neurology, 31*(1), 57–67. doi:10.1177/0883073814543305

Bey, T., & Ostick, B. (2009). Second impact syndrome. *The Western Journal of Emergency Medicine, 10*(1), 6–10.

Broglio, S. P., Sosnoff, J. J., Shin, S., He, X., Alcaraz, C., & Zimmerman, J. (2009). Head impacts during high school football: A biomechanical assessment. *Journal of Athletic Training, 44*(4), 342–349. doi:10.4085/1062-6050-44.4.342

Catroppa, C., Anderson, V. A., Morse, S. A., Haritou, F., & Rosenfeld, J. V. (2008). Outcome and predictors of functional recovery 5 years following pediatric traumatic brain injury (TBI). *Journal of Pediatric Psychology, 33*(7), 707–718. doi:10.1093/jpepsy/jsn006

Centers for Disease Control and Prevention. (2014). *Injury prevention & control: Traumatic brain injury: TBI data and statistics.* Retrieved from www.cdc.gov/traumaticbraininjury/data/index.html

Centers for Disease Control and Prevention. (2016). *Traumatic brain injury & concussion: Resources for health care providers.* Retrieved from www.cdc.gov/traumaticbraininjury/providers.html

Chung, C. Y., Chen, C. L., Cheng, P. T., See, L. C., Tang, S. F., & Wong, A. M. (2006). Critical score of Glasgow Coma Scale for pediatric traumatic brain injury. *Pediatric Neurology, 34*(5), 379–387. doi:10.1016/j.pediatrneurol.2005.10.012

Covassin, T., Elbin, R. J., & Nakayama, Y. (2010). Tracking neurocognitive performance following concussion in high school athletes. *The Physician and Sportsmedicine, 38*(4), 87–93. doi:10.3810/psm.2010.12.1830

Duhaime, A. C., Christian, C. W., Rorke, L. B., & Zimmerman, R. A. (1998). Nonaccidental head injury in infants: The "shaken-baby syndrome". *The New England Journal of Medicine, 338*(25), 1822–1829. doi:10.1056/NEJM199806183382507

Echemendia, R. J., Giza, C. C., & Kutcher, J. S. (2015). Developing guidelines for return to play: Consensus and evidence-based approaches. *Brain Injury, 29*(2), 185–194. doi:10.3109/02699052.2014.965212

Ewing-Cobbs, L., Prasad, M., Kramer, L., Louis, P. T., Baumgartner, J., Fletcher, J. M., & Alpert, B. (2000). Acute neuroradiologic findings in young children with inflicted or noninflicted traumatic brain injury. *Child's Nervous System, 16*(1), 25–33; discussion 34. doi:10.1007/s003810050006

Field, M., Collins, M. W., Lovell, M. R., & Maroon, J. (2003). Does age play a role in recovery from sports-related concussion? A comparison of high school and collegiate athletes. *Journal of Pediatrics, 142*(5), 546–553. doi:10.1067/mpd.2003.190

Gagnon, I., Galli, C., Friedman, D., Grilli, L., & Iverson, G. L. (2009). Active rehabilitation for children who are slow to recover following sport-related concussion. *Brain Injury, 23*(12), 956–964. doi:10.3109/02699050903373477

Gioia, G. A. (2015). Multimodal evaluation and management of children with concussion: Using our heads and available evidence. *Brain Injury, 29*(2), 195–206. doi:10.3109/02699052.2014.965210

Gioia, G. A., Collins, M., & Isquith, P. K. (2008). Improving identification and diagnosis of mild traumatic brain injury with evidence: Psychometric support for the acute concussion evaluation. *Journal of Head Trauma Rehabilitation, 23*(4), 230–242.

Gioia, G. A., Janusz, J., Isquith P., & Vincent, D. (2008). Psychometric properties of the parent and teacher Post-Concussion Symptom Inventory (PCSI) for children and adolescents (Abstract). *Journal of the International Neuropsychological Society, 14*(Suppl. 1), 204.

Gordon, A. L., & di Maggio, A. (2012). Rehabilitation for children after acquired brain injury: Current and emerging approaches. *Pediatric Neurology, 46*(6), 339–344. doi:10.1016/j.pediatrneurol.2012.02.029

Hung, R., Carroll, L. J., Cancelliere, C., Cote, P., Rumney, P., Keightley, M., . . . Cassidy, J. D. (2014). Systematic review of the clinical course, natural history, and prognosis for pediatric mild traumatic brain injury: Results of the International Collaboration on Mild Traumatic Brain Injury Prognosis. *Archives of Physical Medicine and Rehabilitation, 95*(3, Suppl.), S174–S191. doi:10.1016/j.apmr.2013.08.301

Johnson, A. R., DeMatt, E., & Salorio, C. F. (2009). Predictors of outcome following acquired brain injury in children. *Developmental Disabilities Research Reviews, 15*(2), 124–132. doi:10.1002/ddrr.63

Kuppermann, N., Holmes, J. F., Dayan, P. S., Hoyle, J. D., Jr., Atabaki, S. M., Holubkov, R., . . . Pediatric Emergency Care Applied Research Network. (2009). Identification of children at very low risk of clinically-important brain injuries after head trauma: A prospective cohort study. *Lancet, 374*(9696), 1160–1170. doi:10.1016/S0140-6736(09) 61558-0

Langlois, J. A., Rutland-Brown, W., & Thomas, K. E. (2005). The incidence of traumatic brain injury among children in the United States: Differences by race. *The Journal of Head Trauma Rehabilitation, 20*(3), 229–238.

Leddy, J. J., Kozlowski, K., Donnelly, J. P., Pendergast, D. R., Epstein, L. H., & Willer, B. (2010). A preliminary study of subsymptom threshold exercise training for refractory post-concussion syndrome. *Clinical Journal of Sport Medicine, 20*(1), 21–27. doi:10.1097/JSM.0b013e3181c6c22c

Lumba-Brown, A., & Pineda, J. (2014). Evidence-based assessment of severe pediatric traumatic brain injury and emergent neurocritical care. *Seminars in Pediatric Neurology, 21*(4), 275–283. doi:10.1016/j.spen.2014.11.001

McCrea, M., Hammeke, T., Olsen, G., Leo, P., & Guskiewicz, K. (2004). Unreported concussion in high school football players: Implications for prevention. *Clinical Journal of Sport Medicine, 14*(1), 13–17.

McCrory, P., Meeuwisse, W., Aubry, M., Cantu, B., Dvorak, J., Echemendia, R., . . . Turner, M. (2013). Consensus statement on concussion in sport: The 4th International Conference on Concussion in Sport held in Zurich, November 2012. *Physical Therapy in Sport, 14*(2), e1–e13. doi:10.1016/j.ptsp.2013.03.002

Missios, S. (2007). Hippocrates, Galen, and the uses of trepanation in the ancient classical world. *Neurosurgical Focus, 23*(1), E11. doi:10.3171/foc.2007.23.1.11

Mulpuri, K., Slobogean, B. L., & Tredwell, S. J. (2011). The epidemiology of nonaccidental trauma in children. *Clinical Orthopaedics and Related Research, 469*(3), 759–767. doi:10.1007/s11999-010-1565-4

Pearce, M. S., Salotti, J. A., Little, M. P., McHugh, K., Lee, C., Kim, K. P., . . . Berrington de Gonzalez, A. (2012). Radiation exposure from CT scans in childhood and subsequent risk of leukaemia and brain tumours: A retrospective cohort study. *Lancet, 380*(9840), 499–505. doi:10.1016/S0140-6736(12)60815-0

Quayle, K. S., Powell, E. C., Mahajan, P., Hoyle, J. D., Jr., Nadel, F. M., Badawy, M. K., . . . Kuppermann, N. (2014). Epidemiology of blunt head trauma in children in U.S. emergency departments. *The New England Journal of Medicine, 371*(20), 1945–1947. doi:10.1056/NEJMc1407902

Rose, S. C., Weber, K. D., Collen, J. B., & Heyer, G. L. (2015). The diagnosis and management of concussion in children and adolescents. *Pediatric Neurology, 53*(2), 108–118. doi:10.1016/j.pediatrneurol.2015.04.003

Rosema, S., Crowe, L., & Anderson, V. (2012). Social function in children and adolescents after traumatic brain injury: A systematic review 1989–2011. *Journal of Neurotrauma, 29*(7), 1277–1291. doi:10.1089/neu.2011.2144

Silverberg, N. D., & Iverson, G. L. (2013). Is rest after concussion "the best medicine?": Recommendations for activity resumption following concussion in athletes, civilians, and military service members. *The Journal of Head Trauma Rehabilitation, 28*(4), 250–259. doi:10.1097/HTR.0b013e31825ad658

van Tol, E., Gorter, J. W., DeMatteo, C., & Meester-Delver, A. (2011). Participation outcomes for children with acquired brain injury: A narrative review. *Brain Injury, 25*(13/14), 1279–1287. doi:10.3109/02699052.2011.613089

Wing, R., & James, C. (2013). Pediatric head injury and concussion. *Emergency Medicine Clinics of North America, 31*(3), 653–675. doi:10.1016/j.emc.2013.05.007

CHAPTER 14

Acquired Brain Injury in the Elderly

THOMAS J. FARRER
JILL Z. STUART

OVERVIEW

Acquired brain injury (ABI), at any age, is a significant public health concern. It is particularly problematic in the elderly considering the increased rates of mortality and morbidity following ABI in this population. Given the expected age increase in the general population in the next several years, understanding ABI among older adults is critical in successful patient management in neurotrauma and rehabilitation settings. This is especially true given recent population-based research suggesting that as age increases, rates for hospitalization following ABI also increase (Chan, Zagorski, Parsons, & Colantonio, 2013). The following chapter will focus on the unique aspects of ABI among older adults, with a specific focus on prevention and postrehabilitation factors.

HISTORY

ABI consists of traumatic brain injury (TBI) and non-TBI (nTBI). Here, TBI is defined as insult to the brain after the head has been struck by or against another object. For instance, TBIs among older adults are most often caused by falls, but may also include motor vehicle accidents (MVA), assaults, or otherwise being struck by or against another object. Non-TBI is defined as an acquired injury not caused by impact or a degenerative process. This typically includes anoxic or hypoxic injury, stroke, tumor, encephalitis, meningitis, metabolic encephalopathy, and toxic effects of substances (Chan et al., 2013). Historically, ABI literature has focused on general population data and not specifically on older adults. Studies that do focus on older adults typically examine whether injury, particularly TBI, is related to or accelerates the onset of dementia. Additionally, another large portion of studies in the geriatric population is concerned with caregiver factors. Overall, considering older adults will continue to make up larger and larger portions of the population, there is a need for direct research focused in this age group.

PATHOPHYSIOLOGY

The pathophysiology of specific types of ABIs is discussed elsewhere in this book. As such, the focus here will be on the unique aspects of pathophysiology of ABI to elderly populations. First, to understand the physiological disruption of ABI on the aging brain, it is important to understand the natural changes that occur in the brain as healthy older adults age. Research on the aging brain consistently demonstrates that there is a steady rate of volume loss as time goes by, though it is not clear whether this is due to cell death, cell morphological change, or both (Peters, 2006). There are white matter changes with age, with older adults showing signs of loss with myelin sheath deterioration beginning around age 40 (Mukherjee et al., 2002). The aging brain demonstrates changes in the synthesis of key neurotransmitter, including dopamine and serotonin (Mukherjee et al., 2002), and other chemicals important to brain health, such as brain-derived neurotrophic factors (BDNF) (Nugent et al., 2014; Peters, 2006). There is also evidence of changes in glucose metabolism, mitochondrial dysfunction, and calcium dysregulation (Melov, 2004; Peters, 2006). In addition, there are also significant microvascular changes in the aging brain that can impact physiology and cognitive functioning. These changes can lead to attenuated cerebral blood flow, reduced vascularization of brain parenchyma, and increased cerebrovascular risk. With these alterations come natural changes in cognition due to decreased ability of the brain to meet metabolic demands during cognitively demanding tasks. When taken together, natural changes in the adult aging brain—that is, changes in brain volume, white matter integrity, neurotransmitter systems, metabolic processes, and vascular changes—make the pathophysiology of ABI unique in older adults.

ETIOLOGY

In the general adult population, etiology of TBI includes falls (28%), MVA (20%), struck by/against an object (19%), assault (11%), other (13%), and unknown (9%) (Langlois, Rutland-Brown, & Wald, 2006). Falls are the most common cause of TBI in the elderly, accounting for nearly 61% of TBIs among those age 65 and older. A recent, large population-based study by Chan et al. (2013) found that as age increases, the incidence of fall-related TBIs increases whereas MVA-related TBIs decreases. For nTBI, Chan and colleagues (2013) also found that from 2003 to 2009 the most common nTBI for older adults was tumors (44%), followed by anoxia (20%) and stroke (14%). Interestingly, with increased age, the percentage of nTBI due to tumor declines and the percentage of nTBI due to anoxia and stroke increases (Chan et al., 2013). In fact, advancing age is a significant risk factor for fatal stroke, with one study demonstrating that the odds of fatal stroke for adults age 86 and older was seven times that of individuals age 65 to 75 (Clarke, Blount, & Colantonio, 2011).

EPIDEMIOLOGY

In the general population, the incidence of TBI in the United States is somewhere between 1.5 and 2 million cases per year, though these figures do not include individuals in the military or those treated by primary care doctors. This includes 1.4 million ER visits, of which more than 140,000 are from older adults age 65+. In fact, the highest rates of TBI-related ED visits occur among older adults who are age 75+ (Coronado, McGuire, Faul, Sugerman, & Pearson, 2013). From 2002 to 2006, the annual incidence of TBI-related hospital admissions was 275,000 with over 81,000 being older adults age 65+. Dams-O'Connor and colleagues (2013) found a 20% to 25% increase in trauma center admissions for those ≥75 years old relative to the general adult population. Although men are more likely to sustain TBIs than women in the general adult population, the study by Dams-O'Connor et al. suggests that for those age 65+, hospitalization due to TBIs was more common among White women who sustained their injury from a fall. In the general population, approximately one-third of all injury-related deaths are due to TBI (Coronado et al., 2013). The annual incidence of TBI-related deaths is approximately 51,000, with older adults accounting for more than 14,000 of these deaths (Coronado et al., 2013). Dams-O'Connor et al. (2013) demonstrated that the risk of death was greater for TBI patients with hypotension (SBP between 50 and 89 mmHg), for those with lower initial Glasgow Coma Scale (GCS) scores, and for those age 85 and older. In terms of hospitalizations, highest rates are among older adults, with 75 years old and older representing 34% of TBI-related hospitalizations. In a large population-based study in Canada, one study found that the rate of TBI-related hospitalizations increases with age (Chan et al., 2013). Specifically, this study found that for ages 65 to 74, 11% of TBI patients are hospitalized but that this number jumps to 50% for ages 75 to 84 and to 63% for those age 85+. Population data also indicated that from 1995 to 2001 and then from 2002 to 2006, incidence of TBI among older adults has increased.

In addition to age, several other factors are related to TBI risk. For instance, in the general adult population, men are twice as likely to have TBI as women (Frost, Farrer, Primosch, & Hedges, 2013), 3.4 times more likely to sustain fatal TBI, and six times more likely to die from firearm-related injuries (Corrigan, Selassie, & Orman, 2010). There is also evidence for higher rates of TBI among American Indian/Alaska Natives and African Americans relative to other ethnic groups (Corrigan et al., 2010). Alcohol use is also a well-known risk factor of TBI across all ages. Frankel et al. (2006) examined alcohol levels in older adults with TBI (age 55–89) compared with younger adults (age 16–44) and found that the presence of alcohol in the blood was more common in younger adults (44%) relative to older adults (18%), but that when present, blood alcohol levels are equivalent between groups. This study also examined day-of-injury brain CT findings in a subsample of participants and demonstrated that a midline shift of more than 5 mm was more common in older adults (31%) compared with younger adults (14%). In examining postinjury medical complications, Frankel et al. (2006) also reported that older adults had twice the incidence of seizure and urinary tract infection and three times the incidence of cardiopulmonary arrest. Such complications could certainly increase the length of stay (LOS) for older adults. Indeed, this study found that older adults had an average of 5 additional days in acute rehabilitation compared with younger adults and that this was likely responsible for significantly high inpatient rehabilitation charges for older adults. In addition, Dams-O'Connor and colleagues (2013) found that older adults with TBI were more likely to require additional in-hospital procedures such as imaging and surgery.

In terms of the impact of TBI, 43% of TBI survivors released from acute care continue to have life-long TBI-related disability (Selassie et al., 2008). Among older adults, increase in age is associated with increased chance of being released from acute care to a long-term care facility rather than home (Chan et al., 2013), which can contribute to patient and family distress, as well as financial strain. Overall, the medical–legal cost of TBI is estimated to be around US$60 billion annually, with a per-person annual cost estimated around US$45,000 (Corrigan et al., 2010). Note, however, that the cost of TBI among older adults has not been delineated in the research literature. Relatively little is known about the financial impact of nTBI in the United States. However, a large population-based study in Canada found that in the first year postinjury, the per-patient cost of nTBI is estimated to be $38,000 (CAD). The total medical cost for nTBI patients in the first year is estimated at $368 million (CAD), with a majority of the costs being accrued during acute care (Chen et al., 2012).

The incidence and prevalence of ABI among older adults is difficult to define given the variable definition of nTBI-related injuries. However, one study examined both TBI and nTBI population–based statistics from 2003 to 2009 (Chan et al., 2013). Similar to the aforementioned statistics on TBI, this study found that between 2003 and 2009, the rate of nTBI increased among older individuals and hospitalizations due to nTBI also increased with age.

As noted previously in this chapter, age is a significant risk factor for fatal stroke, with the odds of fatal stroke for individuals age 86+ being seven times higher than that of individuals age 65 to 75 (Clarke et al., 2011). The same study, which consisted of over 9,000 adults age 65+, identified education as a significant predictor of fatal stroke among older adults. Those with less than a high school education have a 95% higher odds of fatal stroke relative to older adults with a college education. Not surprisingly, older adults with comorbid diabetes and hypertension have a 50% increase in odds of incidence of stroke when followed longitudinally. In this study, lower baseline cognitive functioning was associated with a two-fold increased risk of fatal stroke, even after controlling for health-related and sociodemographic risk factors. The authors postulated that this was likely due to the fact that those with reduced cognitive functioning at baseline likely already had microvascular and white matter changes that result in reduced cognition and that this poor cerebrovascular health placed them at greater risk of future stroke.

CLINICAL PRESENTATION

The clinical presentation of ABI is varied, depending on the severity of the injury, etiology, and lesion location. The clinical presentation of specific types of ABIs is discoursed elsewhere in this volume. However, a few general points are discussed here. In a neurotrauma or rehabilitation setting, acute presentation of ABI would typically include injuries with acute onset such as TBI, anoxia, and stroke. In such settings, it is important to remember that level of consciousness occurs on a continuum and could include coma, vegetative state, and minimally conscious state (Kwasnica, Brown, Elovic, Kothari, & Flanagan, 2008). In addition, patients with parietal lesions may present with a lack of insight to the nature and severity of their condition. Those with left hemisphere lesions may have aphasia, with greater difficulties in comprehension occurring in posterior temporal and inferior parietal regions and more difficulty with production of speech in anterior regions, namely, the inferior frontal gyrus or Broca's area. Given the high incidence of left middle cerebral artery involvement in stroke, it is important for neurotrauma or rehabilitation clinicians to be aware of language and communication deficits in their patients. Individuals with production aphasia (i.e., impaired expressive language and intact receptive language) tend to be more aware of their impairments and are therefore more vulnerable to depression. Regardless of the type of injury, older adults in an inpatient neurotrauma or rehabilitation setting often have compromised executive functioning (i.e., reduced decision making) and may benefit from a formal mental status or cognitive evaluation. Also, when examining patients' mental status, it is critical to be aware of changes in vision, motor functioning, and language that would only confound test results and make the patients appear more impaired than they truly are. Individuals with TBI or stroke, depending on lesion location, may present with hemiparesis, decreased tone, and/or weakness, which would make them vulnerable to falls in an inpatient setting, especially if insight is compromised. Temporary and intermittent changes in mental status are typical for older adults in acute onset ABI. Mental status can certainly fluctuate on the basis of pain, medication changes, and time of day. Also, TBI and stroke are often associated with mood changes and agitation (Flanagan, Kwasnica, Brown, Elovic, & Kothari, 2008). Further complicating matters, individuals with a preexisting dementia may be poor narrators of their past when discussing the nature of their TBI. Additional information about such factors is discussed in the following section.

DIAGNOSTIC CONSIDERATIONS

Formal diagnosis of various ABI causes may be relatively simple when given proper history and diagnostic tools (i.e., imaging and lab results). However, there are several factors that should be considered when classifying and treating certain ABIs. For example, the severity of the injury needs to be considered in all acute presentations (e.g., GCS scores, NIH Stroke Scale). This allows a treating team to better predict the patient's course and to set realistic outcome expectations with the patient and family members. It is also important to consider the numerous confounding and comorbid factors that can influence outcomes. For example, in TBI, it would be prudent to consider the patient's education, family history (i.e., genetic risk), premorbid functioning, comorbid medical conditions, lesion location and size, psychosocial factors, pharmacotherapy factors, and premorbid substance abuse (Moretti et al., 2012). It is common for older individuals to present in outpatient settings with concerns of memory changes and cognitive impairments, raising concerns of a mild cognitive impairment or dementia process. In this case, it is helpful to have a family member or a person close to the patient provide some history or collateral information. If a patient has a history of a brain injury or small stroke earlier in life, it may be difficult to delineate whether their current presentation is being driven by their ABI or if a new degenerative process is underway. An exacerbated cognitive decline needs to be ruled out in such cases. Here, formal neuropsychological testing and brain imaging may be helpful in determining etiology of cognitive complaints (Moretti et al., 2012).

TREATMENT

One common obstacle in the treatment of individuals with ABI is a lack of insight into their deficits. When a lack of insight, also known as "anosognosia," is present, patients will often refuse treatment because they do not realize the impact their ABI is having on their daily or occupational functioning (Anderson, Doble, Merritt, & Kottorp, 2010). This can be especially true for older adults who may have reduced insight premorbidly owing to a dementia process. In addition, after patients are medically stable and discharged, they are often faced with long-term cognitive sequelae of their injury. In such cases, formal outpatient neuropsychological assessment is encouraged to help establish functional and cognitive needs of the patients and to monitor recovery of cognitive functioning.

Regardless of the etiology, if cognitive impairments arise from the patients' ABIs, cognitive rehabilitation can be helpful. In a meta-analysis of the effectiveness of cognitive rehabilitation in TBI and stroke patients, one study demonstrated a modest but significant overall effect to cognitive rehabilitation, with strongest effects for attention training in TBI and language and visual-spatial training for aphasic and hemi-spatial neglect patients following stroke (Rholing, Faust, Beverly, & Demakis, 2009). In addition to cognitive rehabilitation, multiple studies have demonstrated improved physical, psychological, and cognitive functioning in ABI patients undergoing formal exercise regimens. Evidence from the general population suggests that physical exercise can have positive effects on cognitive, physical, and psychological well-being after ABI (Devine & Zafonte, 2009). There appears to be strong evidence that physical activity is protective in terms of decreasing mortality and morbidity following ABI in older adults, including reduced risk of delirium (Hopkins, Suchyta, Farrer, & Needham, 2012). It is thought that exercise leads to angiogenesis, neurogenesis, increased brain volume, and increased cerebral blood flow (Hopkins et al., 2012). In addition to physical activity, mental engagement is also important. Research indicates that individuals with more cognitive reserve fare better following ABI. For example, individuals who were more academically advanced, cognitively active, and physically active likely have better overall brain health that protects against decline later in life. Continued engagement in a variety of mental and social activities will be helpful in older adulthood. Finally, it is also helpful to reduce factors known to attenuate cognitive reserve, such as alcohol consumption, drug use, polypharmacy, social isolation, and depression (Moretti et al., 2012).

Last, for older adults, prevention of ABI is paramount. The Centers for Disease Control and Prevention (CDC) recommends some simple behavioral and environmental modifications to reduce risk of brain injury. First, regular exercise, as outlined by a physician, is beneficial in reducing falls, especially when the exercise increases balance and flexibility. Next, it is helpful to modify the home environment, including installing hand rails in the bathroom and near stairs; using nonslip surfaces on floors and in the tub; removing unnecessary objects from the floor, such as rugs, books, and furniture; improving lighting; and moving needed objects to lower shelves to reduce the need for step-ladders or overreaching. Patients are also encouraged to review their medications with their physician because some medications, or combinations, can affect psychomotor functioning and suppress the central nervous system. Regular eye exams are also encouraged because poor vision can increase the risk of falls (CDC, 2016).

PROGNOSIS

Prognosis following ABI is largely dependent on the etiology and the severity of injury and lesion location in the brain. Studies of TBI outcome indicate that approximately 43% of TBI survivors continue to have disability at 1 year postinjury. This includes changes in activities of daily living (ADLs) and postinjury symptoms such as seizure, vision changes, paralysis, sensory deficits, mood disruption, cognitive impairment, and other psychosocial changes, such as losing employment, reduced educational opportunity, and so forth. One study found that the odds of long-term disability post-TBI for individuals 65 and older was 3.9 times higher than that for ages 15 to 64. In fact, the estimated rate of disability increases with age, with the highest rate being for individuals age 85 to 89 (Selassie et al., 2008). The same study estimated that women were more likely than men to have TBI-related disability (49% vs. 39%). In a large retrospective study, Frankel et al. (2006) examined functional outcomes of TBI among 273 older adults age 55 to 89 in relation to a younger cohort of adults age 16 to 44. Authors demonstrated that compared with younger adults with TBI, older adults had less overall cognitive independence and older adults were less efficient at making functional gains and recovery across their LOS compared with younger adults. In other words, the older adults with TBI had slower rates of improvement. This is supported by longitudinal studies of older adults with mild to moderate TBI who demonstrate significantly worse processing speed, executive functioning, and memory, as well as worse emotional and psychosocial functioning 1 year postinjury (Rapoport et al., 2006).

Although there continues to be some debate regarding the association between ABI and risk of later dementia, multiple studies find a link indicating an interaction between brain injury and an aging brain or postulate that those who are susceptible to dementia simply have an accelerated course after brain injury (Moretti et al., 2012). In one of the largest studies to date, Gardner and colleagues (2014) compared 164,661 trauma patients (≥55 years old) with a diagnosis of TBI at initial ER visit with an orthopedic injury group and examined the rate of new diagnosis of dementia at 1 year or more postinjury (median follow-up was 6 years). Here, older adults with TBI were more likely to receive a diagnosis of dementia at follow-up relative to individuals with orthopedic injury. The TBI group also received a diagnosis of dementia slightly earlier postinjury compared with the orthopedic injury group. These authors also demonstrated that the severity of injury was also related to dementia onset, with moderate to severe injury increasing risk of dementia in all ages past 55 and mild injury increasing risk of dementia only in the oldest cohort of patients (age 65 and older). In a separate paper, this same group of authors, using similar methodology, documented that TBI also increases the risk of Parkinson's disease (PD). In addition, they found that having more severe injuries had an increased risk relative to mild injuries and that having more than one TBI also increased risk of PD compared with those patients with a single TBI (Gardner et al., 2015). These findings are consistent with recent research indicating that TBI increases the risk of early onset Alzheimer's disease (Mendez, Paholpak, Lin, Zhang, & Teng, 2015).

ABI not only has a direct impact on the well-being of the patient but also has a significant impact on the patient's family. Caregiver burden and distress represents a significant factor in outcomes for ABI. For instance, one study demonstrated that 28.5% of caregivers of ABI patients suffer from severe depression and grief (Calvete & de Arroyabe, 2012). Other literature suggests that the higher the magnitude of impairment of the ABI patient, the higher the caregiver distress (de Arroyabe, Calvete, Hayas, & Zubizarreta, 2013) and that caregivers report more distress for caring for ABI family members than caring for older adults with dementia (Jackson, Turner-Stokes, Murray, Leese, & McPherson, 2009). On the other hand, intervention with caregivers can have a tremendous impact on their response to stress. Specifically, when caregivers have reprieve and acceptance and engage in their own treatment, focus on coping strategies, and utilize cognitive restructuring, they tend to have amelioration of caregiver burden. The most efficacious treatment for caregiver burden has focused on positive aspects of care (PAC) in which caregiving itself is viewed as a positive, rewarding experience, in which family relationships can be strengthened and service is valued. Caregivers with a more positive view on caregiving have a reduced risk of developing depression and burnout. In a general adult population with ABI, the degree of PAC was found to be associated with caregiver satisfaction and reduced caregiver distress (de Arroyabe et al., 2013). The research on caregiver resilience and PAC suggests that rehabilitation services should work within the family unit to increase strategies for caregivers to have positive experiences with care for the ABI family member.

In general, research on discharge destination for older adults with ABI indicates that as age increases, the odds of discharge to long-term care facilities also increases (Chan et al., 2013).

Brown, Colantonio, and Kim (2012) studied factors associated with discharge destination from acute care for older adults with TBI. First, LOS in acute care post-TBI is predictive of discharge destination for older adults; longer LOS is associated with increased odds of discharge to a care facility instead of back home. Second, mechanism of injury is also predictive in that older adults who sustained TBI due to falls are more likely to be discharged to a care facility than are older adults who sustained injury due to MVA. This is ostensibly due to the implied level of functioning for older adults who have falls relative to those who are still able to drive a vehicle. Brown and colleagues (2012) also noted a gender difference in discharge destination for older adults with TBI; women are more likely to be discharged to care facilities than are men. This gender difference is thought to be due to the fact that women are more likely to have outlived their partners and therefore are less likely to have a partner to act as caregiver at home. Also, it is possible that women are differentially impacted by TBI in older adults and thus have poorer recovery relative to their male counterparts. In terms of discharge from acute care for older adults with nTBI, Chan et al. (2013) reported that after acute rehabilitation, a majority of nTBI patients are discharged home (44%), followed by complex continuing care, inpatient rehabilitation, or long-term care facilities (19%); the remainder died in acute care. This study also demonstrated that as age increases for nTBI patients, the rate of discharge to home decreased, although the percentage released to other care facilities increased, and the rate of mortality in acute care increased from 28% for younger older adults (ages 65 to 74) to 36% for nTBI patients age 85+. Similarly, Frankel et al. (2006) demonstrated that older adults with TBI are less likely to discharge to community settings (81%) compared with younger adults with TBI (94%).

CLINICAL SYNOPSIS

- ABI in the elderly will become more of a public health concern with time given the increasing number of elderly individuals in the general populations.
- When considering the pathophysiology of ABI, it is important to consider the natural changes that occur in an aging brain, including general volume loss, myelin sheath deterioration, changes in the synthesis of key neurotransmitter, mitochondrial dysfunction, and calcium dysregulation. Microvascular changes in the aging brain lead to attenuated cerebral blood flow, reduced vascularization of brain parenchyma, and increased cerebrovascular risk.
- For older adults, the most common etiology of TBI is falls and the most common type of non-TBI ABI is tumor.
- The highest rates of TBI-related ED visits occur among older adults who are age 75+.
- In terms of hospitalizations, the highest rates are among older adults, with those 75+ representing 34% of TBI-related hospitalizations.
- Mortality is greater for TBI patients with hypotension, for those with lower initial GCS scores, and for those age 85 and older.
- Although alcohol continues to be a risk factor for TBI in older adults, it is less common than in the general adult population.
- In terms of postinjury medical complications, older adults had twice the incidence of seizure and urinary tract infection, and three times the incidence of cardiopulmonary arrest.
- Older adults have an increased hospital LOS, increased financial changes during hospitalization, and more medical

- procedures than do younger adults with the same types of injuries.
- Among older adults, increase in age is associated with increased chance of being released from acute care to long-term care facility rather than home.
- Depending on lesion location and severity of injury, patients can present with significant motor, cognitive, and neuropsychiatric impairments in an inpatient setting. Poststroke depression and postinjury agitation are common in the acute setting.
- When considering differential diagnosis, it is important to have clear historical data to rule out new-onset cognitive decline against an exacerbated preexisting dementia process.
- There is convincing evidence that TBI increases the risk of later development of dementia, particularly for moderate to severe injuries.
- Treatment is typically multifaceted and may include speech therapy, occupational and physical therapy, neuropsychological testing, cognitive rehabilitation, increased physical activity and exercise, continuation of mental engagement, and consideration of medical and psychosocial factors that may negatively impact recovery (i.e., reducing alcohol and other substances, reducing polypharmacy effects, increasing social support, and monitoring and treatment for mood changes).
- Prevention of TBI for older adults should include behavioral and environmental adjustments to reduce fall risk.
- Long-term disability following ABI is common in older adults and can include changes to ADLs and postinjury symptoms such as seizure, vision changes, paralysis, sensory deficits, mood disruption, cognitive impairment, and other psychosocial changes, such as losing employment and reduced educational opportunity.
- Caregiver burden is a significant problem following ABI. Of caregivers of ABI patients, 28.5% suffer from severe depression and grief. Caregivers with a more positive view on caregiving have a reduced risk of developing depression and burnout.

CASE STUDY

A 72-year-old right-handed, married, White woman with a medical history of type 2 diabetes, hypertension, hyperlipidemia, heart disease, atrial fibrillation, hyperparathyroidism, basal cell carcinoma of the skin, osteopenia, and anxiety presented to the emergency room with a lower gastrointestinal (GI) bleed. During her hospital stay, she suffered two heart attacks and was subsequently admitted to the intensive care unit (ICU). Following successful treatment of GI bleed and medical stabilization, she was discharged home 6 days later. Two days following discharge, she had acute onset left leg and arm weakness, slurred speech, and right gaze deviation. She was transported via EMS to the emergency room as a stroke code. On exam, she also had increased left facial droop, left homonymous hemianopia, and right gaze preference. A CT angiography was done, which demonstrated a right distal middle cerebral artery M1 cutoff. The patient was transferred to the NICU, where endovascular thrombectomy was performed. There was not a symptomatic posttreatment hemorrhage, but the patient had repeat occlusion of the right M1 segment, requiring repeat mechanical thrombectomy. Brain MRI performed during her hospital stay revealed a large region of diffusion restriction involving the posterior right frontal lobe, the right insula, the right temporal lobe, and a small area of restricted diffusion in the medial right occipital lobe. There was also evidence of prior microvascular disease and evidence of a prior infarction in the bilateral basal ganglia and cerebellum. Repeat CT some 4 months later revealed encephalomalacia in the right parietal and temporal regions and moderate small vessel ischemic disease.

Seven months following the stroke, the patient and her husband indicated that she was often confused and disoriented when she was first discharged from the hospital. They observed continued left-sided hemi-spatial neglect and ongoing left upper-limb hemiparesis and gait difficulties. She reported that she slurred her speech and had trouble comprehending her husband. Her husband also indicated that the patient was somewhat disinhibited socially and that she was often confused by the time of day, sometimes waking at 3 a.m. and wanting coffee. Patient reported feeling very tired during the day. Otherwise, she denied difficulties in attention and memory. Changes in ADLs were functional owing to her hemiparesis and not owing to declines in cognitive ability. Comprehensive neuropsychological evaluation 7 months poststroke revealed mild but ongoing left visual field neglect, and impairments in executive functioning and poor visual memory.

Factors to consider in this case include the following:

1. The patient may have had some mild changes in cognitive and functional abilities related to her health status and her imaging findings of chronic microvascular disease and a prior infarction in the bilateral basal ganglia and cerebellum. As such, the difficulties with executive functioning could certainly be related to prior brain health and not completely due to her most recent stroke.
2. Mobility issues are likely going to be an ongoing problem for her.
3. Given her husband is her primary care taker and he too is aging, it is prudent to secure alternate or supplemental supports, such as involving additional family members in her care.
4. Occupational and physical therapy may be beneficial to increase strength, flexibility, and mobility, to reduce risk of falls, and to increase functional capacity and safety at home.
5. Formal neurocognitive testing was helpful in delineating the magnitude of her executive abilities, which led to the recommendation that the patient not return to driving and that she have assistance and monitoring for medication and financial management.
6. Given the patient's ongoing difficulties with spatial neglect, she would also benefit from cognitive rehabilitation to help her attend to her left visual field.
7. Functional and behavioral modifications were also recommended. For example, because of her visual neglect, she was missing food on her plate, was walking into walls on the left, and was driving her supermarket scooter into display counters.
8. In this case, the family was given extensive education about long-term care planning, despite the fact that she was released home. This is prudent because long-term care planning and setting up guardianship and/or power of attorney can be a long and complicated process. When older individuals begin to have medical complications, it is less stressful on both the patient and his or her caregivers for the patient to

already have a plan in place rather than worry over making last-minute plans for the patient's care.
9. Last, this patient was encouraged to minimize loss of cognitive reserve by avoiding alcohol and remaining socially active.

REFERENCES

Anderson, R. L., Doble, S. E., Merritt, B. K., & Kottorp, A. (2010). Assessment of awareness of disability measures among persons with acquired brain injury. *Canadian Journal of Occupational Therapy: Revue Canadienne D'Ergothérapie, 77*(1), 22–29.

Brown, S. B., Colantonio, A., & Kim, H. (2012). Gender differences in discharge destination among older adults following traumatic brain injury. *Health Care for Women International, 33*(10), 896–904. doi:10.1080/07399332.2012.673654

Calvete, E., & de Arroyabe, E. L. (2012). Depression and grief in Spanish family caregivers of people with traumatic brain injury: The roles of social support and coping. *Brain Injury, 26*(6), 834–843. doi:10.3109/02699052.2012.655363

Centers for Disease Control and Prevention. (2016). *Help seniors live better, longer: Prevent brain injury.* Retrieved from https://www.cdc.gov/media/subtopic/matte/pdf/CDCHelpSeniorsLiveBetterPreventBrainInjury.pdf

Chan, V., Zagorski, B., Parsons, D., & Colantonio, A. (2013). Older adults with acquired brain injury: A population based study. *BMC Geriatrics, 13*, 97. doi:10.1186/1471-2318-13-97

Chen, A., Bushmeneva, K., Zagorski, B., Colantonio, A., Parsons, D., & Wodchis, W. P. (2012). Direct cost associated with acquired brain injury in Ontario. *BMC Neurology, 12*, 76. doi:10.1186/1471-2377-12-76

Clarke, P. J., Blount, V., & Colantonio, A. (2011). Cognitive impairment predicts fatal incident stroke: Findings from a national sample of older adults. *Journal of the American Geriatrics Society, 59*(8), 1490–1496. doi:10.1111/j.1532-5415.2011.03494.x

Coronado, V. G., McGuire, L. C., Faul, M., Sugerman, D. E., & Pearson, W. S. (2013). Traumatic brain injury epidemioloogy and public health issues. In N. D. Zasler, D. I. Katz, & R. D. Zafonte (Eds.), *Brain injury medicine: Principles and practice* (2nd ed.). New York, NY: Demos Medical Publishing.

Corrigan, J. D., Selassie, A. W., & Orman, J. A. (2010). The epidemiology of traumatic brain injury. *Journal of Head Trauma Rehabilitation, 25*(2), 72–80. doi:10.1097/HTR.0b013e3181ccc8b4

Dams-O'Connor, K., Cuthbert, J. P., Whyte, J., Corrigan, J. D., Faul, M., & Harrison-Felix, C. (2013). Traumatic brain injury among older adults at level I and II trauma centers. *Journal of Neurotrauma, 30*(24), 2001–2013. doi:10.089/neu.2013.3047

de Arroyabe, E. L., Calvete, E., Hayas, C. L., & Zubizarreta, A. (2013). Distress of the caregiver in acquired brain injury: Positive aspects of care to moderate the effects of psychological problems. *The Australian Journal of Rehabilitation Counselling, 19*(2), 84–99. doi:10.0.1017/jrd.2013.13

Devine, J. M., & Zafonte, R. D. (2009). Physical exercise and cognitive recovery in acquired brain injury: A review of the literature. *PM&R: The Journal of Injury, Function, and Rehabilitation, 1*(6), 560–575. doi:10.1016/j.pmrj.2009.03.015

Flanagan, S. R., Kwasnica, C., Brown, A. W., Elovic, E. P., & Kothari, S. (2008). Congenital and acquired brain injury: 2: Medical rehabilitation in acute and subacute settings. *Archives of Physical Medicine and Rehabilitation, 89*(3, Suppl. 1), S9–S14. doi:10.1016/j.apmr.2007.12.010

Frankel, J. E., Marwitz, J. H., Cifu, D. X., Kreutzer, J. S., Englander, J., & Rosenthal, M. (2006). A follow-up study of older adults with traumatic brain injury: Taking into account decreasing length of stay. *Archives of Physical Medicine and Rehabilitation, 87*(1), 57–62. doi:10.1016/j.apmr.2005.07.309

Frost, R. B., Farrer, T. J., Primosch, M., & Hedges, D. W. (2013). Prevalence of traumatic brain injury in the general adult population: A meta-analysis. *Neuroepidemiology, 40*(3), 154–159. doi:10.1159/000343275

Gardner, R. C., Burke, J. F., Nettiksimmons, J., Goldman, S., Tanner, C. M., & Yaffe, K. (2015). Traumatic brain injury in later life increases risk for Parkinson disease. *Annals of Neurology, 77*(6), 987–995. doi:10.1002/ana.24396

Gardner, R. C., Burke, J. F., Nettiksimmons, J., Kaup, A., Barnes, D. E., & Yaffe, K. (2014). Dementia risk after traumatic brain injury vs. nonbrain trauma: The role of age and severity. *JAMA Neurology, 71*(12), 1490–1497. doi:10.1001/jamaneurol.2014.2668

Hopkins, R. O., Suchyta, M. R., Farrer, T. J., & Needham, D. (2012). Improving post-intensive care unit neuropsychiatric outcomes: Understanding cognitive effects of physical activity. *American Journal of Respiratory and Critical Care Medicine, 186*(12), 1220–1228. doi:10.1164/rccm.201206-1022CP

Jackson, D., Turner-Stokes, L., Murray, J., Leese, M., & McPherson, K. M. (2009). Acquired brain injury and dementia: A comparison of carer experiences. *Brain Injury, 23*(5), 433–444. doi:10.1080/02699050902788451

Kwasnica, C., Brown, A. W., Elovic, E. P., Kothari, S., & Flanagan, S. R. (2008). Congenital and acquired brain injury: 3: Spectrum of the acquired brain injury population. *Archives of Physical Medicine and Rehabilitation, 89*(3, suppl. 1), S15–S20. doi:10.1016/j.apmr.2007.12.006

Langlois, J. A., Rutland-Brown, W., & Wald, M. M. (2006). The epidemiology and impact of traumatic brain injury: A brief overview. *Journal of Head Trauma Rehabilitation, 21*(5), 375–378.

Melov, S. (2004). Modeling mitochondrial function in aging neurons. *Trends in Neurosciences, 27*(10), 601–606. doi:10.1016/j.tins.2004.08.004

Mendez, M. F., Paholpak, P., Lin, A., Zhang, J. Y., & Teng, E. (2015). Prevalence of traumatic brain injury in early versus late-onset Alzheimer's disease. *Journal of Alzheimer's Disease, 47*(4), 985–993. doi:10.3233/JAD-143207

Moretti, L., Cristofori, I., Weaver, S. M., Chau, A., Portelli, J. N., & Grafman, J. (2012). Cognitive decline in older adults with a history of traumatic brain injury. *Lancet Neurology, 11*(12), 1103–1112. doi:10.1016/S1474-4422(12)70226-0

Mukherjee, J., Christian, B. T., Dunigan, K. A., Shi, B., Narayanan, T. K., Satter, M., & Mantil, J. (2002). Brain imaging of 18F-fallypride in normal volunteers: Blood analysis, distribution, test-retest studies, and preliminary assessment of sensitivity to aging effects on dopamine D-2/D-3 receptors. *Synapse, 46*(3), 170–188. doi:10.1002/syn.10128

Nugent, S., Tremblay, S., Chen, K. W., Ayutyanont, N., Roontiva, A., Castellano, C. A., . . . Cunnane, S. C. (2014). Brain glucose and acetoacetate metabolism: A comparison of young and older adults. *Neurobiology of Aging, 35*(6), 1386–1395. doi:10.1016/j.neurobiolaging.2013.11.027

Peters, R. (2006). Aging and the brain. *Postgraduate Medical Journal, 82*(964), 84–88. doi:10.1136/pgmj.2005.036665

Rapoport, M. J., Herrmann, N., Shammi, P., Kiss, A., Phillips, A., & Feinstein, A. (2006). Outcome after traumatic brain injury sustained in older adulthood: A one-year longitudinal study. *American Journal of Geriatric Psychiatry, 14*(5), 456–465. doi:10.1097/01.JGP.0000199339.79689.8a

Rohling, M. L., Faust, M. E., Beverly, B., & Demakis, G. (2009). Effectiveness of cognitive rehabilitation following acquired brain injury: A meta-analytic re-examination of Cicerone et al.'s (2000, 2005) systematic reviews. *Neuropsychology, 23*(1), 20–39. doi:10.1037/a0013659

Selassie, A. W., Zaloshnja, E., Langlois, J. A., Miller, T., Jones, P., & Steiner, C. (2008). Incidence of long-term disability following traumatic brain injury hospitalization, United States, 2003. *Journal of Head Trauma Rehabilitation, 23*(2), 123–131. doi:10.1097/01.HTR.0000314531.30401.39

CHAPTER 15

Psychosocial Characteristics of Acquired Brain Injury

LESLIE GUIDOTTI BRETING
COURTNEY NELSON
THOMAS COTHRAN

OVERVIEW

An acquired brain injury (ABI) not only causes impairment in the areas of motor, cognitive, and other bodily functions, but also can lead to significant psychological distress and impact the patient and support system, including family. Psychosocial problems associated with ABI may actually be one of the major challenges facing rehabilitation and reintegration into one's community.

HISTORY

ABI may result in disability with biological, psychological, and social ramifications. How rehabilitation practitioners conceptualize "disability" has important implications in terms of assessment, treatment planning, service delivery, and outcomes. Furthermore, an understanding and adoption of a model of disability helps the rehabilitation practitioner orient psychosocial topics such as coping, adjustment, social support, and intervention into a broader context. Models of disability (i.e., how disability is understood) have evolved from moral models to the medical model to functional models to social models (Chan, Gelman, Ditchman, Kim, & Chiu, 2009) (see Table 15.1). Moral models tended to view a person's health

TABLE 15.1 DESCRIPTION OF BROAD CATEGORIES OF MODELS OF DISABILITY

Models	Locus of Disability	Positive Outcome	Goals
Charity/moral	Moral failing	Disabled persons provided basic needs	Teach people with disabilities to overcome their personal failings
Medical	Within the body	Health condition is fixed	Treat the health condition
Functional	The interaction of an impairment and task demand	Health condition is fixed	Allocate resources according to the level of functional limitations; provide opportunities to commiserate with functional abilities
Social	Socially constructed restrictions are imposed on the individual with impairments	Impairments are accommodated to allow access to perform social roles in the community	Provide accommodation and modify the environment to support the individual in the social and functional roles of their choosing; address attitudinal and stigma barriers in the community

condition and disability as being indicative of personal failings, or conversely that disability conferred a purified moral superiority (Schillace, 2013). The medical model has traditionally focused almost exclusively on pathology. The primary service providers were physicians who considered the locus of disability as situated entirely within the individual's body (Smart, 2001).

Functional models focused on how the physiological and psychological consequences of a disorder, disease, or injury may incur functional limitations (Livneh & Robert, 1993; Nagi, 1965). A corollary of this definition is that disability is contextually determined. For example, a surgeon may be deemed disabled based on the functional demands of her occupation after evidencing low average attention and processing speed on neuropsychological testing following an ABI. However, another person with the same injury and test results may not be disabled if the cognitive demands of her occupation are less severe.

Social models of disability define disability as the interaction of biological, functional, social, and environmental factors (Brandt & Pope, 1997; Engel, 1977; Tate & Pledger, 2003; Wright, 1960). Purely social models argue disability is a socially constructed phenomenon that results in the imposition of barriers to equal participation and access on individuals with physiological impairments and functional limitations. For example, a person with severe hemiparesis may have physiologic injury to the primary motor cortex that resulted in functional limitations related to ambulation; however, this individual would not be considered disabled in the area of transportation if his vehicle was modified to accommodate his paralysis thereby allowing him to drive. As such, social model theorists place greater responsibility on society for ameliorating disability (Chan et al., 2009).

The medical and functional models are regarded as disablement models because they are focused primarily on impairment and limitations; social models are characterized by enablement (Masala & Petretto, 2008). These models identify enabling factors such as assistive technology, environmental modification, access to health care, medications, and social support that improve the individual's engagement in activities and participation in social roles (Brandt & Pope, 1997).

Currently, the most widely adopted conceptualization of disability is the World Health Organization (WHO) International Classification of Functioning, Disability, and Health (ICF) model, which is a companion to the *International Statistical Classification of Diseases and Related Health Problems*, Tenth Revision (*ICD-10*; World Health Organization [WHO], 1992). The ICF model integrates aspects of the medical, social, and functional models. It encompasses three broad components: (a) body structure and function, (b) activities and participations, and (c) personal and environmental factors (WHO, 2001). In this model, disability is the multifactorial product of a dynamic interplay between a health condition and contextual factors both environmental and personal. Moreover, it enables a biopsychosocial and person-centered perspective on health care (Alford et al., 2015).

From a psychosocial perspective, personal factors, environmental factors, and participation may be particularly relevant. Personal factors are defined as features of the individual that influence his or her performance of activities and participation (Peterson, 2005; WHO, 2001). These include characteristics such as coping style, social background, demographics, personality, and learning history. Environmental factors include the characteristics of the physical layout of the community, as well as the social environment and attitudinal milieu (Peterson, 2005; WHO, 2001). These factors may serve to facilitate inclusion in the community or buttress barriers to participation. Environmental factors include assistive technologies, the physical environment, social support and relationships, attitudes, service delivery systems, and policies. Participation refers to engagement in and fulfillment of life roles in the community (e.g., vocational, relational, recreational roles) (Peterson, 2005; WHO, 2001). The interplay between the individual's health condition, ability to engage in activities, environmental factors, and personal factors impacts participation, which in turn affects quality of life (Chan et al., 2009). Consequently, improved and maintained participation in life roles is the primary goal of rehabilitation.

A qualitative study of persons with ABI demonstrated that issues related to participation and inclusion is a vital concern; moreover, perceived psychosocial and instrumental support from family, friends, and health professionals is important in determining the individual's health status and functioning (Sveen, Ostensjo, Laxe, & Soberg, 2013). However, negative attitudes and beliefs about brain injuries held by the individual's social network may have a detrimental effect. For example, stigmatizing attitudes of friends, colleagues, and acquaintances may be viewed as a barrier to participation, especially when the validity of impairments are questioned because they are "invisible" (Levack, Kayes, & Fadyl, 2010).

In conclusion, disability is a complex and multifactorial phenomenon (Chan et al., 2009). Depending on one's perspective, disability in traumatic brain injury (TBI) can be described exclusively in terms of tissue damage in the brain, or as being derived in the interaction between limitations caused by tissue damage and the contextual demands of performing tasks, or as the restrictions imposed on the person by the surrounding social and physical environment. The ICF attempts to integrate each of these perspectives in its conception of disability (WHO, 2001). As a result, psychosocial aspects of disability become critical in a comprehensive understanding of disability in ABI. Understanding a person's access to social support, family system, coping style, social and vocational roles, personality factors, and cultural background, as well as an appreciation of broader societal attitudes and beliefs, may be just as crucial for the amelioration of disability in ABI as understanding the physiological sequela of brain injury and resultant functional limitations.

PATHOPHYSIOLOGY/ETIOLOGY

Research on the pathophysiology, etiology, and neuroanatomical correlates of psychiatric and psychosocial difficulties due to brain injury is limited; however, the majority of available literature points to a disruption of the frontal subcortical network to explain the behavioral changes. Changes to the frontal region of the brain are often what occur after a brain injury given the bony protuberances in which it sits.

EPIDEMIOLOGY

The incidence of psychological conditions following TBI is often related to pretrauma risk factors, including a history of psychological difficulties and gender. However, posttrauma risk factors also play a role in incidence of psychological conditions. It has been shown that significant life stressors and lack of social support can increase the risk. Clinical research has demonstrated that psychiatric complications are prevalent in ABI, with an incidence of around 40% to 50% for moderate to severe TBI and about 34% after a mild TBI; however, the incidence is not well documented for mild TBI or concussion owing to the fact that many patients at that level do not make it into the health care system (Vaishnavi, Rao, & Fann, 2009).

CLINICAL PRESENTATION/DIAGNOSTIC CONSIDERATIONS

Personality Changes

Up to 60% to 80% of family members report that personality change has occurred in their loved one with a brain injury (Brooks, Campsie, Symington, Beattie, & McKinlayl, 1986; Weddell & Leggett, 2006). Personality changes following an ABI involve three factors: pretrauma patterns of emotion regulation and motivation, neurological disturbances to brain structures involved in emotion regulation and motivation (i.e., damage to the amygdala or higher cortical centers), or reactionary disturbances such as failure to cope with the new environmental demands given reduced resources (Prigatano, 1987). Understanding personality changes following ABI is important because of the inevitable impact on psychosocial adjustment, such as integration into society through employment and maintaining interpersonal relationships (Prigatano, 1987). Personality changes frequently observed in patients with brain injury include the following:

- Emotional lability
- Lack of empathy
- Anger, irritability, and agitation
- Rigidity
- Loss of drive, initiative, and motivation
- Self-directed in motivation
- Loss of spontaneity
- Apathy
- Socially inappropriate behavior
- Impulsivity
- Paranoia
- Lack of insight
- Enhanced sensitivity to distress
- Impaired social awareness and inability to recognize emotional expressions in face and voice

Depression

Many patients experience depression following ABI, with estimated frequencies ranging between 6% and 77% (Jorge & Arciniegas, 2014). Symptoms of depression include sad mood, loss of interest in activities previously enjoyed, feelings of worthlessness and/or guilt, loss of concentration, decreased energy, slowed thinking and movement, appetite loss, and sleep problems. Like personality changes, the pathophysiology of mood disorders following an ABI involves three factors: pretrauma factors such as genetic vulnerability and prior psychiatric history; factors that relate to the injury itself, such as damage to the emotion regulation systems in the brain; and factors associated with recovery, such as social support (Jorge & Arciniegas, 2014). Although it is thought that the risk of developing depression is highest in the first year post injury, research indicates that the risk of depression onset remains high even decades after ABI. Experts on the subject generally accept an estimated first-year post-ABI depression onset frequency between 25% and 50% (Jorge & Arciniegas, 2014). Approximately one-fourth of patients who were not depressed during the first year post injury developed depression during the second year. Approximately two-thirds of patients who were depressed during the first year post injury continued to exhibit significant depressive symptoms, highlighting the perpetual nature of this disorder in ABI patients. Depressive disorders following ABI are strongly associated with the presence of anxiety disorders.

Anxiety

It is estimated that anxiety disorders occur in 24% to 28% of patients with ABI (Warden & Labbate, 2005). Symptoms of anxiety include fear, worry, restlessness, difficulty concentrating, sleep problems, muscle tension, and feelings of panic. Anxiety may be the result of the brain injury directly, such as damage to the neural circuits involved in development of this disorder, or it may manifest due to the postinjury experience, such as worry about physical injury and possible cognitive decline. As a result of physical injury and/or personality and cognitive deficits, self-consciousness may cause anxiety and lead to avoidance of social settings, hindering reintegration into society (Warden & Labbate, 2005).

Posttraumatic Stress Disorder

Reexperiencing the traumatic event through vivid memories or flashbacks, avoidance of situations related to the trauma, and emotional withdrawal following an ABI suggest the presence of a posttraumatic stress disorder (PTSD). This is the most common psychiatric disorder following ABI (Bryant, Marosszeky, Crooks, Baguley, & Gurka, 2001) and is a serious barrier to rehabilitation. It has been suggested that the likelihood of developing PTSD following a brain injury is mediated by the encoding of traumatic memories. Loss of consciousness and poor recall of the event appear to be protective factors against development of PTSD, which explains why PTSD is more commonly seen in patients with mild brain injuries than in those with moderate to severe brain injuries. Even when patients report poor memory of the event, the partial encoding of some details may lead to reexperiencing and hyperarousal (Mallya, Sutherland, Pongracic, Mainland, & Ornstein, 2015). PTSD is associated with anger and increased arousal, which may exacerbate the aggression experienced after ABI and result in reduced impulse control (Chemtob, Novaco, Hamada, Gross, & Smith, 1997). Avoidance behaviors may impede community integration and minimize social activities, contributing to feelings of loneliness, depression, and ultimately reducing the quality of life of these patients.

Communication Disorders

Aphasia is infrequent in patients with ABI; however, deficits in communication skills are not. Many individuals with ABI are described as talkative but inefficient, unable to remain on topic, tangential, and prone to irrelevant comments. Conversational style is slow with incomplete responses, and comprehension may also be impaired. Self-focused conversations, immature humor, frequent interruptions, disinhibited remarks, and inappropriate levels of self-disclosure have been commonly observed (McDonald, Togher, & Code, 2013).

TREATMENT

Initial management of psychological and psychosocial changes post brain injury requires assessment of safety of the patient, patient visitors, and the treatment team. A psychologist can then consider behavioral guidelines for management or use cognitive-behavioral techniques. If the emotional difficulties persist, then a pharmacological management is often considered, which is often prescribed by the treating physiatrist or a psychiatrist. Despite significant efforts, there continues to be a lack of peer-reviewed, empirically supported research studies regarding the treatment of psychiatric complications post brain injury. It seems that more often both pharmacological and talk therapeutic strategies combined are most effective.

Psychosocial Interventions

Effective psychosocial interventions in ABI are informed by models of adaptation to sudden-onset chronic disability. Adaptation and adjustment are different but related concepts (Smedema, Bakken-Gillen, & Dalton, 2009). "Adaptation" refers to the dynamic process whereby a disability, such as an ABI, becomes incorporated into the person's self-concept, identity, and body image and harmonization between the person and environment is reached. In the ideal scenario, "adjustment" refers to this final point of harmony following adaptation. In other words, adaptation leads to adjustment; however, adaptation may not necessarily conclude positively. The process of adaptation represents a continuum that ranges from maladaptive psychosocial functioning to successful adjustment (Livneh & Antonak, 1997).

The goal of psychosocial interventions following an ABI is to promote adaptive functioning and successful adjustment to disability (Smedema et al., 2009). Persons who attain a state of adjustment experience more positive emotions and self-esteem, a healthy self-concept, and an awareness of personal mastery over their limitations. Moreover, they are more likely to overcome challenges in negotiating the physical environment and to participate in social, vocational, and recreational activities. Persons evidencing maladaptive psychosocial functioning are more likely to report negative affect (i.e., depression, anxiety, and anger), to engage in denial of their disability and limitations, to be less engaged in life activities, and to evidence a diminished quality of life. Countless models have been presented to explain the complex process of adaptation (Smedema et al., 2009). Of these, the somatopsychological model, stage models, and ecological models will be discussed.

Somatopsychology

Somatopsychology theorists were greatly influenced by Kurt Lewin's field theory (1935, 1936) that argued behavior was a function of the interaction between person and environment. The somatopsychology perspective (Barker, Wright, Meyerson, & Gonick, 1953; Dembo, Leviton, & Wright, 1956) focused on psychosocial factors that affect how disability is perceived, valued, and reacted to by the self and society. From this perspective, the person's beliefs about individuals with ABI and disability interact with the value their social support network attributes to disability and determines the outcome of adaptation and adjustment. Wright (1960, 1983) argued that positive adjustment occurs when individuals are able to accept the disability as part of their self-concept and do not view their disability as devaluing them as people.

Wright (1960, 1983) proposed a "coping versus succumbing" framework for understanding adjustment to disability. Persons who succumb to disability focus on the negative effects of their limitations, conceptualize disability as a problem rather than a challenge, and expend unreasonable effort hiding their limitations and struggling to achieve unattainable levels of performance. Moreover, they tend to venerate standards of "normal" and base their self-worth on external social comparisons. Persons who cope with disability focus on abilities that have been preserved, conceptualize their limitations as a challenge to be overcome, and base their self-worth on intrinsic characteristics such as their personality, sense of humor, or intelligence. Moreover, Wright (1983) argued that coping is accompanied by a change in values that prevent or limit the internalization of harmful beliefs. For example, the person may begin to de-emphasize the importance of physique and ability and place more value on intrinsic characteristics. Last, Wright argued that persons who succumb to disability evidence "spread," in which the effects of the disability are catastrophized and generalized beyond the scope of the actual injury. Persons who cope limit the effects of their disability to the consequences of the impairment rather than allowing global debilitation.

From a somatopsychology perspective, intervention includes emphasizing preserved abilities and associated activities, encouraging the person's active engagement in shaping his or her life, and underscoring the notion that disability does not preclude a person from living a meaningful and productive life. Wright (1983) suggested interventions that promote mastery such as role-playing and recruiting persons with similar impairments who can role-model successful negotiation of difficult situations in a group therapy session or during excursions in the community. Other focuses of therapy involve minimizing spread of limitations to areas not affected by the injury, clarifying personal values, assisting the person in adopting intrinsic values over physique-based values, and providing validation and encouragement for personal accomplishments (Wright, 1983).

Stage Models

Stage models posit adaptation, and adjustment to disability occurs through a linear process whereby the person with TBI experiences each stage in sequence. A myriad of stage models have been proposed. Livneh (1986) conducted an extensive review of 40 models and concluded that five broad categories were sufficient for describing them. In general, he argued that the stages of the myriad models could be conceived as following a basic sequence characterized by initial impact, defense mobilization, initial realization, retaliation, and reintegration. Initial impact is the stage where the person first realizes an injury has occurred and begins to sense the full scope of it. It is characterized by shock and anxiety. Defense mobilization occurs when the person is not fully able to accept the possibility of disability and its full ramifications. Defense mobilization is characterized by bargaining and denial. Initial realization is when the individual first begins to accept that he or she is disabled and that his or her life is irrevocably changed. This stage is characterized by emotional turmoil, indifference, mourning, grief, depression, and internalized anger expressed as self-hatred and self-blame. During the retaliation stage, the person begins to project anger outward and rebels against the limitations imposed by the disability. He or she may manifest hostility toward others or reminders of his or her disability found in the environment. Passive-aggressive expressions of hostility may take the form of manipulation, subtle abusiveness, and undermining. The final stage is reintegration and is characterized by acknowledgment and acceptance of disability, along with successful adjustment. The disability is fully integrated into the self-concept in a nondevaluing fashion, and the individual manifests self-approval (Livneh, 1986).

Although a tendency toward eventual adjustment is observed in the broad sense and many of the reactions described in stage models are observed (Smedema et al., 2009), critics point out that there is little empirical evidence to support the contention that these stages are universally experienced (Livneh, 1986). Additionally, support for the hypothesis that persons with ABI will pass through stages in a specific order is lacking. However, it may be that stage models are appropriate for a subgroup of people who experience a traumatic injury. For example, Wortman and Silver (1989) examined empirical studies of depression following loss and identified three common patterns of adaptation. Two of the patterns consisted of people who started at low and high levels of distress, respectively, and to a certain degree remained at those levels over time. The third common pattern consisted of individuals who started at a high level of distress that reduced over time. It may be possible that stage models are an appropriate framework for describing adaptation in this subset.

From the perspective of stage models, psychosocial treatment involves matching the intervention to the identified stage (Livneh & Antonak, 2005). Over time, the approach changes from nondirective, supportive therapies (e.g., person-centered therapy) to more directive therapies geared toward prompting action to address symptoms of depression, anxiety, and anger (e.g., cognitive-behavioral therapy) (Livneh & Antonak, 2005).

Ecological Models

Ecological models view the person with disability as nested with multiple systems, including the biological system, the family system, the community, and society, while accounting for the effect of time. Many ecological models of disability have been proposed; however, they may share many conceptual and structural features (Livneh & Antonak, 1997). These models include injury- or disability-related variables, sociodemographic variables, personality and behavioral variables, and variables associated with the external social and physical environment. In ABI, variables related to the injury would include the biomechanical aspects of the injury, type of neural insult, the extent of tissue damage, degree of functional impairment, and whether the impairments were visible (e.g., in the case of paresis). Sociodemographic variables would include gender, age, ethnicity, education, and developmental stage at the time of the injury. Personality and behavior variables would include coping style, defense mechanisms, attitudes, values, and cognitive ability before and after injury. Variables related to the social and physical environment include social support, attitudinal barriers, stigma, the physical layout of living spaces, governmental and institutional policies, and service delivery systems (Livneh & Antonak, 1997).

Injury variables, sociodemographic variables, and personality and behavioral variables all exist within the person with ABI, whereas the social and physical environment variables are external to the person (Livneh & Antonak, 1997). Ecological models maintain that the efficiency of adaptation to disability is the direct result of the interaction between interpersonal and external factors. Like stage models, ecological models also posit a series of reactions. Ecological models describe early reactions being characterized by shock, anxiety, and denial; intermediate reactions being characterized by depression, internalized anger, and externalized hostility; and late reactions being characterized by acknowledgment, acceptance, and adjustment (Livneh & Antonak, 1997).

From the perspective of ecological models, intervention includes addressing intrapersonal factors such as providing information about ABI, constructing positive meaning out of the experience of disability, teaching adaptive coping skills such as assertiveness, decision making, time management, stigma management, relaxation techniques, and stress reduction (Livneh & Antonak, 2005). Additionally, interventions address external factors as well. For example, group therapy with other individuals with ABI and their families may foster social support, insight, and problem-solving skills (Livneh & Antonak, 2005).

PROGNOSIS

Given the complex relationship of frontal brain systems that are functionally and structurally connected, blunt forces that result in ABI lead to variable and overlapping patterns of deficits in cognition, emotion regulation, and behavior. As a result of these deficits, many individuals with ABI find it difficult to maintain interpersonal relationships and employment following rehabilitation. Estimates of the number of patients with ABI who will return to competitive employment are 10% to 70% (Yasuda, Wehman, Targett, Cifu, & West, 2001). The unemployment rate of patients with severe ABI is 60% to 80%. Factors associated with poor employment outcome include severity of injury; degree of cognitive, physical, and psychosocial impairments; and preinjury variables. A premorbid history of substance use disorders is associated with an eight-fold increase in post-ABI unemployment rates. Additionally, limited insight into deficits, depression, and other cognitive barriers are major difficulties in returning to work (Hornstein, 2005).

ABI patients who are unable to return to work must rely on disability insurance for income. The establishment of contact with available sources of funding, the confirmation of eligibility of benefits, and the gathering of necessary data to justify services are vitally important for these individuals and can be a large source of stress for these patients and their caregivers. Additionally, many patients with ABI become involved in litigation, suing either for damages or for wrongful denial of benefits (Miller, 2000; Taylor, 1997). Cases involving brain injury are complex, and finding a lawyer competent and experienced in dealing with the clinical and legal aspects of brain injury can be difficult. Furthermore, the individual with ABI may have cognitive deficits that inhibit the ability to capably participate in the case. Litigation itself can exacerbate anxiety, depression, and psychosocial dysfunction. Despite these potential adverse effects, litigation can sometimes be the only means of financial security for patients with ABI, and it may help alleviate feelings of injustice (Hornstein, 2005).

Social isolation and difficulties integrating into society lead to a renewed dependence on family members for meeting these needs (Morton & Wehman, 1995). Additionally, relatives serve as stand-in decision makers for the critical patient in the hospital. Upon discharge from the hospital, family members may take on the primary caregiver role. Caregiving is a multidimensional responsibility, with assistance being provided at different levels such as eating, bathing, cooking, cleaning, transportation, as well as emotional support. Caregivers of patients with ABI are at risk for depression, anxiety, reduced quality of life, and decreased family functioning (Turner et al., 2010). It is important for caregivers to be aware of the support services and intervention strategies available to them when caring for loved ones with ABI.

Many ABI patients suffer from a lack of insight and may be unrealistic in their self-appraisal of their recovery. Due to the complexity of the brain, it is difficult to provide an accurate prognosis following brain injury. Visible injuries are an unreliable predictor of future recovery, and a positive CT or MRI scan does not necessarily predict how severe the injury is. Although the duration of recovery is difficult to predict, it is important to keep in mind that patients with ABI do get better!

Centers for Independent Living is a community-based agency that provides counseling, information, referrals, training in independent living skills, advocacy, and occasionally housing opportunities for the disabled (Tate Heinrich, Paasuke, & Homa, 1998).

CLINICAL SYNOPSIS

- Psychosocial problems associated with ABI may actually be one of the major challenges facing rehabilitation and reintegration into one's community.
- Most widely adopted conceptualization of disability is the WHO International Classification of Functioning, Disability, and Health (ICF) model. The ICF model integrates aspects of the medical, social, and functional models with three broad components: (a) body structure and function, (b) activities and participations, and (c) personal and environmental factors.
- Incidence of psychiatric complications after ABI is around 40% to 50% for moderate to severe TBI and about 34% after a mild TBI.
- Most common psychosocial difficulties post-ABI include personality changes, depression, anxiety, PTSD, and communication disorders.
- Goal of psychosocial interventions following an ABI is to promote adaptive functioning and successful adjustment to disability (Smedema et al., 2009). Several models are highlighted earlier in this chapter. Oftentimes, treatment requires both pharmacological and nonpharmacological methods.

CASE STUDY

Even though this case occurred over 150 years ago, it continues to be a classic to highlight the psychosocial changes that can occur following a brain injury. Phineas Gage was a 25-year-old, energetic railroad foreman who sustained a left frontal lobe brain injury from an iron tamping bar that passed through his head after an explosion in 1848. Following his brain injury, Dr. Harlow,

Dr. Bigelow, and their colleagues at Harvard examined Mr. Gage's recovery and documented a dramatic change in personality. Prior to the injury, Mr. Gage was described as "reliable, systematic, and hardworking," but afterward was described as "impulsive, disorganized, and stubborn often using profane language" (Damasio, Grabowski, Frank, Galaburda, & Damasio, 1994; Guidotti, 2012). Impressively, Mr. Gage was able to return to work first as a circus act, then as a hand in a livery stable, and lastly as a long-distance stagecoach driver.

REFERENCES

Alford, V. M., Ewen, S., Webb, G. R., McGinley, J., Brookes, A., & Remedios, L. J. (2015). The use of the International Classification of Functioning, Disability, and Health to understand the health and functioning experiences of people with chronic conditions from the person perspective: A systematic review. *Disability and Rehabilitation, 37*(8), 655–666. doi:10.3109/09638288.2014.935875

Barker, R. G., Wright, B. A., Meyerson, L., & Gonick, M. R. (1953). *Adjustment to physical handicap and illness: A survey of the social psychology of physique and disability* (2nd ed.). New York, NY: Social Science Research Council.

Brandt, E. N., & Pope, A. M. (1997). *Enabling America: Assessing the role of rehabilitation science and engineering.* Washington, DC: National Academies Press.

Brooks, D. N., Campsie, L., Symington, C., Beattie, A., & McKinlay, W. (1986). The first year outcome of severe blunt head injury: A relative's view. *Journal of Neurology, Neurosurgery, and Psychiatry, 49*(7), 764–770. doi:10.1136/jnnp.49.7.764

Bryant, R. A., Marosszeky, J. E., Crooks, J., Baguley, I. J., & Gurka, J. A. (2001). Posttraumatic stress disorder and psychosocial functioning after severe traumatic brain injury. *The Journal of Nervous and Mental Disease, 189*(2), 109–113.

Chan, F., Gelman, J. S., Ditchman, N., & Chiu, C.-Y. (2009). The World Health Organization ICF model as a conceptual framework of disability. In F. Chan, E. Da Silva Cardoso, & J. Chronister (Eds.), *Understanding psychosocial adjustment to chronic illness and disability: A handbook for evidence-based practitioners in rehabilitation.* New York, NY: Springer Publishing Company.

Chemtob, C. M., Novaco, R. W., Hamada, R. S., Gross, D. M., & Smith, G. (1997). Anger regulation deficits in combat-related posttraumatic stress disorder. *Journal of Traumatic Stress, 10*(1), 17–36.

Damasio, H., Grabowski, T., Frank, R., Galaburda, A. M., & Damasio, A. R. (1994). The return of Phineas Gage: Clues about the brain from the skull of a famous patient. *Science, 264*(5162), 1102–1105.

Dembo, T., Leviton, G. L., & Wright, B. A. (1956). Adjustment to misfortune: A problem of social-psychological rehabilitation. *Artificial Limbs, 3*(2), 4–62.

Engel, G. L. (1977). The need for a new medical model. *Science, 196*(4286), 129–136. Retrieved from www.jstor.org/stable/1743658

Guidotti, T. L. (2012). Phineas Gage and his frontal lobe—The "American Crowbar Case". *Archives of Environmental & Occupational Health, 67*(4), 249–250. doi:10.1080/19338244.2012.722469

Hornstein, A. (2005). Social issues. In J. M. Silver, T. W. McAllister, & S. C. Yudofsky (Eds.), *Textbook of traumatic brain injury* (2nd ed.). Arlington, VA: American Psychiatric Publishing.

Jorge, R. E., & Arciniegas D. B. (2014). Mood disorders after ABI. *Psychiatric Clinics of North America, 37*(1), 13–29. doi:10.1016/j.psc.2013.1.005

Levack, W. M., Kayes, N. M., & Fadyl, J. K. (2010). Experiences of recovery and outcome following traumatic brain injury: A metasynthesis of qualitative research. *Disability and Rehabilitation, 32*, 986–999. doi:10.3109/09638281003775394

Lewin, K. (1935). *A dynamic theory of personality: Selected papers* (D. K. Adams & K. E. Zener, Trans.). New York, NY: McGraw Hill.

Lewin, K. (1936). *Principles of topological psychology* (F. Heider & G. M. Heider, Trans.). New York, NY: McGraw-Hill.

Livneh, H. (1986). A unified approach to existing models of adaptation to disability: Part 1: A model of adaptation. *Journal of Rehabilitation Counseling, 17*(1), 5–16.

Livneh, H., & Antonak, R. F. (1997). *Psychosocial adaptation to chronic illness and disability* (1st ed.). Gaithersburg, MD: Aspen.

Livneh, H., & Antonak R. F. (2005). Psychosocial aspects of chronic illness and disability: A primer for counselors. *Journal of Counseling and Development, 83*(1), 12–20. doi:10.1002/j.1556-6678.2005.tb00575.x

Livneh, H., & Robert, M. (1993). Functional limitations: A review of their characteristics and vocational impact. *Journal of Rehabilitation, 59*, 44–50.

Mallya, S., Sutherland, J., Pongracic, S., Mainland, B., & Ornstein, T. J. (2015). The manifestation of anxiety disorders after traumatic brain injury: A review. *Journal of Neurotrauma, 32*(7), 411–421. doi:10.1089/neu.2014.3504

Masala, C., & Petretto, D. R. (2008). From disablement to enablement: Conceptual models of disability in the 20th century. *Disability and Rehabilitation, 30*(17), 1233–1244. doi:10.1080/09638280701602418

McDonald, S., Togher, L., & Code, C. (2013). The nature of cognitive deficits and psychosocial function following TBI. In S. McDonald, L. Togher, & C. Code (Eds.), *Social and communication disorders following traumatic brain injury*. New York, NY: Psychology Press.

Miller, L. (2000). Psychological syndromes in traumatic brain injury litigation: Personality, psychopathology, and disability. *Brain Injury Source, 4*, 18–43.

Morton, M. V., & Wehman, P. (1995). Psychosocial and emotional sequelae of individuals with traumatic brain injury: A literature review and recommendations. *Brain Injury, 9*(1), 81–92.

Nagi, S. (1965). Some conceptual issues in disability and rehabilitation. In M. Sussman (Ed.), *Sociology and rehabilitation*. Washington, DC: American Sociological Association.

Peterson, D. B. (2005). International classification of functioning, disability, and health: An introduction for rehabilitation psychologists. *Rehabilitation Psychology, 50*(2), 105–112. doi:10.1037/0090-5550.50.2.105

Prigatano, G. P. (1987). Psychiatric aspects of head injury: Problem areas and suggested guidelines for research. In H. S. Levin, J. Grafman, & H. M. Eisenberg (Eds.), *Neurobehavioral recovery from head injury*. New York, NY: Oxford University Press.

Schillace, B. L. (2013). Curing "moral disability": Brain trauma and self-control in Victorian science and fiction. *Culture, Medicine and Psychiatry, 37*(4), 587–600. doi:10.1007/s11013-013-9339-6

Smart, J. F. (2001). *Disability, society, and the individual*. Austin, TX: Aspen.

Smedema, S. M., Bakken-Gillen, S. K., & Dalton, J. (2009). Psychosocial adaptation to chronic illness and disability: Models and measurement. In E. C. F. Chan & J. A. Chronister (Eds.), *Understanding psychosocial adjustment to chronic illness and disability: A handbook for evidence-based practitioners in rehabilitation*. New York, NY: Springer Publishing Company.

Sveen, U., Ostensjo, S., Laxe, S., & Soberg, H. L. (2013). Problems in functioning after a mild traumatic brain injury within the ICF framework: The patient perspective using focus groups. *Disability and Rehabilitation, 35*(9), 749–757. doi:10.3109/09638288.2012.707741

Tate, D. G., Heinrich, R. K., Paasuke, L., & Homa, D. (1998). Vocational rehabilitation, independent living, and consumerism. In J. A. DeLisa & B. M. Gans (Eds.), *Rehabilitation medicine: Principles and practice* (3rd ed.). Philadelphia, PA: Lippincott-Raven.

Tate, D. G., & Pledger, C. (2003). An integrative conceptual framework of disability: New directions for research. *American Psychologist, 58*(4), 289–295.

Taylor, J. S. (1997). *Neurolaw: Brain and spinal cord.* Washington, DC: ATLA Press.

Turner, B., Fleming, J., Parry, J., Vromans, M., Cornwell, P., Gordon, C., & Ownsworth, T. (2010). Caregivers of adults with traumatic brain injury: The emotional impact of transition from hospital to home. *Brain Impairment, 11*(3), 281–292. doi:10.1375/brim.11.3.281

Vaishnavi, S., Rao, V., & Fann, J. R. (2009). Neuropsychiatric problems after traumatic brain injury: Unraveling the silent epidemic. *Psychosomatics, 50*(3), 198–205. doi:10.1176/appi.psy.50.3.198

Warden, D. L., & Labbate, L. A. (2005). Posttraumatic stress disorder and other anxiety disorders. In J. M. Silver, T. W. McAllister, & S. C. Yudofsky (Eds.), *Textbook of traumatic brain injury.* Arlington, VA: American Psychiatric Publishing.

Weddell, R. A., & Leggett, J. A. (2006). Factors triggering relatives' judgements of personality change after traumatic brain injury. *Brain Injury, 20*(12), 1221–1234. doi:10.1080/02699050601049783

World Health Organization. (1992). *International statistical classification of disease and related health problems, tenth revision (ICD-10).* Geneva, Switzerland: Author.

World Health Organization. (2001). *International classification of functioning, disability, and health (ICF).* Geneva, Switzerland: Author.

Wortman, C. B., & Silver, R. C. (1989). The myths of coping with loss. *Journal of Consulting and Clinical Psychology, 57*(3), 349–357.

Wright, B. (1960). *Physical disability: A psychological approach.* New York, NY: Harper & Row.

Wright, B. (1983). *Physical disability: A psychosocial approach* (2nd ed.). New York, NY: Harper & Row.

Yasuda, S., Wehman, P., Targett, P., Cifu, D., & West, M. (2001). Return to work for persons with traumatic brain injury. *American Journal of Physical Medicine and Rehabilitation, 80*(11), 852–864.

CHAPTER 16

Acquired Brain Injury Rehabilitation: Clinical Essentials

SILKE BERNERT
DONG (DAN) Y. HAN

NEUROREHABILITATION

In order to highlight intervention models for conditions mentioned in previous chapters, this chapter is formulated differently from the rest of this book. Paradigms of neurorehabilitation are explained, and the interdisciplinary and transdisciplinary nature of brain injury rehabilitation is explored.

Because acquired brain injury (ABI) is a concept inclusive of many types of injuries, the definition can differ between clinical and pedagogical models, rendering it rather controversial. For the purpose of this chapter, we will use definitions published by the Commission on Accreditation of Rehabilitation Facilities (CARF) and the World Health Organization (WHO):

> *Acquired Brain Injury is an insult to the brain that affects its structure or function, resulting in impairments of cognition, communication, physical function or psychosocial behavior. ABI includes both traumatic and nontraumatic brain injury. . . . Nontraumatic brain injuries may include those caused by strokes, nontraumatic hemorrhages (AVM, Aneurysm), tumors, infectious disease,*

> hypoxic injuries, metabolic disorders, toxin exposure. ABI does not include brain injuries that are congenital, degenerative, or induced by birth trauma. (CARF International, 2016)
>
> Damage to the brain, which occurs after birth and is not related to a congenital or a degenerative disease. These impairments may be temporary or permanent and cause partial or functional disability or psychosocial maladjustment. (WHO, 1996)

ABI in this context is nonprogressive, and it does not include degenerative brain diseases such as Alzheimer's dementia, Parkinson's disease, motor neuron disease, or multiple sclerosis. As illustrated in prior chapters, ABI:

- Is heterogeneous in cause, pathophysiology, affected brain areas, and presentation
- Affects all body systems
- Causes physical, cognitive, behavioral, or emotional impairments
- Can result in fundamental functional impairments causing social changes for the individual

Optimal rehabilitation of ABI requires a multidisciplinary approach of trained rehabilitation specialists at appropriate timing and with appropriate intensity. Not only is brain injury an acute event but it also needs to be understood as a chronic condition with often acute onset. Promoting optimal rehabilitation for ABI throughout this entire chronologic span is a critical component of the discipline of physical medicine and rehabilitation.

A definition of physical medicine and rehabilitation is:

> Medical Specialty involved in diagnosis and treatment of patients with painful or functionally limiting conditions, the management of comorbidities and co-impairments, diagnostic and therapeutic injection procedures, electrodiagnostic medicine, and emphasis on prevention of complications of disability from secondary conditions. (American Board of Physical Medicine and Rehabilitation [ABPMR], n.d.)

Brain Injury

ABI results in:
- Loss of function by direct injury of brain areas
- Loss of function by diaschisis—neurophysiological changes of one brain area caused by injury to a second remote area, resulting in deafferentation and alteration of the neuronal network

Recovery and Neuroplasticity

Early Recovery
- Resolution of local brain edema
- Improvement of local circulation
- Recovery of injured neurons

Plasticity
Influenced by environment: Stimulation, repetition, intensity, and motivation
- Neuronal regeneration, collateral sprouting, and synaptogenesis (Nudo et al., 2001)
- Reversal of diaschisis
  - May enhance functional recovery or result in maladaptive response (Carrera et al., 2014)
- Functional learning-associated reorganization/unmasking
- Redundancy: Recovery of function due to uninjured areas involved in specific function now becoming more active
- Vicariation: Healthy neural structures assume function of damaged areas
- Substitution: Development of new strategies to compensate for deficits

Rehabilitation
Brain injury rehabilitation requires a comprehensive treatment program to:
- Reduce impairments
- Restore function
- Restore participation
- Restore quality of life

Comprehensive Neurorehabilitation/Transdisciplinary Team

Members

Rehabilitation physician/physiatrist
Medical specialty concerned with diagnosis, evaluation, and management of persons of all ages with physical and/or cognitive impairment and disability

- "Leads multidisciplinary teams concerned with maximal restoration or development of physical, psychological, social, occupational and vocational functions in persons whose abilities have been limited by disease, trauma, congenital disorders or pain to enable people to achieve their maximum functional abilities" (ABPMR, 2015)

Rehabilitation nurse
- Builds therapeutic relationship with patient and family
- Responsible for medical monitoring and behavioral management
- Reinforces use of skills learned during therapies and facilitates reemergence of patient independence
- Assists with maintenance of motivation and education for patient and family

Neuropsychologist
- "Uses psychological, neurological, cognitive, behavioral and physiologic principles, techniques and tests to evaluate patient's neurocognitive, behavioral, and emotional strengths and weaknesses and their relationship to normal and abnormal central nervous system functioning" (National Academy of Neuropsychology, 2001)
- Assists in diagnosis and treatment
- Implements therapy plans for groups, individuals, and family

Clinical psychologist
- Evaluates and treats mental and emotional conditions after ABI
- Assists individuals and their families with adjustment to the disability
- Assists the individual in achieving optimal physical, psychological, and interpersonal functioning

- Provides services consistent with the level of impairment, disability, and handicap relative to the personal preferences, needs, and resources of the individual (American Board of Professional Psychology, n.d.)

Physical therapist
- Examines each individual and develops a plan, using treatment techniques to promote the ability to move, reduce pain, restore function, and prevent disability
- Works with individuals and their families to prevent the loss of mobility
- Assesses individuals for appropriate mobility devices
- Teaches individuals and their families how to manage their condition for long-term health benefits
- Assists in education of individual and family (American Physical Therapy Association, 2016)

Occupational therapist
- Examines each individual and develops a plan to enable people to participate in the activities of everyday life
- Works with individuals and communities to enhance an individual's ability by teaching the use of assistive devices and modifying the occupation or the environment to better support the occupational engagement
- Assists in education of individual and family (World Federation of Occupational Therapists, 2013)

Speech-language pathologist
- Assesses, diagnoses, and treats cognitive, communication, and swallowing disorders
- Develops communication strategies
- Teaches use of assistive devices
- Assists in education of individual and family

Orthotist
- Makes and fits orthoses
- Manages comprehensive orthotic patient care

Case manager
- Assesses, plans, and facilitates comprehensive patient care services
- Assesses the needs and strengths of the individuals and their families or support systems
- Develops personalized goals
- Identifies resources for services
- Monitors progress toward goals

Recreational therapist
- Assists individuals and their families in the development of skills, knowledge, and behaviors for daily living and community involvement
- Improves the physical, cognitive, emotional, social, and leisure capabilities (American Therapeutic Recreation Association, 2004)

Vocational rehabilitation specialist
- Assesses an individual's functional level and vocational potentials
- Sets goals and plans interventions
- Provides career (vocational) counseling, job analysis, and development as well as placement services
- Coordinates individual and group counseling focused on facilitating adjustments to the medical and psychological impact of disability
- Provides case management, referral, and service coordination
- Implements interventions to remove environmental, employment, and attitudinal obstacles
- Provides consultation about and access to rehabilitation technology (NHS Health Scotland, 2013)

Dietician
- Assesses nutritional status and needs of individuals with various comorbidities, manages food services, and optimizes nutritional programs to promote health and control of diseases
- Provides nutritional counseling to individuals and families

Physical and Cognitive Rehabilitation

- Enhances intracortical reorganization to develop adaptive connection patterns while suppressing maladaptive responses
- Rehabilitation professionals use a variety of techniques to specifically manipulate behavior and thereby modulate the neuronal network (Cramer et al., 2011)

Psychosocial Rehabilitation

- Goal of optimal rehabilitation is the reintegration into family and community at the functionally highest level possible
- Optimal rehabilitation of brain injury requires a team approach of a variety of experts

Guiding Principles for Rehabilitation

Guiding principles for rehabilitation include all areas of therapy, namely, physical, occupational, cognitive, and speech-language therapy.

Graduated Approach
- Activities will gradually be adjusted on the basis of progress, starting with easier tasks or successive approximation graduating to more complex tasks.

Intensity
- This is the amount of time the individual is engaged in active, goal-directed, face-to-face rehabilitation therapy over time.
- More intensive training in animals resulted in increased brain reorganization.
- Lack of training causes a decrease of reorganization (Jette et al., 2005).

Repetition
- Appropriate amount of repetition is necessary to stimulate functional recovery.

Saliency
- New task or goal must be pertinent to the individual.
- Successful therapy requires an interactive, patient-directed approach.

Task Specificity
- Task-specific training improves motor learning (Cramer et al., 2011).

Timing of Rehabilitation
- Very early mobility after ABI may prevent medical complications (Klein et al., 2015; Titsworth et al., 2012).
- Early functional rehabilitation in poststroke and traumatic brain injury (TBI) patients has been shown to improve functional outcomes and may decrease "learned nonuse" (Taub et al., 2006).
- There may be an early optimal time window after the injury to achieve maximal neuroplasticity (Bernhardt, Dewey, Thrift, Collier, & Donnan, 2008; Biernaskie, Chernenko, & Corbett, 2004; Craig, Bernhardt, Langhorne, & Wu, 2010; Cumming et al., 2011; Griesbach, Gomez-Pinilla, & Hovda, 2007; Hu, Hsu, Yip, Jeng, & Wang, 2010; Maulden, Gassaway, Horn, Smout, & DeJong, 2005).

(Functional) Transference
- Change in function in one task or area may improve function in a second area.

Interference
- Plasticity in response to experience can interfere with improvement in function in a different area (Kleim & Jones, 2008; Lenze et al., 2012).

MODALITIES

Traditional Approaches

- Brunnstrom approach: Use of primitive synergistic patterns to improve motor control
- Bobath approach: Suppression of abnormal behavioral patterns and mass synergies; aims to regain motor control and function and includes task-specific practice (Kollen et al., 2009)
- Rood approach: Sensory stimulation of muscles and joints to normalize tone and produce desired movement

- Proprioceptive neuromuscular facilitation: Use of spiral and diagonal components of movements to facilitate more functional movement patterns
- Carr and Shepherd approach: Emphasis on functional training tasks and teaching of general strategies

An integrated therapeutic approach using a combination of the traditional approaches listed is more effective than no treatment. Data are limited in inferring that any one approach is more effective in promoting recovery than any of the other approaches (Pollock, Baer, Langhorne, & Pomeroy, 2007).

Functional Electrical Stimulation (FES)

- FES is an application of electrical current to activate nerves and achieve functional muscle contractions and sensory awareness and enhance motor control.
- FES treatment improves upper and lower extremity function in acute stroke as well as in chronic stroke.
- FES can also play a role in reduction of subluxation of the plegic shoulder (Daly et al., 2011; Powell, Pandyan, Granat, Cameron, & Stott, 1999).

Mirror Therapy

- Mirror is placed in the patient's mid-sagittal plane, reflecting movements of the nonparetic side as if it were the affected side.
- Mirror conveys visual stimuli to the brain through observation of the unaffected limb performing prescribed actions (Thieme, Mehrholz, Pohl, Behrens, & Dohle, 2012).

Constraint-Induced Movement Therapy (CIMT)

- Individuals need at least 20 degrees of active wrist extension and 10 degrees of active finger extension.
- Only minimal cognitive or sensory deficits can be present.
- Intensive upper extremity training program for affected limb is employed while the unaffected side is restrained (Mark,

Taub, & Morris, 2006; Suputtitada, Suwanwela, & Tumvitee, 2004; Wolf et al., 2010).

Locomotor Training

- Based on the idea of a central pattern generator in the spinal cord
- Uses body weight support systems in conjunction with a treadmill
- Provides task-oriented training for ambulation and sensorimotor feedback (Pohl et al., 2007)

Virtual Reality

- Virtual reality may be used for motor and cognitive rehabilitation; visual learning.
- Visual information can present as a potent inducer for reorganization of the sensorimotor network.
- It involves the immersion of a person in a computer-generated, three-dimensional environment.
- It has the potential to provide individualized repetitive, task-specific therapy (Adamovich, Fluet, Tunik, & Merians, 2009; Goodman, Zou, Dascalu, 2008).

Robotics in Rehabilitation

- Sensorimotor training with robotic devices; may incorporate virtual reality
- Delivers highly repetitive and reproducible training
- Can simulate functional tasks and ambulation (Schwartz et al., 2009)

Brain–Computer Interfaces

- Data still limited
- Computer communication software and hardware allowing cerebral activity to control computers or external devices

- Capture neuronal signals in real time and deliver sensory feedback
- May directly activate movements through functional electrical stimulation by peripheral or central mechanisms (Boninger, Wechsler, & Stein, 2014; Chung, Kim, Park, & Lee, 2015; Nicolas-Alonso & Gomez-Gil, 2012)

MEDICATION MANAGEMENT

Medication management is based on comprehensive history and physical examination of all organ systems, including neurocognitive and neuropsychiatric evaluations. General guiding principles for providers tasked with medication management include the following:

- Stop before you start; evaluate current medications.
- **DO NO HARM!** Anticipate and weigh benefits against possible side effects and drug–drug interactions; define treatment goal and outcome expectation.
- Start low and go slow.
- Initiate serially, not concurrently.
- Allow for an adequate trial.
- Continuously reassess management.
- Monitor for side effects and drug–drug interactions.
- Use medications for augmentation.
- Consider medications that can multitask.

REHABILITATION SETTINGS

Early Acute Care Rehabilitation

Rehabilitation services in the acute care hospital
- Need close management because early acquired compensatory behavior patterns may suppress neurological and functional recovery

- Occur at a variety of timing and intensity across the United States, without uniform approach
- May reduce mortality and long-term disability; exact timing for provision remains controversial
- May reduce length of stay and accelerate functional restoration

Post–Acute Rehabilitation

Acute Inpatient Rehabilitation

- Inpatient rehabilitation facility that provides intensive comprehensive treatment for neurologic dysfunction as well as patient and family education
- Requirements for admission:
  - In need of at least two skilled rehabilitation services (services include physical, occupational, or speech therapy)
  - Able to participate in and benefit from at least 3 hours of therapy per day, 5 days a week
  - Medically and psychologically stable
  - Expected to improve on the basis of measurable program goals
  - Patient will be evaluated by a physician at least three times per week, often on a daily basis

Subacute Rehabilitation

- If the individual cannot tolerate the intensity delivered at an acute inpatient rehabilitation facility; he or she does not or no longer requires therapy at this intensity level; is still unable to return home
- Frequently housed in skilled nursing facilities or in skilled nursing units
- Generally, receives only 1 or 2 hours of therapy per day
- Seen by his or her physician on a monthly basis
- Average length of stay generally longer than at an acute rehabilitation center

Home Rehabilitation Services

- Focuses on rehabilitation in the home of the individual

- Decreased intensity and supervision compared with inpatient rehabilitation services
- To qualify:
  - Individual must be unable to leave home because of the medical condition
  - Individual must be unable to leave home without help (is using a wheelchair or walker, requires special transportation, requires help by another person)
  - Leaving home must take a considerable and taxing effort

Outpatient Rehabilitation Services
- Rehabilitation needs often more specifically delineated for individuals who no longer require more comprehensive treatment

Specialized outpatient program: Community reentry
- Focused on higher level motor, social, and cognitive skills; prepares for a return to independent living and potentially work; may involve vocational evaluation and training

Neurobehavioral Facility
- Inpatient facility with close supervision and active behavioral and pharmacological management

Residential Care
- Safe environment for patients with behavioral or physical impairments who require 24-hour-7-days-per-week supervision and support

Holistic Day Care Program
- Comprehensive interdisciplinary day program in structured group setting

COMMUNITY (RE)INTEGRATION

Preparation
- Increasing independence in the rehabilitation facility
- Patient and family education

- Community outings, home visits, therapeutic day passes

Challenges of Return to Home

- Change in living situation due to need for additional physical or financial support, for example, moving in with children or parents
- Gradual emergence of frustration, anxiety due to increasing awareness of persisting or only slowly improving physical, cognitive, and behavioral impairments and inability to resume prior independence and social roles
- Development of depression and anxiety
  - Risk factors: Preinjury depression, level of self-reported impairment at discharge from the rehabilitation facility, limited family support, other social factors, localization of brain injury

Goals for Community Reintegration

- Regain independence in the home
- Regain independence for community access
- Return to work or education, driving, health and leisure, general life/personal goals

Assisted by rehabilitation services as indicated: Home health services, outpatient rehabilitation services, holistic day programs, neurobehavioral inpatient programs, residential programs, vocational rehabilitation services

SELECT REHABILITATION TOPICS

- Disorders of consciousness:
  - Coma
  - Vegetative state or unresponsive wakefulness
  - Minimally conscious state
- Leading cause: TBI

Coma

- Caused by severe, diffuse, bihemispheric lesions of the cortex or underlying white matter, bilateral thalamic damage, focal lesions of the paramedian tegmentum (Giacino, Fins, Laureys, & Schiff, 2014)
- Characterized by:
  - Loss of spontaneous or stimulus-induced arousal
  - Loss of sleep–wake cycle; eyes closed
  - Lack of purposeful movement or communication
  - Primitive reflexes
  - Reduced autonomous function; require respiratory assistance (Laureys, Perrin, Schnakers, Boly, & Majerus, 2005)

Vegetative State or Unresponsive Wakefulness

- Caused by severe, diffuse cortical injury or underlying white matter, often with bilateral thalamic damage, but with recovery of the reticular activating system
- Most commonly associated with severe diffuse axonal injury, also with vascular damage to the paramedian thalamus, with associated diffuse laminar necrosis after anoxic brain injury
- Characterized by:
  - Spontaneous or stimulus-induced arousal
  - Spontaneous eye opening
  - Lack of language comprehension or expression
  - Lack of purposeful behavior; involuntary movement only (stereotyped or reflexive)
  - Respiratory function usually occurring without assistance (Laureys et al., 2004, 2005, 2010)

Minimally Conscious State

- Severely altered state of consciousness, often transitional

- Caused by typical lesions including diffuse axonal injury with multifocal cortical involvement; can occur with thalamic lesions with greater sparing of corticocortical and corticothalamic connections
- Characterized by:
  - Minimal and inconsistent, but definite, behavioral evidence of self-awareness or environmental awareness
  - Evidenced by reproducible and recognizable command following, yes–no responses, visual tracking, situation-appropriate emotional response (crying or smiling), reaching for objects, manipulation of objects (Bruno, Vanhaudenhuyse, Thibaut, Moonen, & Laureys, 2011; Laureys et al., 2000; Laureys et al., 2005)

Emergence

- Reemergence of cortical connectivity
- Characterized by:
  - Reliable and consistent evidence of self-awareness and meaningful environmental interaction
  - Assessed by functional object use and interactive communication (Giaicino, Fins, Laureys, & Schiff, 2014)

Behavioral Assessment for Disorders of Consciousness

- Neurobehavioral rating scales:
  - Coma Recovery Scale–Revised (CRS-R)
  - Disorders of Consciousness Scale (DOCS)
  - Western Neuro Sensory Stimulation Profile (WNSSP)
  - Sensory Modality Assessment and Rehabilitation Technique (SMART)
  - Wessex Head Injury Matrix (WHIM)
  - Sensory Stimulation Assessment Measure (SSAM)

The CRS-R received the strongest recommendations for use from the DOC task force of the American Congress of Rehabilitation

(Giacino et al., 2014). Up to 40% of patients may be misdiagnosed due to inexperience and failure to use standardized scales (Schnakers et al., 2009).

Disorders of Consciousness Rehabilitation

Usually occurs in specialized neurorehabilitation programs with the following goals:

- Prevention of secondary medical complications, often related to immobility
  - Medical and neurological stabilization
  - Assessment and optimization of pharmacological management
  - Assessment and optimization of nutritional status
  - Prevention of contractures
  - Management of muscular hypertonicity
  - Prevention of skin break down
  - Prevention of infectious complications, especially urinary tract infections and pneumonias
- Restoration of cognitive and behavioral function
  - Physical modalities
  - Neuropharmacological enhancement
- Family education

Neurorehabilitation is a highly multidisciplinary, interdisciplinary, and transdisciplinary process, involving a team of experts from many different subspecialties. It is important to remember that the rehabilitation process should not be seen only as an acute process, but as a long-term investment for patient care because it involves a long road to full functional recovery. Many may not reach baseline status. However, many modalities are used to ensure continued progress in the field of neurorehabilitation. Neurorehabilitation in the context of ABI continues to be a demanding challenge, which requires clinical translational approaches involving a multidisciplinary team.

REFERENCES

Adamovich, S. V., Fluet, G. G., Tunik, E., & Merians, A. S. (2009). Sensorimotor training in virtual reality: A review. *NeuroRehabilitation, 25*(1), 29–44. doi:10.3233/NRE-2009-0497

American Board of Physical Medicine and Rehabilitation. (n.d.). *Definition of physical medicine and rehabilitation.* Retrieved from www.abpmr.org/consumers/pmr_definition.html

American Board of Professional Psychology. (n.d.). *Rehabilitation psychology.* Retrieved from www.abpp.org/i4a/pages/index.cfm?pageid=3361

American Physical Therapy Association. (2016). *Who are physical therapists?* Retrieved from www.apta.org/AboutPTs/

American Therapeutic Recreation Association. (2004). *The recreational therapy professional.* Retrieved from www.healthpronet.org/ahp_month/07_04.html

Bernhardt, J., Dewey, H., Thrift, A., Collier, J., & Donnan, G. (2008). A very early rehabilitation trial for stroke (AVERT): Phase II safety and feasibility. *Stroke, 39,* 390–396.

Biernaskie, J., Chernenko, G., & Corbett, D. (2004). Efficacy of rehabilitative experience declines with time after focal ischemic brain injury. *Journal of Neuroscience, 24*(5), 1245–1254. doi:10.1523/JNEUROSCI.3834-03.2004

Boninger, M. L., Wechsler, L. R., & Stein, J. (2014). Robotics, stem cells, and brain-computer interfaces in rehabilitation and recovery from stroke: Updates and advances. *American Journal of Physical Medicine and Rehabilitation, 93*(11, Suppl. 3), S145–S154. doi:10.1097/PHM.0000000000000128

Bruno, M. A., Vanhaudenhuyse, A., Thibaut, A., Moonen, G., & Laureys, S. (2011). From unresponsive wakefulness to minimally conscious PLUS and functional locked-in syndromes: Recent advances in our understanding of disorders of consciousness. *Journal of Neurology, 258*(7), 1373–1384. doi:10.1007/s00415-011-6114-x

Bureau of Labor Statistics, U.S. Department of Labor. (2016, September 17). *Occupational outlook handbook, 2016-17 edition, speech-language pathologists.* Retrieved from www.bls.gov/ooh/healthcare/speech-language-pathologists.htm

CARF International. (2016). *CARF accreditation focuses on quality, results.* Retrieved from www.carf.org/home

Carrera, E., & Tononi, G. (2014). Diaschisis: Past, present, future. *Brain, 137*(Pt. 9), 2408–2422. doi:10.1093/brain/awu101

Chung, E., Kim, J. H., Park, D. S., & Lee, B. H. (2015). Effects of brain-computer interface-based functional electrical stimulation on brain activation in stroke patients: A pilot randomized controlled trial. *Journal of Physical Therapy Science, 27*(3), 559–562. doi:10.1589/jpts.27.559

Craig, L. E., Bernhardt, J., Langhorne, P., & Wu, O. (2010). Early mobilization after stroke: An example of an individual patient data meta-analysis of a complex intervention. *Stroke, 41*(11), 2632–2636. doi:10.1161/STROKEAHA.110.588244

Cramer, S. C., Sur, M., Dobkin, B. H., O'Brien, C., Sanger, T. D., Trojanowski, J. Q., . . . Vinogradov, S. (2011). Harnessing neuroplasticity for clinical applications. *Brain, 134*(Pt. 6), 1591–1609. doi:10.1093/brain/awr039

Cumming, T. B., Thrift, A. G., Collier, J. M., Churilov, L., Dewey, H. M., Donnan, G. A., & Bernhardt, J. (2011). Very early mobilization after fast-tracks return to walking: Further results from the phase II AVERT randomized controlled trial. *Stroke, 42*(1), 153–158.

Daly, J. J., Zimbelman, J., Roenigk, K. L., McCabe, J. P., Rogers, J. M., Butler, K., . . . Ruff, R. L. (2011). Recovery of coordinated gait: Randomized controlled stroke trial of functional electrical stimulation (FES) versus no FES, with weight-supported treadmill and overground training. *Neurorehabilitation and Neural Repair, 25*(7), 588–596. doi:10.1177/1545968311400092

Giacino, J. T., Fins, J. J., Laureys, S., & Schiff, N. D. (2014). Disorders of consciousness after acquired brain injury: The state of the science. *Nature Reviews: Neurology, 10*(2), 99–114. doi:10.1038/nrneurol.2013.279

Goodman, P. H., Zou, Q., & Dascalu, S. M. (2008). Framework and implications of virtual neurorobotics. *Frontiers in Neuroscience, 2*(1), 123–129. doi:10.3389/neuro.01.007.2008

Griesbach, G. S., Gomez-Pinilla, F., & Hovda, D. A. (2007). Time window for voluntary exercise-induced increases in hippocampal neuroplasticity molecules after traumatic brain injury is severity dependent. *Journal of Neurotrauma, 24*(7), 1161–1171. doi:10.1089/neu.2006.0255

Hu, M. H., Hsu, S. S., Yip, P. K., Jeng, J. S., & Wang, Y. H. (2010). Early and intensive rehabilitation predicts good functional outcomes in patients admitted to the stroke intensive care unit. *Disability and Rehabilitation, 32*(15), 1251–1259. doi:10.3109/09638280903464448

Jette, D. U., Warren, R. L., & Wirtalla, C. (2005). The relation between therapy intensity and outcomes of rehabilitation in skilled nursing facilities. *Archives of Physical Medicine and Rehabilitation, 86*(3), 373–379.

Kleim, J. A., & Jones, T. A. (2008). Principles of experience dependent neural plasticity: Implications for rehabilitation after brain damage. *Journal of Speech, Language, and Hearing Research, 51*(1), S225–S239.

Klein, K., Mulkey, M., Bena, J. F., & Albert, N. M. (2015). Clinical and psychological effects of early mobilization in patients treated in a neurologic ICU: A comparative study. *Critical Care Medicine, 43*(4), 865–873.

Kollen, B. J., Lennon, S., Lyons, B., Wheatley-Smith, L., Scheper, M., Buurke, J. H., ... Kwakkel, G. (2009). The effectiveness of the Bobath concept in stroke rehabilitation: What is the evidence? *Stroke, 40*(4), e89–e97. doi:10.1161/STROKEAHA.108.533828

Laureys, S., Celesia, G. G., Cohadon, F., Lavrijsen, J., Leon-Carrion, J., Sannita, W. G., ... European Task Force on Disorders of Consciousness. (2010). Unresponsive wakefulness syndrome: A new name for the vegetative state or apallic syndrome. *BMC Medicine, 8*, 68. doi:10.1186/1741-7015-8-68

Laureys, S., Faymonville, M. E., De Tiege, X., Peigneux, P., Berre, J., Moonen, G., ... Maque, P. (2004). Brain function in the vegetative state. *Advances in Experimental Medicine and Biology, 550*, 229–238.

Laureys, S., Faymonville, M. E., Luxen, A., Lamy, M., Franck, G., & Maquet, P. (2000). Restoration of thalamocortical connectivity after recovery from persistent vegetative state. *Lancet, 355*(9217), 1790–1791.

Laureys, S., Perrin, F., Schnakers, C., Boly, M., & Majerus, S. (2005). Residual cognitive function in comatose, vegetative and minimally conscious states. *Current Opinion in Neurology, 18*(6), 726–733.

Lenze, E. J., Host, H. H., Hildebrand, M. W., Morrow-Howell, N., Carpenter, B., Freedland, K. E., ... Binder, E. F. (2012). Enhanced medical rehabilitation increases therapy intensity and engagement and improves functional outcomes in postacute rehabilitation of older adults: A randomized-controlled trial. *Journal of the American Medical Directors Association, 13*(8), 708–712. doi:10.1016/j.jamda.2012.06.014

Mark, V. W., Taub, E., & Morris, D. M. (2006). Neuroplasticity and constraint-induced movement therapy. *Europa Medicophysica, 42*(3), 269–284.

Maulden, S. A., Gassaway, J., Horn, S. D., Smout, R. J., & DeJong, G. (2005). Timing of initiation of rehabilitation after stroke. *Archives of Physical Medicine and Rehabilitation, 86*(12, Suppl. 2), S34–S40. doi:10.1016/j.apmr.2005.08.119

National Academy of Neuropsychology. (2001). *NAN definition of a clinical neuropsychologist*. Retrieved from www.nanonline.org/docs/PAIC/PDFs/NANPositionDefNeuro.pdf

NHS Health Scotland. (2013). *What is vocational rehabilitation?* Retrieved from www.healthyworkinglives.com/advice/Legislation-and-policy/work-related-illness-injury/vocational-rehabilitation/definition

Nicolas-Alonso, L. F., & Gomez-Gil, J. (2012). Brain computer interfaces: A review. *Sensors, 12*, 1211–1279.

Nudo, R. J., Plautz, E. J., & Frost, S. B. (2001). Role of adaptive plasticity in recovery of function after damage to motor cortex. *Muscle and Nerve, 24*(8), 1000–1019.

Pohl, M., Werner, C., Holzgraefe, M., Kroczek, G., Mehrholz, J., Wingendorf, I., . . . Hesse, S. (2007). Repetitive locomotor training and physiotherapy improve walking and basic activities of daily living after stroke: A single-blind, randomized multicentre trial (DEutsche GAngtrainerStudie, DEGAS). *Clinical Rehabilitation, 21*(1), 17–27. doi:10.1177/0269215506071281

Pollock, A., Baer, G., Langhorne, P., & Pomeroy, V. (2007). Physiotherapy treatment approaches for the recovery of postural control and lower limb function following stroke: A systematic review. *Clinical Rehabilitation, 21*(5), 395–410. doi:10.1177/0269215507073438

Powell, J., Pandyan, A. D., Granat, M., Cameron, M., & Stott, D. J. (1999). Electrical stimulation of wrist extensors in post stroke hemiplegia. *Stroke, 30*(7), 1384–1389.

Schnakers, C., Vanhaudenhuyse, A., Giacino, J., Ventura, M., Boly, M., Majerus, S., . . . Laureys, S. (2009). Diagnostic accuracy of the vegetative and minimally conscious state: Clinical consensus versus standardized neurobehavioral assessment. *BMC Neurology, 9*, 35. doi:10.1186/1471-2377-9-35

Schwartz, I., Sajin, A., Fisher, I., Neeb, M., Shochina, M., Katz-Leurer, M., & Meiner, Z. (2009). The effectiveness of locomotor therapy using robotic-assisted gait training in subacute stroke patients: A randomized controlled trial. *PM&R: The Journal of Injury, Function, and Rehabilitation, 1*, 516–523.

Suputtitada, A., Suwanwela, N. C., & Tumvitee, S. (2004). Effectiveness of constraint-induced movement therapy in chronic stroke patients. *Journal of the Medical Association of Thailand, 87*(12), 1482–1490.

Taub, E., Uswatte, G., Mark, V. W., & Morris, D. M. (2006). The learned nonuse phenomenon: Implications for rehabilitation. *Europa Medicophysica, 42*(3), 241–256.

Thieme, H., Mehrholz, J., Pohl, M., Behrens, J., & Dohle, C. (2012). Mirror therapy for improving motor function after stroke. *Cochrane Database of Systematic Reviews, 3*, CD008449. doi:10.1002/14651858.CD008449.pub2

Titsworth, W. L., Hester, J., Correia, T., Reed, R., Guin, P., Archibald, L., . . . Mocco, J. (2012). The effect of increased mobility on morbidity in the neurointensive care unit. *Journal of Neurosurgery, 116*(6), 1379–1388. doi:10.3171/2012.2.JNS111881

Wolf, S. L., Thompson, P. A., Winstein, C. J., Miller, J. P., Blanton, S. R., Nichols-Larsen, D. S., . . . Sawaki, L. (2010). The EXCITE stroke trial: Comparing early and delayed constraint-induced movement therapy. *Stroke, 41*(10), 2309–2315. doi:10.1161/STROKEAHA.110.588723

World Federation of Occupational Therapists. (2013). *Resource Centre.* Retrieved from www.wfot.org/ResourceCentre.aspx

World Health Organization. (1996). *World health report 1996—Fighting disease, fostering development.* Retrieved from www.who.int/whr/1996/en

CHAPTER 17

Feigning Issues in Brain Injury

DAVID T. R. BERRY
BRITTANY D. WALLS
CHELSEA M. BOUQUET
ELIZABETH R. WALLACE

OVERVIEW

"Malingering" is defined by the *Diagnostic and Statistical Manual of Mental Disorders* (fifth edition; *DSM-5*; American Psychiatric Association [APA], 2013) as ". . . the intentional production of false or grossly exaggerated physical or psychological symptoms, motivated by external incentives such as avoiding military duty, avoiding work, obtaining financial compensation, evading criminal prosecution, or obtaining drugs" (p. 726). Malingering must be distinguished from factitious disorder (see section Diagnostic Considerations) and conversion disorder (functional neurological symptom disorder; see section Diagnostic Considerations). This diagnostic framework has been carried over virtually unchanged since *DSM-III* (APA, 1980) and has been criticized for requiring extremely challenging distinctions, such as discriminating voluntary versus involuntary control and internal versus external motivations (Berry & Nelson, 2010). Nevertheless, the *DSM-5* malingering framework is enshrined in the current psychiatric nosology and thus cannot be ignored.

As discussed in previous chapters, mild traumatic brain injury (mTBI) is the most common form of traumatic brain injury (TBI), representing approximately 80% of TBIs (Kraus & Chu, 2005). Because by definition, mTBI involves only a brief loss or alteration of consciousness and no findings of pathology on neuroimaging of the brain, patients with this diagnosis have limited means to document their injury in litigation or disability proceedings. This may be at least a partial cause of reports that a significant proportion of mTBIs undergoing neuropsychological evaluation in compensation-seeking circumstances have been found to have evidence of poor effort and cooperation using objective procedures. As reviewed in the following sections, approximately 40% of compensation-seeking mTBI cases are thought to feign during neuropsychological evaluations. These findings suggest that complaints of long-term cognitive and behavioral deficits in a compensation-seeking mTBI patient should have careful and formal consideration given to the possibility of feigned symptoms.

HISTORY

Vickery, Berry, Inman, Harris, and Orey (2001) meta-analytically reviewed published studies on the detection of feigned deficits during neuropsychological testing. They characterized the extant literature to that date as having undergone three major phases. Initially, the forensic neuropsychology community was resistant to the notion that clients could convincingly feign deficits on testing. However, influential papers by Faust, Hart, and Guilmette (1988) and Heaton, Smith, Lehman, and Vogt (1978) conclusively demonstrated that relatively naive individuals instructed to fake neuropsychological deficits could successfully do so and escape detection by clinical judgment. In the subsequent second phase, several procedures introduced by Rey (1964) and popularized by Lezak (1983) began to be used by many neuropsychologists.

In the third phase, the symptom validity paradigm (more recently, widely known as Performance Validity Tests or PVTs) described by Binder (1990) and Hiscock and Hiscock (1989) began to gain wide acceptance by neuropsychologists. In the most popular format, a patient who is claiming memory deficits is given a series of trials, as shown in Figures 17.1 and 17.2, in which he or she is first shown a simple stimulus (5-digit number) to remember, followed by a blank delay, and then asked to choose between two alternative 5-digit numbers, one of which was given to remember. Because of the dichotomous choice involved, the binomial theorem may be used

52942

Figure 17.1. Digit memory test stimulus card.

A: 52942   **B: 83914**

Figure 17.2. Digit memory test answer card.

to calculate the probability of making a given number of correct choices in the face of no retained ability (random guessing). If a test-taker scored statistically significantly below chance, this was taken as clear evidence of suppressed ability, because in order to perform this poorly, the correct answer must have been recognized.

Subsequently, it was determined that instructed or simulating malingerers rarely performed this poorly. Thus, the threshold was later revised to compare a test-taker's performance to a "normative group" of non–compensation-seeking patients with a severe level of the same pathology. The "normative group" performance was used to determine a cutting score, usually set to correctly identify 90% of the normative group, to identify feigned deficits. Vickery et al. (2001) reported that the latter approach resulted in an overall specificity rate of 0.957 (percentage of honest test-takers correctly classified) and a sensitivity rate of 0.560 (percentage of malingering test-takers correctly classified). These authors concluded that such procedures should be used in all evaluations of compensation-seeking neuropsychological evaluees. These findings were updated and substantially replicated a decade later in a follow-up meta-analysis by Sollman and Berry (2011).

Results from these meta-analyses as well as numerous independent supportive studies led professional organizations to recommend the use of symptom validity tests in all neuropsychological evaluations, particularly those in a compensation-seeking context. For example, the National Academy of Neuropsychology published a position paper that stated, ". . . the assessment of symptom validity is an essential part of a neuropsychological evaluation (and) the clinician should be prepared to justify a decision not to assess symptom validity as part of a neuropsychological evaluation" (Bush et al., 2005, p. 421).

PATHOPHYSIOLOGY/ETIOLOGY

The pathophysiology and etiology of malingering are not well understood. The *DSM-5* conceptualization of this condition has been criticized as having a strong moral overtone in that it posits bad people (antisocial personality disorder) in bad circumstances (legal procedures) doing bad things (feigning). An alternative perspective is that feigning is simply in service of a desired goal (compensation) and maintained by progress toward that end. In clinical practice, malingering cases often present as having multiple determinants including both unconscious and conscious components as well as both internal and external goals.

EPIDEMIOLOGY

Because malingerers actively avoid detection, the prevalence of the condition is difficult to determine. One approach has been to survey forensic neuropsychologists for their estimates. Mittenberg, Patton, Canyock, and Condit (2002) reported results from such a study with an estimated prevalence of 41% in litigating mild head injury cases. Larrabee (2003) meta-analytically reviewed published data on feigning in compensation-seeking mild head injury cases, with 40% determined to be malingering based on objective tests. A useful rule of thumb is that as the "stakes" contingent on an evaluation increase, the probability of feigning increases in proportion.

CLINICAL PRESENTATION

In cases of mTBI, a period of several days to a few weeks of decreased attention, memory, and problem-solving skills is common, along with symptoms such as headache, irritability, and sensitivity to noise and light. However, longitudinal studies of non–compensation-seeking mTBI cases strongly suggest resolution of these problems by 3 months postinjury (Schretlen & Shapiro, 2003). Thus, continuing severe complaints in an mTBI case, particularly if compensation-seeking is involved, should raise the index of suspicion for malingering and trigger administration of objective instruments such as the aforementioned PVTs. Other factors often present in these cases include inconsistencies in self-report, lack of independent corroboration of injury circumstances, and unusual symptom complaints such as reports of triple-vision.

DIAGNOSTIC CONSIDERATIONS

Generally speaking, malingering should not be aggressively considered until a thorough medical workup has excluded known physical explanations for symptom complaints. As alluded to in the Overview section, the *DSM-5* framework for "diagnosing" malingering is complex and implicitly requires determination of conscious versus unconscious intent (to discriminate malingering from conversion disorder) as well as internal versus external goals (to discriminate malingering from factitious disorder). Rather than attempt to make these inherently difficult distinctions, it is recommended that invalid performance deficits be documented through administration of PVTs, with multiple failures leading to a conclusion that the impairments are invalid.

TREATMENT/PROGNOSIS

There is virtually no published literature on successful "treatments" for malingering. A feedback meeting explaining the failure to exert adequate effort during testing with an admonition to apply oneself fully during future evaluations seems logical, but no data on the success of this approach are available in the published literature. No published long-term follow-ups of malingering individuals are available to inform prognostic considerations.

CLINICAL SYNOPSIS

- Malingering is the deliberate fabrication or exaggeration of symptoms and performance deficits.
- In certain populations, such as compensation-seeking mTBI patients, the base rate of feigned symptoms and deficits is thought to be as high as 40%.
- Performance Validity Tests have been shown to be easily passed by patients with moderate to severe TBI who are not compensation seeking. These may assist in objectively documenting feigned deficits.
- Malingering should not be considered until a thorough and appropriate medical evaluation has ruled out physical causes for complaints and deficits.

CASE STUDY

In the following case study, which involves apparent feigning in a case of mTBI, several details have been altered to maintain the privacy of the patient. Dr. Q was a 47-year-old, White, male physician who was referred by his insurer for evaluation secondary to claimed disability secondary to a head injury. Dr. Q reported that he was no longer able to practice medicine because of cognitive and emotional deficits secondary to a head injury. On clinical interview, it emerged that Dr. Q had a long history of stormy interpersonal relationships, anxiety and mood disorders, and unsuccessful psychiatric treatment. Approximately 2 years before the evaluation, Dr. Q was involved in a motor vehicle accident in which his car was hit from behind and he reportedly struck his head on the driver's side window. He reported probable loss of consciousness for an unspecified period, which he estimated at 10 to 15 minutes. He was evaluated in an emergency department with no focal neurologic signs and negative neuroimaging. He was diagnosed with concussion and told to stay home for a few days until he felt ready to return to work. By his report, he suffered headache, dizziness, problems with attention and memory, difficulty "keeping my thoughts straight," and emotional lability. When he attempted to return to his practice of medicine 2 weeks later, he could not remember several clinical and administrative procedures, which his support staff noticed and commented on. This increased his anxiety, which in turn further interfered with his ability to function professionally. He was worked up by several medical providers who variously diagnosed cognitive disorder not otherwise specified, generalized anxiety disorder, major depression, and posttraumatic stress syndrome. It was determined that he was disabled from his occupation and he began to receive payments from his private disability carrier. This insurance company referred him for a neuropsychological evaluation.

Dr. Q was late for his appointment but called to explain that he was lost. He was guided to the office over a cell phone. He presented as somewhat disheveled, emotionally labile, and apologetic over his problems. Following the clinical interview, testing was initiated with performance validity tests mixed in with standard neuropsychological tests. During the first scheduled break period, the neuropsychometrist reported that Dr. Q had failed the two PVTs administered to that point. She was instructed to give a third PVT and to break again if it was failed. When it emerged that this third test was also failed, neuropsychological testing was suspended in favor of evaluating his psychological conditions. Dr. Q completed the Personality Assessment Inventory (PAI) (Morey, 1991), a multiscale test of psychopathology. When this was scored, it emerged that the Negative Impression Management (NIM) scale was extremely elevated, which invalidated this instrument. Dr. Q. was next administered the Structured Inventory of Reported Symptoms (Rogers, Kropp, Bagby, & Dickens, 1992), a procedure for evaluating the validity of psychological symptoms. He elevated one scale into the "Definite Feigning" range and two others into the "Probable Feigning" range, which was strongly suggestive of malingered psychiatric complaints. At this point, the evaluation was suspended and Dr. Q left the evaluation.

A report was prepared, which indicated that it was highly likely that Dr. Q was feigning cognitive deficits as well as psychological symptoms. It was recommended that he be referred to another provider for evaluation with a strong admonition to exert strong effort on cognitive testing and to be careful not to overemphasize his psychological complaints.

This case was somewhat unusual in that blatant feigning was documented across all relevant instruments and apparently included false cognitive deficits as well as exaggerated psychological complaints. Although broad-spectrum malingering such as this is not unheard of, clinical experience suggests that most feigning evaluees seem to "specialize" in either neuropsychological impairment or psychiatric exaggeration.

REFERENCES

American Psychiatric Association. (1980). *Diagnostic and statistical manual of mental disorders* (3rd ed.). Washington, DC: Author.

American Psychiatric Association. (2013). *Diagnostic and statistical manual of mental disorders* (5th ed.). Arlington, VA: American Psychiatric Publishing.

Berry, D. T. R., & Nelson, N. W. (2010). DSM-5 and malingering: A modest proposal. *Psychological Injury and Law, 3*(4), 11–18.

Binder, L. M. (1990). Malingering following minor head trauma. *The Clinical Neuropsychologist, 4*, 25–36.

Bush, S. S., Ruff, R. M., Troster, A. I., Barth, J. T., Koffler, S. P., Pliskin, N. H., ... Silver, C. H. (2005). Symptom validity assessment: Practice issues and medical necessity NAN policy & planning committee. *Archives of Clinical Neuropsychology, 20*(4), 419–426. doi:10.1016/j.acn.2005.02.002

Faust, D., Hart, K., & Guilmette, T. J. (1988). Pediatric malingering: The capacity of children to fake believable deficits on neuropsychological testing. *Journal of Consulting and Clinical Psychology, 56*(4), 578–582.

Heaton, R. K., Smith, H. H., Jr., Lehman, R. A., & Vogt, A. T. (1978). Prospects for faking believable deficits on neuropsychological testing. *Journal of Consulting and Clinical Psychology, 46*(5), 892–900.

Hiscock, M., & Hiscock, C. K. (1989). Refining the forced-choice method for the detection of malingering. *Journal of Clinical and Experimental Neuropsychology, 11*(6), 967–974. doi:10.1080/01688638908400949

Kraus, J. F., & Chu, L. D. (2005). Epidemiology. In J. M. Silver, T. W. McAllister, & S. C. Yudofsky (Eds.), *Textbook of traumatic injury* (pp. 3–26). New York, NY: Oxford University Press.

Larrabee, G. J. (2003). Detection of malingering using atypical performance patterns on standard neuropsychological tests. *The Clinical Neuropsychologist, 17*, 410–425.

Lezak, M. D. (1983). *Neuropsychological assessment* (2nd ed.). New York, NY: Oxford University Press.

Mittenberg, W., Patton, C., Canyock, E. M., & Condit, D. C. (2002). Base rates of malingering and symptom exaggeration. *Journal of Clinical and Experimental Neuropsychology, 24*(8), 1094–1102. doi:10.1076/jcen.24.8.1094.8379

Morey, L. C. (1991). *Personality assessment iventory manual*. Odessa, FL: Psychological Assessment Resources.

Rey, A. (1964). *The clinical examination in psychology*. Paris, France: Press Universitaire de France.

Rogers, R., Kropp, P. R., Bagby, R. M., & Dickens, S. E. (1992). Faking specific disorders: A study of the Structured Interview of Reported Symptoms (SIRS). *Journal of Clinical Psychology, 48*(5), 643–648.

Schretlen, D. J., & Shapiro, A. M. (2003). A quantitative review of the effects of traumatic brain injury on cognitive functioning. *International Review of Psychiatry, 15*(4), 341–349. doi:10.1080/09540260310001606728

Sollman, M. J., & Berry, D. T. (2011). Detection of inadequate effort on neuropsychological testing: A meta-analytic update and extension. *Archives of Clinical Neuropsychology, 26*(8), 774–789. doi:10.1093/arclin/acr066

Vickery, C. D., Berry, D. T., Inman, T. H., Harris, M. J., & Orey, S. A. (2001). Detection of inadequate effort on neuropsychological testing: A meta-analytic review of selected procedures. *Archives of Clinical Neuropsychology, 16*(1), 45–73.

Index

ABI. *See* acquired brain injury
abnormal brain MRI findings, 82
abortive medications, 192–193
abstinence, 179
accident neurosis, 3
ACE. *See* Acute Concussion Evaluation
acoustic schwannomas, 62
acquired brain injury (ABI), 203
  in children
    case study of, 256
    clinical presentation of, 247–250
    clinical synopsis of, 256
    diagnostic considerations of, 250–251
    epidemiology of, 247
    etiology of, 246–247
    history of, 245
    overview of, 245
    pathophysiology of, 245–246
    prognosis of, 255–256
    treatment of, 251–255
  common sequelae of, 204
  in elderly
    case study of, 274–276
    clinical presentation of, 266–267
    clinical synopsis of, 272–273
    diagnostic considerations of, 267
    epidemiology of, 263–266
    etiology of, 263
    history of, 261–262
    overview of, 261
    pathophysiology of, 262
    prognosis of, 269–272
    treatment of, 267–269
  psychosocial characteristics of
    case study of, 293–294
    clinical presentation of, 284–285
    clinical synopsis of, 293
    diagnostic considerations of, 284–285
    epidemiology of, 283
    etiology of, 283
    history of, 279–283
    overview of, 279
    pathophysiology of, 283
    posttraumatic stress disorder (PTSD), 286
    prognosis of, 291–293
    treatment of, 286–291
acquired brain injury (ABI) rehabilitation
  behavioral assessment for disorders of consciousness, 314–315
  coma, 313
  community (re)integration, 311–312
  disorders of consciousness rehabilitation, 315
  emergence, 314
  medication management, 309
  minimally conscious state, 313–314

acquired brain injury (ABI) *(continued)*
  modalities
    brain–computer interfaces, 308–309
    constraint-induced movement therapy (CIMT), 307–308
    functional electrical stimulation (FES), 307
    locomotor training, 308
    mirror therapy, 307
    robotics in rehabilitation, 308
    traditional approaches, 306–307
    virtual reality, 308
  neurorehabilitation, 299–300
  brain injury, 301
  comprehensive neurorehabilitation/transdisciplinary team, 302–304
  guiding principles for rehabilitation, 305–306
  physical and cognitive rehabilitation, 305
  psychosocial rehabilitation, 305
  recovery and neuroplasticity, 301
  settings, 309–311
  vegetative state/responsive wakefulness, 313
acquired epilepsy, 203, 206, 216
acquired prothrombotic states, 48
activities of daily living (ADLs), 269
acute acquired brain injury symptoms, 237–238
acute and short-term cognitive effects, 175
acute benzodiazepine intoxication, 175
Acute Concussion Evaluation (ACE), 250
  inhibitors, 55
acute confusional states, 109
acute effects
  cocaine, 176
  methamphetamine, 177
acute encephalitis, 83
acute inpatient rehabilitation, 310
acute intoxication of toluene, 175
acute neurocognitive deficits, 174
acute pharmacologic treatment, 191
acute stroke management
  hemorrhagic stroke, 53–54
  ischemic stroke, 51–53
  rehabilitation, 54–55
  secondary stroke prevention, 55–57
  venous sinus thrombosis, 54
acute treatment of post–acquired brain injury headaches, 192–193
AD. *See* Alzheimer's disease
adaptation, 287
adenosine triphosphate (ATP) production, 129
adjustment, 287
ADLs. *See* activities of daily living
advanced MRI approach, 5
aging brain, 262
AIDS, 88
alcohol
  clinical presentation of, 174–175
  pathophysiology of, 169–170
alertness/coma, level of, 29
Alzheimer, Alois, 98
Alzheimer's disease (AD), 209
  clinical presentation of, 108
  clinical synopsis of, 117
  diagnostic considerations of, 110–111
  epidemiology of, 105–106
  etiology of, 102–103
  history of, 98

overview of, 96
pathophysiology of, 100
prognosis of, 115
treatment of, 113
unequivocal diagnosis of, 111
American Cancer Society, 65
American Congress of Rehabilitation Medicine Mild Traumatic Brain Injury Committee (1993), 9
American Diabetes Association, 56
American Heart Association (AHA) guidelines, for blood pressure, 53
amino acid methionine, 102
ammonia neurotoxicity, 99
amphetamine, 171–174
amyloid angiopathy, 46
anaplastic astrocytomas, 62
animal models, 209
anosognosia, 267
anoxia
  case study of, 138–139
  clinical presentation of, 131–132
  clinical synopsis of, 136–138
  diagnostic considerations of, 133–134
  epidemiology of, 130–131
  etiology of, 130
  history of, 128
  overview of, 127–128
  pathophysiology of, 129–130
  prognosis of, 135–136
  treatment of, 134–135
anoxic brain injuries, 131, 137, 171
anticancer drug therapies, 68
anticholinergic medications, 236
anticoagulation, 48
antiphospholipid antibodies, 48
antiplatelet therapy, 56
antiviral drugs, 85
anxiety, 285
anxiolytics

clinical presentation of, 175–176
pathophysiology of, 171
aphasia, 286
apoplexy, 43
Aretaeus of Cappadocia, 43
aseptic meningitis, 81
astrocytomas, 62, 211
ataxia, 111
atheromatous debris, embolization of, 46
atherosclerosis, 46
atrial fibrillation, 45
avoidance behaviors, 286

Backer, George, 99
bacteria, 78
bacterial meningitis, 75–76, 80, 82, 85–87
bacterial neuroinfections, 89
baseline neuropsychological testing, 251
behavior variable, 291
behavioral assessment for disorders of consciousness, 314–315
behavioral issues, 32
benign versus malignant, 63
benzodiazepines, 173, 175
blood, 45, 48
blood pressure, American Heart Association (AHA) guidelines for, 53
blood tests, 110
blood vessels, 44, 46–48
  tearing of, 24
blunt-force trauma, 5–6
BDNF. *See* brain-derived neurotropic factors
Bobath approach, 306
bony skull protuberances, 23
boundary-zone
  infarctions, 136
brain imaging, for anoxic/hypoxic injuries, 132, 137

brain injury, 301. *See also specific entries*
feigning issues in
case study of, 326–327
clinical presentation of, 324
clinical synopsis of, 325
diagnostic considerations of, 325
epidemiology of, 324
etiology of, 324
history of, 322–323
overview of, 321–322
pathophysiology of, 324
prognosis of, 325
treatment of, 325
brain tumors, 210, 216
case study of, 70–71
clinical presentation of, 66
clinical synopsis of, 69–70
diagnostic considerations of, 67
epidemiology of, 65
etiology of, 64–65
history of, 63–64
overview of, 61–63
pathophysiology of, 64
prognosis of, 68–69
treatment of, 67–68
brain–computer interfaces, 308–309
brain-derived neurotropic factors (BDNF), 262
Brunnstrom approach, 306
burns, 157

calcifications, 62
calvarium, 61
carbamazepine, 214
cardiovascular and pulmonary diseases, 137
caregivers, 273
CARF. *See* Commission on Accreditation of Rehabilitation Facilities
Carr and Shepherd approach, 307

cART. *See* combination antiretroviral therapy
case manager, 304
case study
of acquired brain injury
in children, 256
in elderly, 274–276
of anoxia, 138–139
of brain tumors, 70–71
of cerebrovascular injuries, 58–59
of feigning issues in brain injury, 326–327
of hypoxia, 138–139
of mild traumatic brain injury, 13–15
of moderate to severe brain injury, 34–35
of neuroinfection, 90–91
of post–acquired brain injury
epilepsy, 217–218
headaches, 198–199
movement disorders, 239
of psychosocial characteristics of acquired brain injury, 293–294
cellular cholesterol levels, 103
Centers for Disease Control and Prevention (CDC), 1, 7, 21, 33, 81, 268
central nervous system (CNS)
depressant, 169–170
infection, 211, 216
cerebellar hemorrhages, 54
cerebral venous thrombosis, 50
cerebrospinal fluid (CSF), 25, 76
markers, 84–85
cerebrovascular disease, 187
diagnostic considerations of, 190
cerebrovascular injuries
case study of, 58–59
clinical presentation of, 49–50
clinical synopsis of, 58

diagnostic considerations of, 50
epidemiology of, 49
etiology of
 blood, 48
 blood vessels, 46–48
 heart, 45–46
history of, 43–44
overview of, 41–42
pathophysiology of, 44–45
prognosis of, 57
treatment of, 50–51
 acute stroke management, 51–57
cerebrovascular system, components of, 44–45
cervicogenic HA, 187, 189
CHE. *See* chronic hepatic encephalopathy
chemotherapy, 68
children, acquired brain injury in
 case study of, 256
 clinical presentation of, 247–250
 clinical synopsis of, 256
 diagnostic considerations of, 250–251
 epidemiology of, 247
 etiology of, 246–247
 history of, 245
 overview of, 245
 pathophysiology of, 245–246
 prognosis of, 255–256
 treatment of, 251–255
cholinergic system, 31
cholinesterase inhibitors, 108, 118
chronic complications, of traumatic brain injury (TBI), 25
chronic encephalitis, 83
chronic hepatic encephalopathy (CHE)
 clinical presentation of, 107–108
 clinical synopsis of, 116–117
 diagnostic considerations of, 110
 epidemiology of, 105

etiology of, 102
history of, 97
overview of, 95
pathophysiology of, 99
prognosis of, 115
treatment of, 112
chronic obstructive pulmonary disease (COPD), 128
chronic pesticide, 116
chronic traumatic encephalopathy (CTE), 230, 231
CIMT. *See* constraint-induced movement therapy
clinical psychologist, 302–303
clots, 47
clotting factors, 54
cocaine, 171, 176–177
cognitive disturbances, 159
cognitive recovery, 33
cognitive rehabilitation, 30, 305
cognitive screening, 216
cognitive-behavioral processes, 111
coma, 313
 level of, 29
combination antiretroviral therapy (cART), 86
Commission on Accreditation of Rehabilitation Facilities (CARF), 30, 299
common sequelae of acquired brain injuries, 204
commotio cerebri, 2
communication disorders, 286
community (re)integration, 311–312
community-acquired bacterial meningitis, 77
comorbidities, 198
complex pathophysiological process, 247
complicated mild traumatic brain injury, 5

comprehensive neuropsychological evaluation, 154–155
comprehensive neurorehabilitation/transdisciplinary team, 302–304
comprehensive rehabilitation therapies, 34
computed tomography (CT), 22, 154, 251
concurrent dexamethasone therapy, 86
concussion, 2–3, 245, 247
confusion, 111
consciousness rehabilitation, disorders of, 315
consistent medication adherence, 86
constraint-induced movement therapy (CIMT), 307–308
controlling type 2 diabetes, 113
contusions, 23–24
convulsions, 215
COPD. *See* chronic obstructive pulmonary disease
countless models, 287
course of recovery, 29
cranial cavity, abnormal growths of cells in, 69
cranium, 63
cryptococcal meningitis, 81
CSF. *See* cerebrospinal fluid
CT. *See* computed tomography
CTE. *See* chronic traumatic encephalopathy
current, type of, 145–146
current flow, path of, 147
Cushing, Harvey, 63

DAI. *See* diffuse axonal injury
DASH. *See* Dietary Approach to Stop Hypertension
decompressive craniotomy, 24–25
defense mobilization, 289
degenerative brain diseases, 300

delayed neurologic sequelae, 152
delayed posthypoxic leukoencephalopathy, 136
dementia pugilistica, 230
Department of Veterans Affairs, 1
depression, 285
diabetes mellitus, 56
diagnosed concussion, management of, 254
Diagnostic and Statistical Manual of Mental Disorders, Fifth Edition (DSM-5; APA, 2013), 9, 167, 178, 321, 324
Diagnostic and Statistical Manual of Mental Disorders, Fourth Edition, Text Revision (DSM-IV-TR, APA, 2000), 11
dialyzable uremic toxins, 100
Dietary Approach to Stop Hypertension (DASH), 56
dietician, 304
diffuse axonal injury (DAI), 24
diffuse electrical injuries, 157
digit memory test answer card, 323
disability, 280, 283
  social models of, 281
disordered methionine–homocysteine metabolism, 113
dissection, 47
disturbed methionine metabolism, 102
diuretics, 55
dopaminergic medications, 236
drug-resistant epilepsy (DRE), 213, 215
dyskinesia, 230
dyslipidemia, 113
dystonia, 136, 230, 234

early acute care rehabilitation, 309–310
ecological models, 290–291

electrical and lightning brain injuries
  case study of, 159–162
  clinical presentation of, 150–153
  clinical synopsis of, 157–159
  diagnostic considerations of, 153–155
  epidemiology of, 148–150
  etiology of, 148
  history of, 144–145
  injury characteristics of, 153
  overview of, 143–144
  pathophysiology of, 145–147
  prognosis of, 156–157
  treatment of, 155–156
elevated plasma homocysteine levels, 108
emotional disturbances, 159
EMU. *See* epilepsy-monitoring unit
encephalitis
  clinical presentation of, 81–82
  diagnostic considerations of, 83–84, 191
  epidemiology of, 79
  etiology of, 77, 187–188
  pathophysiology of, 75
  prognosis of, 87
  treatment of, 85
encephalopathy, 83
endocarditis, 45–46
end-stage renal disease (ESRD), 105
environmental factors, 282
ependymal cells, 62
ependymomas, 62
epidural hemorrhage, 58
epilepsy, 204–205
  case study of, 217–218
  clinical presentation of, 212
  clinical synopsis of, 216–217
  definition of, 205
  diagnostic considerations of, 213

  epidemiology of, 205–207
  etiology of, 205–207
  overview of, 203
  pathophysiology of, 208–210
  postinfectious, 211–212
  poststroke, 210–212
  prognosis of, 215–216
  treatment of, 213–215
  tumor-associated, 210–211
epilepsy-monitoring unit (EMU), 213
epileptogenesis, 204, 206, 208, 216
episodic tension–type HA, 186
ESRD. *See* end-stage renal disease
Essay on the Shaking Palsy (Parkinson), 229

feigning issues in brain injury
  case study of, 326–327
  clinical presentation of, 324
  clinical synopsis of, 325
  diagnostic considerations of, 325
  epidemiology of, 324
  etiology of, 324
  history of, 322–323
  overview of, 321–322
  pathophysiology of, 324
  prognosis of, 325
  treatment of, 325
FES. *See* functional electrical stimulation
FIM. *See* Functional Independence Measure
fMRI research, 5
focal cerebral ischemia, 42
focal neurological deficits, 50
focal seizures, 212
  onset, 212
focal syndrome, 41
4th Concussion in Sport Group meeting, 247
frontal brain systems, 291

functional electrical stimulation (FES), 307
Functional Independence Measure (FIM), 23
functional models, 281
functional MRI, 251
functional neuroimaging, 85
functional stereotactic surgery, 236

GABA. *See* gamma-aminobutyric acid
Galen, 43, 97
gamma-aminobutyric acid (GABA), 31
GBM. *See* glioblastoma multiforme
GCS. *See* Glasgow Coma Scale
generalized seizures, 212
GFAP. *See* glial fibrillary acidic protein
Glasgow Coma Scale (GCS), 8–9, 22, 28, 134
glial cells, 62–63
glial fibrillary acidic protein (GFAP), 209
glioblastoma multiforme (GBM), 211
glioblastomas, 62
gliomas, 62–63
globus pallidus internus (GPi), 236
glutamine, 99
GPi. *See* globus pallidus internus
gut-derived ammonia, 102

HA. *See* headache
HAART. *See* highly active antiretroviral therapy
HAND (HIV-associated neurocognitive disorder), 83
Hcy. *See* homocysteine
headache (HA), 66, 185–186
heart, 44–46
hematomas, 24
hemorrhages, 23, 51, 54, 58
hemorrhagic strokes, 42, 49, 53–55, 57, 58
hepatic portal system, 102
hereditary thrombophilias, 48
herpes simplex virus (HSV), 79, 82, 87
HHcy. *See* hyperhomocysteinemia
highly active antiretroviral therapy (HAART), 86
high-voltage electrical injuries, 155
Hippocrates, 43, 63, 97, 186
writings, 43
HIV. *See* human immunodeficiency virus
holistic day care program, 311
home rehabilitation services, 310–311
homocysteine (Hcy), 96
hostility, passive-aggressive expressions of, 289
HSV. *See* herpes simplex virus
human immunodeficiency virus (HIV)
clinical presentation of, 83
diagnostic considerations of, 84–85
epidemiology of, 81
etiology of, 78–79
pathophysiology of, 76–77
prognosis of, 88
transmission, increased risk of, 78
treatment of, 86
human "PTE" model, 208
hydrocephalus, 25
hypercholesterolemia, 55, 103
hyperhomocysteinemia (HHcy)
clinical presentation of, 108
clinical synopsis of, 117
diagnostic considerations of, 110–111

etiology of, 102–103, 105–106
history of, 98
overview of, 96
pathophysiology of, 100
prognosis of, 115
treatment of, 113
hyperinsulinemia, 103
hyperinsulinemic brain, 103
hyperkinetic movement symptoms, 237
hypnotics
   clinical presentation of, 175–176
   pathophysiology of, 171
hypothermia, 215
hypoxia
   case study of, 138–139
   clinical presentation of, 131–132
   clinical synopsis of, 136–138
   diagnostic considerations of, 133–134
   epidemiology of, 130–131
   etiology of, 130
   history of, 128
   overview of, 127–128
   pathophysiology of, 129–130
   prognosis of, 135–136
   treatment of, 134–135
hypoxic brain injuries, 127, 129, 136, 137
hypoxic–ischemic brain injury, 130
ICH forms. *See* intracerebral hematoma forms
ICP. *See* increased intracranial pressure
IEDs. *See* improvised explosive devices
ILAE. *See* International League Against Epilepsy
ILAE Diagnostic Methods Commission, 213
improvised explosive devices (IEDs), 6
inadequate vitamin D levels, 103

increased intracranial pressure (ICP), 24–25, 49
increased proinflammatory cytokines, 104
infarction, 42
infective debris, 45–46
infective endocarditis, 45
inhalants
   clinical presentation of, 175
   pathophysiology of, 170–171
injury, severity of, 27–28
innovative technology, 4
INRs. *See* international normalized ratios
insulin resistance, 103
interdisciplinary brain injury rehabilitation programs, 22
International Classification of Functioning, Disability, and Health (ICF) model, 281–282, 293
International League Against Epilepsy (ILAE), 204–205, 212, 213
international normalized ratios (INRs), 54
International Society for Hepatic Encephalopathy and Nitrogen Metabolism (ISHEN), 110
International Statistical Classification of Diseases and Related Health Problems, Tenth Revision *(ICD-10),* 281–282
intestinal flora, 102
intracardiac tumor, 46
intracerebral hematoma (ICH) forms, 24
intravenous tissue plasminogen activator (IV-tPA), 51–53
involuntary muscle contractures, 234
ischemic lacunar strokes, 57
ischemic strokes, 42, 49, 51–55, 58

ISHEN. *See* International Society for Hepatic Encephalopathy and Nitrogen Metabolism
isolated hypoxia/anoxia, 127, 130, 136–137
isolated hypoxic brain injuries, 130
IV-tPA. *See* intravenous tissue plasminogen activator

Jennett, Bryan, 22

keraunoparalysis, 152
ketogenic diet, 215
knowledge of prognosis, 34
Kurt Lewin's field theory, 288

lactulose, 112
large vessel strokes, 57
"latency period" concept, 208
late-onset AD (LOAD), 96
LDL. *See* low-density lipoproteins
lead ingestion, 105
lead poisoning
 clinical presentation of, 109
 clinical synopsis of, 119
 diagnostic considerations of, 112
 epidemiology of, 107
 etiology of, 105
 history of, 99
 overview of, 97
 pathophysiology of, 102
 prognosis of, 116
 treatment of, 114
Libman–Sacks endocarditis, 46
lightning injury, 144, 146. *See also* electrical and lightning brain injuries
 case study of, 159–160
 victims of, 155
lipohyalinosis, 46
LOAD. *See* late-onset AD

LOC. *See* loss of consciousness
locomotor training, 308
long-term disability, 273
long-term effects
 of benzodiazepine, 176
 cocaine, 176–177
 methamphetamine, 178
long-term neurocognitive deficits, 174–175
loss of consciousness (LOC), 9
low-density lipoproteins (LDL), 55
low-grade gliomas, 65

magnetic resonance imaging (MRI), 251
malignancy, 48
 benign versus, 63
marantic endocarditis, 46
M-CHE. *See* mild chronic hepatic encephalopathy
medical model, 281
medication management, 113, 309
medication-overuse HA, 191
Mediterranean diets, 56
meningiomas, 62–63, 65, 211
meningitis
 clinical presentation of, 82
 diagnostic considerations of, 84
 epidemiology of, 80
 etiology of, 77–78
 pathophysiology of, 75–76
 prognosis of, 87–88
 treatment of, 85–86
meningoencephalitis, 187–188
 diagnostic considerations of, 191
metabolic encephalopathies, 97, 104
metabolic syndrome hypercholesterolemia, 113
methamphetamine, 177–178
microglial activation, 209
migraine phenotype, 189

mild chronic hepatic encephalopathy (M-CHE), 95
mild traumatic brain injury (mTBI), 188, 321–322
  case study of, 13–15
  clinical presentation of, 8
  clinical synopsis of, 13
  diagnostic considerations of, 8–9
  epidemiology of, 6–8
  etiology of, 5–6
  history of, 2–4
  overview of, 1–2
  pathophysiology of, 4–5
  prognosis of, 10–12
  treatment of, 9–10
minimally conscious state, 313–314
mirror therapy, 307
modalities
  brain–computer interfaces, 308–309
  constraint-induced movement therapy (CIMT), 307–308
  functional electrical stimulation (FES), 307
  locomotor training, 308
  mirror therapy, 307
  robotics in rehabilitation, 308
  traditional approaches, 306–307
  virtual reality, 308
moderate and mild acquired brain injury, 232
moderate to severe acquired brain injuries, 231
moderate to severe brain injury
  acute pathophysiology of, 23
  case study of, 34–35
  clinical presentation and diagnostic considerations of
    complication factors in recovery, 29–30
    course of recovery, 29
    physical and emotional symptoms, 28–29
    severity of injury, 27–28
    typical cognitive deficits, 28
  clinical synopsis of, 33–34
  epidemiology of, 26–27
  etiology of, 25–26
  history of, 22–23
  overview of, 21
  pathophysiology of, 23
    chronic complications of TBI, 25
    primary injury, 23–24
    secondary injury, 24–25
  prognosis of, 32–33
  treatment of
    pharmacotherapy, 31
    psychotherapy and neurobehavioral interventions, 31–32
    rehabilitation therapy, 30–31
moderate traumatic brain injury, 9
mortality for bacterial meningitis, 87
motor vehicle accidents (MVAs), 26, 261
motor-related symptoms, 28–29
movement disorders, 136
MR CLEAN (Multicenter Randomized Clinical Trial of Endovascular Treatment for Acute Ischemic Stroke in the Netherlands), 52
MRI. *See* magnetic resonance imaging
mTBI. *See* mild traumatic brain injury
multiple brain neurotransmitter systems, 31
MVAs. *See* motor vehicle accidents
myoclonus, 233
myoglobinuria, 154
myriad of stage models, 289

National Academy of Neuropsychology, 323
National Health and Nutrition Examination Survey, 107
National Institute of Disability and Rehabilitation Research (NIDRR), 22
National Institutes of Health (NIH), 130
National Institute on Drug Abuse (NIDA), 170
National Survey on Drug Use and Health, 174
NCD. *See* neurocognitive disorder
neuroanatomical damage, 129
neurobehavioral facility, 311
neurobehavioral interventions, 31–32
neurobehavioral rating scales, 314
neurobehavioral symptoms, 29
neurobiological mechanisms, mTBI, 2
neurocognitive disorder (NCD), 83, 85
neurocognitive evaluation, during subacute phase, 134
neurocognitive symptoms, 13
neurodegenerative disorders, 232–233
neurodegenerative movement disorder, 238
neurodiagnostic imaging, 154
neurofibrillary tangles (NFTs), 100–101
neuroimaging, 197
neuroinfection, 74–75
  case study of, 90–91
  clinical presentation of
    encephalitis, 81–82
    HIV, 83
    meningitis, 82
  clinical synopsis of, 88–90
  diagnostic considerations of
    encephalitis, 83–84
    HIV, 84–85
    meningitis, 84
  epidemiology of
    encephalitis, 79
    HIV, 81
    meningitis, 80
  etiology of
    encephalitis, 77
    HIV, 78–79
    meningitis, 77–78
  history of, 74
  overview of, 73–74
  pathophysiology of, 74–75
    encephalitis, 75
    HIV, 76–77
    meningitis, 75–76
  prognosis of, 87–88
  treatment of, 85–86
neurons, 127
neuroplasticity, 301
neuropsychiatric symptoms, 104
neuropsychological assessment, 154–155, 213
neuropsychological deficits, 8, 83
neuropsychological evaluation, 10
neuropsychological testing, 197, 251, 281
neuropsychologist, 302
Neuropsychology Task Force, 213
neurorehabilitation, 299–300, 315
  brain injury, 301
  comprehensive neurorehabilitation/transdisciplinary team, 302–304
  guiding principles for rehabilitation, 305–306
  physical and cognitive rehabilitation, 305
  psychosocial rehabilitation, 305
  recovery and neuroplasticity, 301
neurosurgeons, 30
neurotoxic and metabolic injuries
  clinical presentation of, 107–109

clinical synopsis of, 116–119
diagnostic considerations of, 110–112
epidemiology of, 105–107
etiology of, 102–105
history of, 97–99
overview of, 95–97
pathophysiology of, 99–102
prognosis of, 115–116
treatment of, 112–114
New England Journal of Medicine, 214
NFTs. *See* neurofibrillary tangles
NIDA. *See* National Institute on Drug Abuse
NIDRR. *See* National Institute of Disability and Rehabilitation Research
NIH. *See* National Institutes of Health
nonalcohol substance use, 173
nondegenerative movement disorders, 233
nonfatal electrical injuries, 149
noninfective endocarditides, 46
nonpharmacologic interventions of post-ABI HA, 193, 195–196
nontraumatic brain injury (nTBI), 261–262, 263
"normative group" performance, 323
Nymman, 44

obstructive sleep apnea (OSA), 128
occupational therapist, 303
ocular injuries, 151
ocular signs, 111
OEF. *See* Operation Enduring Freedom
OIF. *See* Operation Iraqi Freedom
oligodendrogliomas, 62, 211

Operation Enduring Freedom (OEF), 6
Operation Iraqi Freedom (OIF), 6
opiates, 191
Optimal Rehabilitation of ABI, 300
organic solvent exposure, 171
organophosphates
 clinical presentation of, 108–109
 clinical synopsis of, 118
 diagnostic considerations of, 111
 epidemiology of, 106
 etiology of, 104
 history of, 98
 overview of, 96
 pathophysiology of, 101
 prognosis of, 116
 treatment of, 114
orthopedic injury group, 270
orthotist, 303
OSA. *See* obstructive sleep apnea
outpatient rehabilitation services, 311

PAC. *See* positive aspects of care
pain, 189
parkinsonian symptoms, 136
partial seizures, 212
passive-aggressive expressions of hostility, 289
patent foramen ovale (PFO), 45
PCS. *See* postconcussion syndrome
PECARN. *See* Pediatric Emergency Care Applied Research Network
Pediatric and Standard Glasgow Coma Scale, 249
Pediatric Emergency Care Applied Research Network (PECARN), 251, 252
permanent brain dysfunction, 87
personality changes, 284

personality variable, 291
pesticides
　chemicals, 104
　clinical presentation of, 108–109
　clinical synopsis of, 118
　diagnostic considerations
　　of, 111
　epidemiology of, 106
　etiology of, 104
　history of, 98
　overview of, 96
　pathophysiology of, 101
　prognosis of, 116
　treatment of, 114
petechial hemorrhage, 24
PFO. *See* patent foramen ovale
pharmacological therapy, 34, 254
pharmacotherapy, 31
phenobarbital, 214
phenytoin, 214
PHES. *See* Psychometric Hepatic
　　Encephalopathy Score
physical and cognitive rehabilitation, 305
physical therapist, 303
pituitary tumors, 67
plaques of Aβ protein, 209
pneumococcal meningitis, 82
poor oxygenation, 170
positive aspects of care (PAC), 271
post–acquired brain injury
　epilepsy, 204–205
　　case study of, 217–218
　　clinical presentation of, 212
　　clinical synopsis of, 216–217
　　diagnostic considerations
　　　of, 213
　　epidemiology of, 205–207
　　etiology of, 205–207
　　overview of, 203
　　pathophysiology of, 208–210
　　post stroke, 210–212
　　prognosis of, 215–216
　　treatment of, 213–215

　movement disorders,
　　229, 230, 238
　　case study of, 239
　　clinical presentation of,
　　　232–234
　　clinical synopsis of, 238–239
　　diagnostic considerations of,
　　　234–235
　　epidemiology of, 231–232
　　etiology of, 231
　　history of, 229–230
　　overview of, 229
　　pathophysiology of, 230–231
　　prognosis of, 237–238
　　treatment of, 235–237
　movement symptoms, 233
　tremors, 233–234, 237
post–acquired brain injury
　　headache (post-ABI HA),
　　197–198
　acute treatment of, 192–193
　case study of, 198–199
　clinical presentation of, 188–189
　clinical synopsis of, 197–198
　diagnostic considerations of,
　　189–191
　epidemiology of, 188
　etiology of, 187–188
　history of, 186
　overview of, 185–186
　pathophysiology of, 186–187
　prognosis of, 196–197
　prophylactic medications for,
　　194–195
　semiologies of, 189
　treatment of, 191–196
post–acute rehabilitation, 310–311
Post-Concussion Symptom Inventory (PCSI)–child, 250
postconcussion syndrome (PCS),
　11, 12, 185, 256
posterior fossa tumors, 65
postinfectious epilepsy,
　211–212

postinjury neurocognitive performance, 3
postinjury performances, 10
postinjury symptoms, 269
poststroke epilepsy
  tumor-associated epilepsy, 210–211
  postinfectious epilepsy, 211–212
posttraumatic amnesia (PTA), 27
posttraumatic dystonia, 236–238
posttraumatic epilepsy (PTE), 25, 205–207, 215–216
posttraumatic headache (PTH), 185
  clinical presentations of, 188–189
  prevalence of, 188
posttraumatic hyperkinesias, 234, 237, 238
posttraumatic parkinsonism, 236, 238
posttraumatic seizures, 211–212, 214
posttraumatic stress disorder (PTSD), 8, 286
posttraumatic symptoms, 235
posttraumatic tics, 237
posttraumatic tremor, 237
pregnancy, 48
premorbid psychiatric condition, 8
primary absolute contraindication, 51
primary brain tumors, risk of, 64–65
primary encephalitis, 83
primary injury, 23–24, 245
primary service providers, 281
prophylactic medications, 213–214
  for post–acquired brain injury headache, 194–195
proprioceptive neuromuscular facilitation, 307

protein metabolism, 102
prothrombotic drugs, 48
psychoeducation, 10
Psychometric Hepatic Encephalopathy Score (PHES), 110
psychosocial characteristics of acquired brain injury
  case study of, 293–294
  clinical presentation of, 284–285
  clinical synopsis of, 293
  diagnostic considerations of, 284–285
  epidemiology of, 283
  etiology of, 283
  history of, 279–283
  overview of, 279
  pathophysiology of, 283
  posttraumatic stress disorder (PTSD), 286
  prognosis of, 291–293
  treatment of, 286–291
psychosocial interventions, in acquired brain injury, 287
psychotherapeutic techniques, use of, 32
psychotherapeutic treatments, 34
psychotherapy, 31–32
PTA. See posttraumatic amnesia
PTE. See posttraumatic epilepsy
PTH. See posttraumatic headache
PTSD. See posttraumatic stress disorder
PubMed search of "anoxic brain injury," 128
"punch drunk" syndrome, 230
pure hypoxic brain injury, 131

quantitative meta-analysis, 178

radiation therapy, 65
radiotherapy, 68
raised intracranial pressure
  acute management for, 70
  treatment for, 67

RBANS. *See* Repeated Battery for Assessment of Neuropsychological Status
RCVS. *See* reversible cerebral vasoconstriction syndrome
recovery, 301
  complication factors in, 29–30
  course of, 29
  and neuroplasticity, 301
recreational therapist, 304
rehabilitation, 51, 54–55, 58, 90
  guiding principles for, 305–306
  nurse, 302
  physician/physiatrist, 302
  programs, 23
  robotics in, 308
  settings, 309–311
  therapy, 30–31
Repeated Battery for Assessment of Neuropsychological Status (RBANS), 110
resection surgery, 215
residential care, 311
resistance, 146–147
resuscitation, 134
retrievable stent, 52
reversible cerebral vasoconstriction syndrome (RCVS), 47
rifaximin, 112
robotics in rehabilitation, 308
Rood approach, 306

saccular aneurysm, 46–47
SAH. *See* subarachnoid hemorrhage
SAMHSA. *See* Substance Abuse and Mental Health Services Administration
SCAT3. *See* Sport Concussion Assessment Tool
school-aged children, 247
Schwann cells, 62
schwannomas, 62
SDH. *See* subdural hematoma

secondary encephalitis, 83
secondary injury, 24–25, 246
secondary stroke prevention, 55–58
sedatives
  clinical presentation of, 175–176
  pathophysiology of, 171
seizures, 136, 204, 210. *See also* epilepsy
  acute and late, 209
  clinical presentation of, 212
  focal, 212
  focal onset, 212
  generalized, 212
  genesis of, 215
  posttraumatic, 214
  prophylaxis of, 213–214
  spontaneous, 208
  traumatic brain injury and, 207
  types of, 211–212
  unpredictable, impact in epilepsy, 205, 206
  unprovoked, 204–205, 216
selective serotonin reuptake inhibitors (SSRIs), 31
serotonergic pathway activation, 31
severe acquired brain injury, 231–232
severe traumatic brain injury, 9, 185, 217
severity of injury, 27–28
Shepherd approach, 307
shorter term deficits, 180
short-term effects
  cocaine, 176–177
  methamphetamine, 177
short-term neurocognitive deficits, 174
skeletal system, 151
sleep hygiene, 255
social models of disability, 281
sociodemographic variables, 290–291

somatopsychology, 288–289
somatosensory evoked potentials (SSEPs), 133
SPARCLE trial. *See* Stroke Prevention by Aggressive Reduction in Cholesterol Levels trial
spasticity, 233
speech-language pathologist, 303
spontaneous burst discharges, 208
spontaneous subarachnoid hemorrhage, 42
sporadic Alzheimer's disease, metabolic risk factors of
    clinical presentation of, 108
    clinical synopsis of, 117–118
    diagnostic considerations of, 111
    epidemiology of, 106
    etiology of, 103–104
    history of, 98
    overview of, 96
    pathophysiology of, 100–101
    prognosis of, 115
    treatment of, 113–114
Sport Concussion Assessment Tool (SCAT3), 250
sports-related concussion (SRC), 5, 7, 11
sports-related traumatic brain injury, 26
SRC. *See* sports-related concussion
SSEPs. *See* somatosensory evoked potentials
SSRIs. *See* selective serotonin reuptake inhibitors
stage models, 289–290
stereotactic ablative surgery, 237
stimulants, 173–174
    clinical presentation of, 176–178
    pathophysiology of, 171–172
stroke, 41, 44, 58, 210, 216
    symptoms of, 42, 49
    treatment of, 50–57
Stroke Prevention by Aggressive Reduction in Cholesterol Levels (SPARCLE) trial, 55–56
subacute phase, neurocognitive evaluation during, 134
subacute rehabilitation, 310
subarachnoid hemorrhage (SAH), 24, 47, 54, 58
subdural hematoma (SDH), 24
subdural hemorrhage, 58
subsequent injuries, 148
Substance Abuse and Mental Health Services Administration (SAMHSA), 168
substance misuse/abuse, 180
substance use disorder, acquired brain injury secondary to
    case study of, 181–182
    clinical presentation of, 174–178
    clinical synopsis of, 180
    diagnostic considerations of, 178–179
    epidemiology of, 172–174
    etiology of, 172
    history of, 168–169
    overview of, 167–168
    pathophysiology of, 169–172
    prognosis of, 179–180
    treatment of, 179
subthalamic deep brain stimulation, 236
supratentorial brain tumors, risk of, 65
surgical resection, 68
suspected concussion, management of, 254
suspected delirium, 119

TAE. *See* tumor-associated epilepsy
TAI. *See* traumatic axonal injury
TBI. *See* traumatic brain injury

Teasdale, Graham, 22
tension-type HA, 189
tension-type phenotype, 189
temporal lobe epilepsy (TLE), 213
thalamic deep brain stimulation, 235
Theiler's murine encephalomyelitis virus (TMEV), 209
thiamine, 101
  deficiency, 169
tissue, type of, 62–63
TLE. See temporal lobe epilepsy
TME. See toxic metabolic encephalopathy
TMEV. See Theiler's murine encephalomyelitis virus
toluene, 170
  acute intoxication of, 175
toxic metabolic encephalopathy (TME)
  clinical presentation of, 109
  clinical synopsis of, 118–119
  diagnostic considerations of, 112
  epidemiology of, 107
  etiology of, 104
  history of, 99
  overview of, 97
  pathophysiology of, 101
  prognosis of, 116
  treatment of, 114
transdisciplinary team, 302–304
transient ischemic attack, 42
trauma, 48
trauma surgeons, 30
traumatic axonal injury (TAI), 24
traumatic brain injury (TBI), 5–7, 204
  Centers for Disease Control and Prevention, 21
  chronic complications of, 25
  definition of, 206
  diagnostic considerations of, 190, 213

  early medical interventions for, 22
  etiology of, 25, 187
  growing awareness of, 26
  injury severity, 8
  Model Systems programs, 22
tremor, 230, 235–236, 238
tumor-associated epilepsy (TAE), 210–211
typical cognitive deficits, 28
typical symptoms, 28–29

UE. See uremic encephalopathy
unresponsive wakefulness, 313
upper extremity flexors, 146
uremic encephalopathy (UE)
  clinical presentation of, 108
  clinical synopsis of, 117
  diagnostic considerations of, 110
  epidemiology of, 105
  etiology of, 102
  history of, 97
  overview of, 95–96
  pathophysiology of, 99–100
  prognosis of, 115
  treatment of, 112–113

valproate, 214
vascular imaging, 44, 54
vascular malformation, 47
vasculitis, 47–48
vasospasm, 47
vegetative state/responsive wakefulness, 313
venous sinus thrombosis, 54
ventricular thrombosis, 45
Vietnam War era, 22
viral meningeal infection, 78
viral meningitis, 76, 80, 82, 86
  CSF examination, 84
viremia, 75
virtual reality, 308
vitamin D_3 insufficiency, 103

vitamin therapy, 113
vocational rehabilitation specialist, 304
voltage, 146

warfarin, 56–57
watershed, 136
WE. *See* Wernicke's encephalopathy
Wepfer, 44
Wernicke–Korsakoff's syndrome, 169
Wernicke's encephalopathy (WE)
  clinical presentation of, 109
  clinical synopsis of, 118
  diagnostic considerations of, 111
  epidemiology of, 106–107
  etiology of, 104
  history of, 98
  overview of, 96
  pathophysiology of, 101
  prognosis of, 116
  treatment of, 114
Wilson, Kinnier, 99
World Health Organization, 9, 172–173, 281, 299

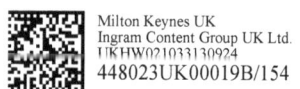

Milton Keynes UK
Ingram Content Group UK Ltd.
UKHW021033130924
448023UK00019B/154